T0179772

# Statistical Methods for Evaluating Safety in Medical Product Development

**STATISTICS IN PRACTICE**

*Series Advisors*

**Human and Biological Sciences**
Stephen Senn
*CRP-Santé, Luxembourg*

**Earth and Environmental Sciences**
Marian Scott
*University of Glasgow, UK*

**Industry, Commerce and Finance**
Wolfgang Jank
*University of Maryland, USA*

**Founding Editor**
Vic Barnett
*Nottingham Trent University, UK*

---

*Statistics in Practice* is an important international series of texts which provide detailed coverage of statistical concepts, methods and worked case studies in specific fields of investigation and study.

With sound motivation and many worked practical examples, the books show in down-to-earth terms how to select and use an appropriate range of statistical techniques in a particular practical field within each title's special topic area.

The books provide statistical support for professionals and research workers across a range of employment fields and research environments. Subject areas covered include medicine and pharmaceutics; industry, finance and commerce; public services; the earth and environmental sciences; and so on.

The books also provide support to students studying statistical courses applied to the above areas. The demand for graduates to be equipped for the work environment has led to such courses becoming increasingly prevalent at universities and colleges.

It is our aim to present judiciously chosen and well-written workbooks to meet everyday practical needs. Feedback of views from readers will be most valuable to monitor the success of this aim.

A complete list of titles in this series appears at the end of the volume.

# Statistical Methods for Evaluating Safety in Medical Product Development

Editor

**A. Lawrence Gould**

*Merck Research Laboratories, USA*

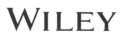

This edition first published 2015
© 2015 John Wiley and Sons Ltd

**Registered office**
John Wiley & Sons Ltd, The Atrium, Southern Gate, Chichester, West Sussex, PO19 8SQ, United Kingdom

For details of our global editorial offices, for customer services and for information about how to apply for permission to reuse the copyright material in this book please see our website at www.wiley.com.

The right of the author to be identified as the author of this work has been asserted in accordance with the Copyright, Designs and Patents Act 1988.

All rights reserved. No part of this publication may be reproduced, stored in a retrieval system, or transmitted, in any form or by any means, electronic, mechanical, photocopying, recording or otherwise, except as permitted by the UK Copyright, Designs and Patents Act 1988, without the prior permission of the publisher.

Wiley also publishes its books in a variety of electronic formats. Some content that appears in print may not be available in electronic books.

Limit of Liability/Disclaimer of Warranty: While the publisher and author have used their best efforts in preparing this book, they make no representations or warranties with respect to the accuracy or completeness of the contents of this book and specifically disclaim any implied warranties of merchantability or fitness for a particular purpose. It is sold on the understanding that the publisher is not engaged in rendering professional services and neither the publisher nor the author shall be liable for damages arising herefrom. If professional advice or other expert assistance is required, the services of a competent professional should be sought.

*Library of Congress Cataloging-in-Publication Data*

Statistical methods for evaluating safety in medical product development / [edited by] Lawrence Gould.
    p. ; cm.
  Includes bibliographical references and index.
  ISBN 978-1-119-97966-1 (cloth)
  I. Gould, Lawrence (A. Lawrence), editor.
  [DNLM: 1. Drug Evaluation–methods.   2. Clinical Trials as Topic.   3. Models, Statistical.   4. Pharmacovigilance.
5. Safety Management–methods.   6. Technology, Pharmaceutical–standards.   QV 771]
  R853.C55
  615.5072′4 – dc23
                                                                                                    2014025599

A catalogue record for this book is available from the British Library.

ISBN: 9781119979661

Typeset in 10/12pt Times by Laserwords Private Limited, Chennai, India
Printed and bound in Malaysia by Vivar Printing Sdn Bhd

1   2015

# Contents

# Preface

This is a book about statistical methods that are useful for evaluating safety at all stages of medical product development. It is not a book about statistical methods or theory as such: many excellent texts address these topics. Indeed, it is assumed that the reader either is familiar with the various statistical methods or has access to literature and other resources that can provide needed descriptions of the methods. Rather, the focus is on how existing methods can be applied effectively to provide insight into the existence and perhaps even cause of potential safety issues associated with medical products. To this end, the emphasis has been on modern statistical techniques that have not yet been widely accepted in practice, with brief descriptions of how they work and a selective bibliography to guide the reader to more extensive descriptions of the methods. In addition, a concerted effort has been made to supply or identify sources for software for carrying out the calculations, in order to facilitate application of the methods.

Medical product development engages many different biological and medical specialties and areas of expertise. Every stage of product development requires the evaluation of quantitative information obtained from experiments or trials, for which statistical methods are crucial. For example, developments in computational toxicology over the past decade or so have raised the possibility of identifying molecular structural characteristics that might lead to toxic effects even before experiments in animals (let alone people) are undertaken, thus avoiding waste of resources and subjecting volunteers or patients to unnecessary risks. The statistical issues have been discussed in the toxicology literature, but not in the statistical literature to any extent. Likewise, statistical issues associated with the evaluation of hepatotoxicity and neurotoxicity are discussed in the application area literature, but not very extensively in the statistical literature. The primary aim of this book is to provide understanding of, and some practical guidance on, the application of contemporary statistical methods to contemporary issues in safety evaluation throughout medical product development.

A. LAWRENCE GOULD

# List of Contributors

**Ismaïl Ahmed, Ph.D.**
Biostatistics Team, Centre for Research in Epidemiology and Population Health
UMRS U1018 Inserm – Université Paris Sud
F-94807, Villejuif
France

**Bernard Bégaud, M.D., Ph.D.**
U657 – Pharmacoepidemiology, Inserm – Université de Bordeaux
F-33000, Bordeaux
France

**Jie Chen, M.D., M.Ph., Ph.D.**
Merck Serono (Beijing) R&D Hub
9 Jian Guo Road, Chaoyang
Beijing 100022
China

**Richard J. Cook, Ph.D.**
Department of Statistics and Actuarial Science
University of Waterloo
200 University Avenue West
Waterloo, ON
Canada N2L 3G1

**Liqun Diao, Ph.D**
Department of Statistics and Actuarial Science
University of Waterloo
200 University Avenue West
Waterloo, ON
Canada N2L 3G1

**A. Lawrence Gould**
Merck Research Laboratories
770 Sumneytown Pike, West Point, PA 19486
USA

**Jay Herson, Ph.D.**
Johns Hopkins Bloomberg School of Public Health
Baltimore, MD 21205
USA

**Ker-Ai Lee, M.Sc.**
Department of Statistics and Actuarial Science
University of Waterloo
200 University Avenue West, Waterloo, ON
Canada N2L 3G1

**Andy Liaw, M.Sc.**
Biometrics Research
Merck & Co., Inc
Rahway, NJ 07065
USA

**Arne Ring, Ph.D.**
Leicester Clinical Trials Unit
University of Leicester
LE5 4PW
UK

Department of Mathematical Statistics and Actuarial Science
University of the Free State
205 Nelson Mandela Drive, Bloemfontein 9301
South Africa

**Robert Schall, Ph.D.**
Department of Mathematical Statistics and Actuarial Science
University of the Free State
205 Nelson Mandela Drive, Bloemfontein 9301
South Africa

Quintiles Biostatistics, Bloemfontein 9301
South Africa

**Stephen Senn, Ph.D.**
Competence Center for Methodology and Statistics
Strassen
Luxembourg

**Vladimir Svetnik, Ph.D.**
Biometrics Research
Merck & Co., Inc
Rahway, NJ 07065
USA

**Donald C. Trost, M.D., Ph.D.**
Director, Intelligent Systems, Ativa Medical
1000 Westgate Drive, Suite 100
St Paul, MN, 55114
USA

**Pascale Tubert-Bitter, Ph.D.**
Biostatistics Team, Centre for Research in Epidemiology and Population Health
UMRS U1018, Inserm – Université Paris Sud
F-94807, Villejuif
France

# 1

# Introduction

## A. Lawrence Gould

*Merck Research Laboratories, 770 Sumneytown Pike, West Point, PA 19486, USA*

## 1.1 Introduction

Many stakeholders have an interest in how pharmaceutical products are developed. These include the medical profession, regulators, legislators, the pharmaceutical industry, and, of course, the public who ultimately will use the products. The expectations of these stakeholders have become more demanding over time, especially with regard to product safety. The public perception of the safety of pharmaceutical products often is driven by publicity about the occurrence of adverse events among patients using the products that has on occasion led to withdrawal of the products from the market [1]. This circumstance usually pertains to products that have reached the marketplace and have had sufficient exposure among patients for rare and potentially serious harmful events to occur frequently enough to cause concern. However, the development of products can be suspended or terminated before they ever reach the market because of toxicities discovered during development [2–6]. These situations may or may not be made the object of intense public scrutiny, but they are important because failed products can have consumed possibly considerable resources that might have been allocated more productively to the development of products more likely to succeed by virtue of being less toxic or more beneficial.

Any biologically active pharmaceutical product potentially can harm as well as benefit its users. This can happen because a drug or biological agent has multiple mechanisms of action besides those involved in the therapeutic target, or idiosyncratically, possibly because of an immune response. It also can happen because of how the body reacts to non-pharmaceutical products, especially indwelling medical devices such as cardiovascular stents or artificial joints. Understanding how these potential harms can manifest themselves and at what stages of product development the potential for harm can be identified is critical to the development

*Statistical Methods for Evaluating Safety in Medical Product Development*, First Edition.
Edited by A. Lawrence Gould.
© 2015 John Wiley & Sons, Ltd. Published 2015 by John Wiley & Sons, Ltd.

of products that provide real benefits to patients. Many potential products that enter development fail because of unanticipated safety issues. Some of these occur early in development, but some occur very late in development. It is important to be able to predict the likelihood of harm from potential products as early as possible in the development process, and certainly before they reach the marketplace and present unnecessary risks to large numbers of patients.

## 1.2    Background and context

The safety of drugs, vaccines, and medical devices has become the Pole Star of product development. Discovery and development of drugs and other pharmaceutical products takes a long time, costs a lot of money, and has a low probability of success [7]. Failures can occur often during the development process, especially for novel drugs [2, 3]. Product withdrawals also can occur after products have been approved for marketing although, adverse publicity notwithstanding, these are relatively rare. Of the 740 new molecular entities (NMEs) approved by the Food and Drug Administration (FDA) in the USA between 1980 and 2009, 118 were withdrawn from the market. Most of these withdrawals were for reasons other than safety. Only 26 NMEs (3.5% of the approvals during this period) were withdrawn for safety reasons [8].

Safety issues arising consequent to chronic treatment do not always appear evident during drug development, either by preclinical assays or in the clinical phase of development. At least for cardiovascular events there is a need for understanding of fundamental mechanisms of cardiovascular liability that provide a way to detect potential toxicities during development [9]. The possibility of using biomarkers as leading indicators of potential safety issues has become a subject of discussion in the recent literature [10, 11]. There also has emerged in recent years an increasing interest in the application of methods for preclinical safety pharmacology and computational toxicology [12–16].

There is an increasing appreciation and availability of sophisticated means for making measurements early in the drug development process to identify potential safety issues that may emerge later on. There also is a need for means to provide more realistic assessments of risks of adverse events than are provided by clinical trials that do not, ordinarily cannot, include patients across the spectrum of potential susceptibility to adverse events [17–19].

Advances in the sophistication of measurement and interpretation of data make it appropriate to consider how recent developments in statistical methods for modeling, design, and analysis can contribute to progress in drug development, especially with regard to evaluating safety. Many books, and many more articles, describe conventional strategies for evaluating the safety of pharmaceutical products at various stages of development. Balakrishnan *et al.* [20] provide an exhaustive collection (86 chapters) of statistical methods but without a focus on safety. Chow and Liu [21] focus on the design of clinical trials, but do not address safety in depth or describe the implementation of novel methods for dealing with new types of complex data. Everitt and Palmer [22] provide an exhaustive collection of statistical essays intended to give medical researchers and clinicians readable accounts statistical concepts as they apply in various areas of medical research, especially in various therapeutic areas. Gad [23] focuses primarily on non-clinical pharmacology and toxicology studies needed to support product development with some attention to safety assessment in humans during and after the clinical development process, but does not appear to be directed toward statistical methods that can be applied, except possibly for conventional methods; there do not appear to be any references to the statistical literature past 1994. Lachin [24] describes standard tools and more recent likelihood-based theories for assessing risks and relative risks in clinical investigations, especially two-group comparisons, sample size considerations, stratified-adjusted analyses, case–control and matched studies, and logistic regression. Moyé [25] covers a number of topics, but addresses safety fairly briefly from a monitoring point of view. Proschan *et al.* [26] address the theoretical and practical aspects of monitoring clinical trials, primarily with the aim of assessing efficacy, but also with recommendations for monitoring safety in ongoing trials. The book edited by Rao *et al.* [27] covers a substantial range of methods for addressing various aspects of the design and analysis of clinical trials, including early phase trials and post-marketing trials, but does not address safety as such. Senn [28] identifies and addresses various issues, including (briefly) safety.

## 1.3 A fundamental principle for understanding safety evaluation

The evaluation of efficacy differs fundamentally from the evaluation of safety of medical products, that is, drugs, vaccines, and medical devices. To simplify the presentation in what follows, the term "drug" or "therapy" generally be used; however, statements using these terms generally will apply to any medical product.

Efficacy is at least conceptually easy to evaluate because the criteria for assessing efficacy in a trial need to be specified explicitly at the outset. A trial is designed with the expectation that one or more specific null hypotheses of no difference between the effect of the test therapy and a control will be rejected on the basis of the observations made during the trial. An antidiabetic drug may be assessed in terms of change in HbA1c over a defined period of time, an antiarrhythmic drug may be assessed in terms of survival, an antidepressant may be assessed in terms of change in Hamilton Depression Rating Score after a few months of treatment, and so on. If there is more than one hypothesis to be tested, some adjustment for the fact that multiple tests are performed is made in the statistical analysis so that the probability of concluding that a test therapy is efficacious when it is not can be controlled at an acceptable level. What constitutes efficacy and what the expectations are at the outset are known. That is how the sample size for the trial is determined. This is the same whether the aim of the trial is to prove that a new therapy is superior to a control or, if not, that it is not materially inferior to the control.

Safety is different. Although a few hypotheses about specific safety issues can be identified at the outset of a trial, and are treated in the statistical analysis similarly (but not identically) to hypotheses about efficacy, most safety issues are not identified at the outset of the trial. Consequently, the basis for determining that a test therapy is or is not acceptably "safe" generally cannot be identified before undertaking the trial. The inference about safety rests on interpretation of the observations. This can be problematic for at least two reasons. Firstly, it amounts to using the same observations to generate and to test hypotheses, which violates a basic scientific principle [29]. Secondly, attempts to adjust for the multiplicity of tests that are carried out for the often substantial number of adverse events that emerge during a trial using the same approaches that would apply for evaluating efficacy can decrease the sensitivity of any comparison so much that no difference in toxicity risk can be detected. However, not adjusting for multiplicity means that the chance of finding a material difference between the test and control therapies becomes appreciable even when the therapies pose the same risks.

How is one to interpret a "significant" increase in cardiac arrhythmias on a test therapy when perhaps 50 different adverse events that were not identified at the outset emerge during the trial? Is this a real effect, or is it a statistical artifact due to the fact that 50 tests were carried out? Clearly, a test of the null hypothesis that there is no additional risk of arrhythmia cannot by itself *confirm* an elevated risk of arrhythmia, but the way the findings from the trial usually are presented to the medical world at large invites a statistically significant finding to be (mis)interpreted as demonstrating at least association if not outright causality [30–32].

## 1.4 Stages of safety evaluation in drug development

Consideration of the potential toxicity of a potential drug or vaccine occurs at every stage of development:

1. Preclinical (efficacy, toxicity, pharmacokinetics, and epidemiology)

    a. *In silico* (computational toxicology, quantitative structure–activity relationship, and chemometrics)

    b. *In vitro* studies

    c. *In vivo* studies

2. Phase 1 (first in humans, healthy populations – toxicity and pharmacokinetics/ pharmacodynamics)

3. Phase 2 (toxicity and efficacy)

    a. Proof of concept studies

    b. Dose ranging studies

4. Phase 3 (toxicity and efficacy)

    a. Randomized controlled trials

    b. Confirmation of hypotheses generated in Phase 2

5. Post-approval

    a. Phase 4 studies

    b. Post-marketing safety surveillance

    c. Pharmacoepidemiology.

At every stage, the aims are to identify and characterize potential safety problems, understand the risk–benefit balance, and (especially at later stages) plan for risk management and mitigation.

While toxicity may be manifested in a variety of ways, certain key potential safety issues pervade the developmental process. These include cardiotoxicity, especially alterations of the electrical activity of the heart as manifested on electrocardiograms (ECGs), hepatotoxicity, nephrotoxicity, and bone marrow toxicity. Drugs in particular can be metabolized in different ways, and can have effects that depend on, that is, interact with, other co-administered drugs, the patient's disease state, and the general environment of the patient's life. Many adverse events can occur, but serious adverse events are potentially of most concern, particularly death, life-threatening events (e.g., bone marrow suppression), events leading to hospitalization, events leading to significant, persistent, or permanent disability, and congenital anomalies and other birth defects.

## 1.5     National medical product safety monitoring strategy

The National Medical Product Safety Monitoring Strategy that is part of the FDA Sentinel Initiative [33] aims to provide an integrated approach to monitoring pharmaceutical product safety throughout the entire life cycle of a product. The strategy seeks to combine an understanding of the underlying disease states with new methods of signal detection, data mining, and analysis. The Organizational Medical Outcomes Partnership, established under the Foundation of the National Institutes of Health, unites regulatory, industrial, and academic contributors in the development and implementation of tools for carrying out the monitoring strategy on marketed products using medical information accumulated in a variety of databases.

The overall strategy is implemented through an interdisciplinary team approach including geneticists, cell biologists, clinical pharmacologists, statisticians, epidemiologists, and informatics experts. The teams are charged with generating and confirming hypotheses about causal factors of safety problems among product users.

## 1.6     Adverse events vs adverse drug reactions, and an overall view of safety evaluation

Adverse events are not the same as adverse drug reactions. The ICH Guidelines (E6) define an *adverse event* as "any untoward medical occurrence in a patient or subject administered in a pharmaceutical product" [34]. Untoward medical occurrences include any unfavorable and unintended sign, symptom, or disease temporally associated with the use of the product. It is only the occurrences that matter, without a judgment about causality. The same guidelines define *adverse drug reactions* as either all noxious and unintended responses at least possibly causally related to a new medicinal product or usage, or a noxious and unintended response that occurs to patients on a marketed medicinal product at doses normally used in man. The element of possible causality is the key difference between these two concepts. There is, in addition, an extensive set of safety guidelines [35].

Risks associated with medicinal products arise from a number of sources, diagrammed in Figure 1.1. Some risks are known consequences of administration of medicinal products due to the disease treated or to the mechanism of action. Of these, some are unavoidable consequences that can lead to injury or death, and are part of the cost of the potential benefits of the product. Others are avoidable by appropriate choice of dosage or identification of patients who should or should not receive the product. Avoidable adverse events are in principle at least preventable, so that a key focus of safety evaluation is determining how characteristics of patients and dosage strategies are related to the risk of preventable adverse events. However, adverse events can occur for other than predictable reasons, especially when usage of the product is extended to wider patient populations than were studied during product development, or to uses not included in the originally approved set of indications.

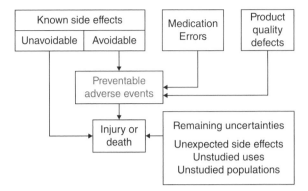

**Figure 1.1**  Sources of risk from medicinal products.

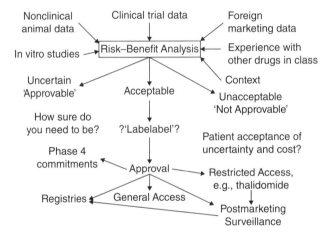

**Figure 1.2**  Overview of the components of the risk–benefit evaluation process in a regulatory context.

The evaluation of medicinal product safety occurs in the larger context of risk management and risk–benefit assessment. Figure 1.2 provides an outline of the context. The evaluation of risk and benefit incorporates information from clinical trials, but also information from non-clinical animal and *in vitro* studies that may provide insights into mechanisms of action, experience from other drugs in the same class, and the context for the use of the drug. Risk–benefit analyses lead to recommendations for further actions. If the risks are unacceptable, then the drug will be deemed "not approvable." If the risks are acceptable then the approval process can proceed to the next steps. If there is uncertainty about the risks, then further evaluation or trials may be needed. Once a drug has reached the point of possible approval, further decisions are in order, for example, whether the drug should be approved for general access or restricted access because there is a subpopulation for which the risk is unacceptable. In addition, approval may be granted conditional on further studies to assure that important, but rare, risks are not overlooked. In some cases, registries may be set up to follow specific subgroups of patients, for example, women who become pregnant. For most

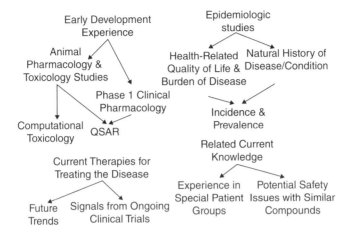

**Figure 1.3**   Elements of strategies for safety evaluation.

drugs, post-marketing surveillance of at least spontaneous reports will be required as part of periodic safety updates.

As the overview in Figure 1.2 makes clear, the evaluation of safety for any medicinal product needs to be considered in a fairly wide context and, therefore, must be the consequence of a well-thought-out strategy. Figure 1.3 illustrates some of the considerations that drive strategies for evaluating safety.

## 1.7   A brief historical perspective on safety evaluation

The discovery, testing, and utilization of medicines to treat human and animal ailments is as ancient as human history. Every human culture has its pharmacopeia based on extensive, if haphazard, trial and error [36–44]. Not all medications are derived from herbs. Some are derived from animals [40], some from marine fauna [44], and some from minerals and metals [45, 46]. Many ancient medicines whose effectiveness rests on long traditions of observation present potential health issues because of their pharmacologic effects, so that their use often traditionally has been restricted to physicians or trained healers [47]. Most traditional medicines have not been assessed by the standards employed for more conventional modern therapies so that even though they may be effective for specific purposes, they also may be toxic or may interact with conventional therapies in ways injurious to a patient [47–55].

The need to assure the safety of medicines and medical devices, a key objective of modern product development, has been recognized for centuries [56, 57]. For example, of the components that traditional Chinese medicine principles identify for a medicinal compound, one (the "adjuvant") is specifically intended to neutralize any side effects of the effective moieties (the "monarch" and the "minister") and another (the "guide") is intended essentially to enhance their bioavailability [39]. However, effective attempts to provide this assurance by government regulation of these products, at least in the West, date back, with apparently one exception, only to the late eighteenth and nineteenth centuries [58]. The exception, which addresses quality control of the preparation process rather than potential toxicity, is a pair of compounds formulated in the second century BCE, mithridatium and theriac, collectively known as "Venetian treacle," that led to a series of statutes in England dating from 1540 through 1799 for the regulation of the production of pharmaceuticals [47].

Although every national government includes a ministry of health (possibly with a different name) whose responsibilities include some form of evaluation of medicinal products, oversight of drug product safety is (or, at least until recently, has been) essentially non-existent in many parts of the Third World [59].

In the United States, the Biologics Control Act of 1902 authorized the regulation of the sale of biologic agents (viruses, sera, toxins, etc.); this Act required licensing of manufacturers and manufacturing establishments, established standards for safety, purity, and potency of biologics, and gave the federal government inspection authority. The Pure Food and Drug Act of 1906 culminated over 40 years of effort and various Acts of Congress to produce effective regulatory oversight of food and medicines; this Act prohibited interstate commerce in misbranded and adulterated foods, drinks, and drugs [60]. The 1906 legislation had a number of legal and regulatory shortcomings and was superseded by the Federal Food, Drug, and Cosmetic Act of 1938 after five years of legislative struggle, largely in response to a scandal resulting from the deaths of 107 children due to a lethal diluent used in a preparation of sulfanilamide elixir marketed by the Massengill Corporation [60, 61]. The new legislation required that new drugs be shown to be safe before marketing, extended regulatory control to cosmetics and therapeutic devices, and added the remedy of court injunctions to previous penalties, among other provisions. The legislation was amended several times in subsequent years. The most significant changes were implemented in 1962 with the Kefauver–Harris Drug Amendments that required drug manufacturers to prove the effectiveness of their products to the FDA before marketing. The Medical Device Amendments were passed in 1976, to assure safety and effectiveness of medical devices and diagnostic products.

The Council for International Organizations of Medical Sciences (CIOMS) was established jointly by WHO and UNESCO in 1949 as an umbrella organization for facilitating and promoting international biomedical science activities, especially those requiring the participation of international associations and national institutions. CIOMS has initiated and coordinated various long-term programs pertaining to drug development and use. CIOMS working groups have covered a broad range of drug safety topics, including consensus guidelines for reporting adverse drug reactions, drug safety update summaries, development safety update reports, core clinical safety information on drugs, terminology of adverse drug reactions, standardized MedDRA queries, and pharmacogenetics [62].

## 1.8    International conference on harmonization

The importance of independent evaluation of medicinal products before release to the public was reached at different times in different regions. Laws, regulations, and guidelines for reporting and evaluating data on safety, quality, and efficacy of new medicinal products increased rapidly in the 1960s and 1970s for most countries. Although the medicinal products industry was becoming more international, variations in technical and regulatory requirements among countries made it necessary for producers to duplicate time-consuming and expensive test procedures in order to market new products internationally. Concerns over rising costs of healthcare, escalation of the cost of research and development (R&D), and the need to meet the public expectation of rapid availability of safe and efficacious new treatments drove an urgent need to rationalize and harmonize regulatory requirements.

The European Community (now the European Union) pioneered the harmonization of regulatory requirements in the 1980s, concurrently with the evolution of a single market for medical products. Discussions initiated at the WHO Conference of Drug Regulatory Authorities in 1989 led to the establishment of a joint regulatory-industry initiative involving representatives of regulatory agencies and industry associations from Europe, Japan, and the United States that became the International Conference on Harmonisation (ICH) in 1990 [63]. The ICH steering committee decided to focus on harmonization of requirements for establishing the safety, quality, and efficacy of new medical products, leading to the ICH Harmonised Tripartite Guidelines. The effort to implement the guidelines and recommendations in the initial ICH regions and to extend the benefits to other regions has continued in the decades since the establishment of the ICH.

## 1.9    ICH guidelines

The safety guidelines provide detailed descriptions of the kinds of information that need to be obtained to evaluate various aspects of safety, as indicated in Table 1.1 [64, 65]. They often provide specific recommendations for specific kinds of experiments or trials, including recommendations about how doses should be selected. However, in contrast to considerable discussion of design and analysis considerations for evaluating efficacy, no details are provided about appropriate statistical designs as such or analytic methods, although Guideline S5 provides valuable insights:

> "Significance" tests (inferential statistics) can be used only as a support for the interpretation of results. The interpretation itself must be based on biological plausibility. It is unwise to assume that a difference from control values is not biologically relevant simply because it is not "statistically significant". To a lesser extent it can be unwise to assume that a "statistically significant" difference must be biologically relevant. … Confidence intervals for relevant quantities can indicate the likely size of the effect.

**Table 1.1**    ICH safety guidelines.

| Guideline | Addresses | Guideline | Addresses |
| --- | --- | --- | --- |
| S1A, S1B, S1C | Carcinogenicity | S6 | Biotechnology-derived pharmaceuticals |
| S2A, S2B | Genotoxicity | S7A | Safety pharmacology studies for human pharmaceuticals |
| S3A | Toxicokinetics | S7B | QT interval prolongation for human pharmaceuticals |
| S3B | Repeated dose tissue distribution | S8 | Immunotoxicity studies |
| S4 | Chronic toxicity testing in animals | S9 | Non-clinical evaluation for anticancer pharmaceuticals |
| S5 | Detection of reproductive toxicity | M3 | Non-clinical safety studies to support human clinical trials |

The efficacy guidelines are more extensive, and consider many statistical issues relevant to the evaluation of efficacy in detail. However, they are not very informative about how to address the evaluation of safety. Guideline E1 (Population exposure for assessing safety of chronic treatments for non-life-threatening conditions) provides recommendations as to the number of patients to treat (300–500) for at least 6 months in prospective studies and the number to treat for at least a year (100 patients or more). Guideline E2 (Safety data management: Expedited reporting and individual case reports) provides specific definitions of "adverse event," "adverse drug reaction," "unexpected drug reaction," and "serious adverse event or drug reaction," but no guidance on statistical design or analysis issues. Guideline E2E (Pharmacovigilance planning) briefly mentions methods for evaluating spontaneous reports, including Bayesian methods and data mining techniques for evaluating drug–drug interactions, but does not provide details. The guideline also includes a brief summary of epidemiologic methods that could be useful for evaluating adverse events. Guideline E3 (Structure and content of clinical study reports) provides some general comments, but no specific recommendations about evaluating safety. For example, when discussing exposure, "the more common adverse events, laboratory test changes etc. should be identified, classified in some reasonable way, compared for treatment groups, and analysed, as appropriate, for factors that may affect the frequence of adverse reactions/events" (p. 19). There appears to be a recognition that some focus generally is well advised; for example, "[i]t is not intended that every adverse event be subjected to rigorous statistical evaluation" (p. 22). Guideline E5 (Ethnic factors), which is primarily concerned with bridging studies, recommends evaluating rates of common adverse events in an efficacy bridging study or a separate safety study (p. 6), with no recommendations as to appropriate designs or analysis methods. Guideline E9 (Statistical principles for clinical trials) addresses safety only briefly (pp. 28–29), recommending that comprehensive safety and tolerability measures should be collected, including type, severity, onset, and duration of adverse events. However,, it is "not always self-evident how to assess incidence" and, in fact, "[i]n most trials the safety and tolerability implications are best addressed by applying descriptive statistical methods to the data, supplemented by calculation of confidence intervals whenever this aids interpretation" (p. 29). The guideline comes closest to recommending specific statistical analysis approaches on p. 32 when discussing the evaluation of information from a safety database: "The evaluation should also make appropriate use of survival analysis methods to exploit the potential relationship of the incidence of adverse effects to duration of exposure and/or follow-up. The risks associated with identified adverse effects should be appropriately quantified to allow a proper assessment of the risk/benefit relationship." Guideline E14 (The clinical evaluation of QT/QTc interval prolongation and proarrhythmic potential for non-antiarrhythmic drugs) provides some general recommendations, but no methodologic specifics. There is a need for a negative thorough QT/QTc study showing that the upper bound of a 95% one-sided confidence interval excludes 10 ms, and the guideline recommends carrying out analyses using uncorrected ECG values and values corrected using Bazett, Fridericia, and possibly linear approximation corrections to adjust for heart rate differences.

It is clear that there is a need for more definitive guidance on the use of statistical methods for assessing safety, for designing trials to provide useful clinical perspective about safety, and for making most effective use of new technologies that may be appropriate for very early identification of potential toxicity issues. The objective of this book is to provide recommendations and guidance for the effective application of statistical methods, both old and new, to the evaluation of drug and other medical product safety.

# References

[1] Olsen, A.K. and Whalen, M.D. (2009) Public perceptions of the pharmaceutical industry and drug safety. *Drug Safety*, **32**, 805–810.

Surveys conducted in 2006–2007 identified concerns about the effectiveness of drug companies and the FDA in assuring drug safety during development and after approval. This article addresses reforms aimed at addressing the concerns, including promoting a "safety culture throughout the health system" as a goal of every corporate and organizational entry, bringing stakeholders together to work towards achieving such a safety culture via public–private partnerships such as the FDA Sentinel Network and encouraging all healthcare professionals to track and report adverse events, and identifying a key role for pharmacovigilance professionals in promoting the understanding of the importance of cooperative activity in implementing the activities necessary to assure drug safety.

[2] Arrowsmith, J. (2011) Phase III and submission failures: 2007–2010. *Nature Reviews Drug Discovery*, **10**, 87–87.

This article summarizes reasons for failure of compounds during Phase 3 and after submission. The safety failure rate was 21% of 83 products that failed. One conclusion from the entire review: many failures occurred with drugs having novel mechanisms of action in areas of high unmet medical need.

[3] Arrowsmith, J. (2011) Phase II failures: 2008–2010. *Nature Reviews Drug Discovery*, **10**, 328–329.

Summary of reasons for failure of compounds during Phase 2; 19% (17 of 87) failed for safety.

[4] Kola, I. and Landis, J. (2004) Can the pharmaceutical industry reduce attrition rates? *Nature Reviews Drug Discovery*, **3**, 711–715.

Most pharmaceutical products (about 90%) were observed to fail in development between 1991 and 2000, with some variation by therapeutic area. About 25% were observed to fail during the registration review period, when almost all development costs had been incurred. Major causes of attrition in 2000 were lack of efficacy and safety (toxicology and clinical safety), both accounting for about 30% of failures. The high attrition rate is not economically sustainable for the industry. A number of proposals are presented to address the problem, including implementing testing methods that can effectively eliminate compounds with potential toxicity, especially mechanism-based toxicity, early in the development process.

[5] Walker, D.K. (2004) The use of pharmacokinetic and pharmacodynamic data in the assessment of drug safety in early drug development. *British Journal of Clinical Pharmacology*, **58**, 601–608.

It is important to assure that the target therapeutic free drug concentration required for efficacy, which often can be estimated from in vitro studies, is likely to be achieved by a realistic dosage regimen. This is extendable to assess potential safety risk when plasma free concentration is predictive of compound safety. However, many limiting safety findings, for example, hepatotoxicity, are unrelated to systemic concentrations. Pharmacogenetic considerations also are important, for example, dependence on CYP2D6 or CYP2C19 metabolism may present an undesirable safety risk. Single-dose pharmacokinetic data can provide guidance for deciding about the further development of a compound when there is information relating predictability of free drug concentration for efficacy or safety.

[6] Williams, R. (2011) Discontinued drugs in 2010: oncology drugs. *Expert Opinion on Drug Discovery*, **20**, 1479–1496.

This paper reviews the reasons for discontinuation of 28 oncology drugs dropped from the worldwide pipeline in 2010. Most discontinuations were for strategic or unspecified reasons, probably reflecting lack of resources or of evidence that the drug could be differentiated from or represent an improvement over current therapies. Three were dropped for safety-related reasons.

[7] DiMasi, J.A., Hansen, R.W. and Grabowski, H.G. (2003) The price of innovation: new estimates of drug development costs. *Journal of Health Economics*, **22**, 151–185.

Comprehensive analysis of the costs of drug development for 68 "randomly selected" products from 10 companies, updating a similar study published 12 years earlier. Average estimated total R&D cost is about $800 million (actually closer to $900 million counting post-approval R&D cost) as opposed to $231 million from the previous study. A number of factors contribute to increased cost, including more difficult therapeutic targets and more comprehensive studies. Most of the increase in cost comes at the clinical development as opposed to preclinical stage.

[8] Qureshi, Z.P., Seoane-Vazquez, E., Rodriquez-Monguio, R. and Stevenson, K.R. (2011) Market withdrawal of new molecular entities approved in the United States from 1980 to 2009. *Pharmacoepidemiology and Drug Safety*, **20**, 772–777.

This paper examines the bases for withdrawal of new molecular entities from the market between 1980 and 2009 based on data from FDA and other sources. During the period 740 NMEs were approved by FDA, and 118 (16%) were withdrawn. Withdrawal rates varied across categories of NME. Safety was the primary reason for withdrawal for 26 products (22% of withdrawals). About half of the discontinuations were for drugs approved in the 1980s, about 40% for drugs approved in the 1990s, and about 10% for drugs approved from 2000 on. Among safety withdrawals, about half occurred for drugs approved in the 1990s, 40% for drugs approved in the 1980s, and about 10% for drugs approved from 2000 on.

[9] Laverty, H., Benson, C., Cartwright, E.J. *et al.* (2011) How can we improve our understanding of cardiovascular safety liabilities to develop safer medicines? *British Journal of Pharmacology*, **163**, 675–693.

This is a report from a workshop hosted by the MRC Centre for Drug Safety Science to address issues retarding cardiovascular safety, focusing on three questions: (a) What are the key cardiovascular safety liabilities in drug discovery and development, and clinical practice? (b) How good are preclinical and clinical strategies for detecting these liabilities? (c) Is there a mechanistic understanding of the liabilities? With respect to (a), most adverse events (AEs) reported in the FDA's Adverse Event Reporting System often are not well described, nor are the AE–drug relationships established. AEs leading to discontinuation or withdrawal can be rare, for example, less than 10 per million patients for Torsade des Pointes arrhythmias. Myocardial ischemia or necrosis, heart failure, and coronary artery disorders often are not reported early in drug development, suggesting that they are not being captured by preclinical assays or during development. However, drugs with drug-induced vascular injury have been successfully developed. With regard to (b), it was observed that preclinical safety evaluation generally is conducted in young healthy animals lacking the pathophysical background underlying these disease conditions, so it is not clear whether the usual preclinical models accurately reflect the patient population ultimately to be exposed to drug. QT-related assays appear to be good, but not perfect, predictors of arrhythmia in clinical setting. The picture is much less clear for other AEs such as myocardial ischemia. Certain aspects of drug-induced cardiovascular (CV) disturbances are not routinely addressed during preclinical development. With regard to (c), although the mechanism for QT prolongation is known, arrhythmias account for only a small proportion of drug withdrawals due to CV safety issues. The mechanism for most of these is unclear. Targeted cancer therapies, particularly protein kinase inhibitors, also can lead to CV toxicity because they inhibit kinases necessary for maintaining homeostasis in cardiac tissue, so that risk must be balanced against benefit. Two key points from the report are the need for approaches that discover the fundamental mechanisms of CV liability to allow a step change in the detection of CV liability early in drug development, and that current understanding about mechanisms resulting in CV dysfunction is inadequate.

[10] Rolan, P., Danhof, M., Sanski, D. and Peck, C. (2007) Current issues relating to drug safety especially with regard to the use of biomarkers: a meeting report and progress update. *European Journal of Pharmaceutical Sciences*, **30**, 107–112.

This paper is a summary of the discussion at a meeting of an expert group to review the state of the art in detecting drug-related safety problems and the role of biomarkers and modeling techniques in improving the ability to detect toxicity issues early in drug development. Without a causal mechanism linking a biomarker with a clinical endpoint and toxicity it is difficult to distinguish between a biomarker change reflecting exposure and a change reflecting toxicity. Even for hepatotoxic drugs, it is difficult to predict whether a patient demonstrating a change will go on to experience toxicity. There are few useful skin-based biomarkers for prediction/development of toxicity. There are also few new biomarkers of hepatotoxicity; current ones have poor specificity. Hemotoxicity and immunotoxicity are usually easy to detect in development of oncology drugs, less successful for non-cytotoxic and non-immunosuppressive drugs. Many drugs are toxic to bone marrow through non-humoral mechanisms, but current diagnostic tests have poor diagnostic properties. Preclinical models are not very useful for predicting behavioral toxicity. Simple behavioral toxicities like sedation are easy to detect early, but toxicities affecting complex behavior (e.g., depression) are difficult to detect. Modeling biological systems/responses mechanistically may be useful for predicting subtle toxicities.

[11] Marrer, E. and Dieterle, F. (2010) Impact of biomarker development on drug safety assessment. *Toxicology and Applied Pharmacology*, **243**, 167–179.

This article addresses considerations about the role and objectives of safety biomarkers at each stage of drug development. Effective biomarkers can enable the therapeutic use even of drugs that may be toxic if the toxicity potential can be recognized early and managed clinically. The article provides an overview of safety biomarkers for specific organ systems (kidney, liver, heart, vascular system) along with evidence supporting their use in preclinical and clinical development. Current standards for monitoring renal safety are late in identifying toxicity, insensitive, and not very specific. However, a number of new protein-based biomarkers have promise for early detection of acute kidney injury. The picture is similar for liver toxicity; a number of biomarkers used together may help in early prediction of hepatotoxicity. Cardiac troponins are recently studied biomarkers for damage to heart muscle that have reasonable specificity and sensitivity. Vascular safety is a major concern because of a lack of diagnostic markers and gaps in understanding of pathogenesis and mechanisms of vascular lesion development. The article discusses issues related to stages of development of biomarkers: identification, preclinical qualification, and clinical qualification and diagnostic use.

[12] Bass, A.S., Cartwright, M.E., Mahon, C. *et al.* (2009) Exploratory drug safety: a discovery strategy to reduce attrition in development. *Journal of Pharmacological and Toxicological Methods*, **60**, 69–78.

This paper describes a number of areas of study aimed at mitigating risk of failure during development, with primary emphasis on preclinical and early clinical development stages. These include pre-development safety pharmacology to ascertain pharmacodynamic properties of test molecules on major organ system function, genetic toxicology to evaluate potential genotoxicity of active constituents, metabolites, and excipients, exploratory drug metabolism and pharmacokinetic studies, studies aimed at evaluating potential for off-target activity of a test molecule that could present potential safety liabilities, Also important are exploratory drug safety studies aimed at identifying toxic effects that may be evident in extended administration (up to 14 days), to identify issues that would be likely to emerge in longer-term chronic studies.

[13] Benbow, J.W., Aubrecht, J., Banker, M.J. *et al.* (2010) Predicting safety toleration of pharmaceutical chemical leads: cytotoxicity correlations to exploratory toxicity studies. *Toxicology Letters*, **197**, 175–182.

Cytotoxicity assessments are used to conduct high-throughput safety screening for evaluating compounds considered for further development. Difficulties in extrapolating *in vitro* cytotoxicity to *in vivo* effects have been reported due to direct correlations or limitations caused by confounding factors of the whole organism. Moreover, relationships found on a limited set of compounds may not apply for a wider set of compounds. This article addresses the hypothesis that compounds with less cytotoxic potential would have fewer safety findings in short-term rat exploratory toxicity studies using a wide range of pharmaceutically relevant compounds (72 compounds). A composite safety score was generated for each compound based on the incidence and severity of adverse outcomes using a scoring algorithm based on systemic toleration, organ functional assessment, and multiorgan pathology. Results indicate that a simple cytotoxicity assessment can be a useful addition to the battery of information usually obtained during lead development.

[14] Merlot, C. (2010) Computational toxicology – a tool for early safety evaluation. *Drug Discovery Today*, **15**, 16–22.

This insightful review focuses on recent developments in computational toxicology aimed at predicting the toxicity of a molecule from a representation of its chemical structure. Algorithms for the computations mostly invoke expert systems or statistical modeling. There are a number of key issues associated with either approach. One of these is the reliability of a prediction for one or more compounds, and much effort has been devoted to defining the applicability of computational models. The methods work best when the test compounds are similar to the compounds used to train the model; failures of the approaches can be due to differences between the test compounds and the set of training compounds. However, even being close to the training set does not guarantee correct prediction because small structural differences can have substantial toxicological effects. Complex endpoints are difficult to predict, and carcinogenicity, liver toxicity, and developmental toxicity are complex endpoints whose prediction by current models is inadequate. The role of computational toxicology is to shift compound attrition early in the development cycle, to fail cheaply. While computer screens can identify many false positives, they can be used as a preliminary screening device and followed up by *in vitro* or *in vivo* testing.

[15] Nigsch, F., Macaluso, N.J.M., Mitchell, J.B.O. and Zmuidinavicius, D. (2009) Computational toxicology: an overview of the sources of data and of modelling methods. *Expert Opinion on Drug Metabolism & Toxicology*, **5**, 1–14.

Computational toxicology presents an opportunity to save time and expense in evaluating the toxic potential of drugs and their metabolites, but is limited by the need for comprehensive and extensive data in structured, machine-accessible form. Included within this purview is the emerging field of toxicogenomics driven by the possibility of extensive genome-wide expression analyses, although its practical application remains in doubt. The goals are much clearer than the current ability to achieve them. The article provides an overview of commonly used toxicity assays and discusses a number of kinds of computational approaches, including quantitative structure–activity relationships, target prediction models, and protein target and structure-based methods. Computational methods usually are knowledge-based, relying on a substantial body of expert opinion, or statistically based, relying on substantial data mining activity.

[16] Nigsch, F., Lounkine, E., McCarren, P. *et al.* (2011) Computational methods for early predictive safety assessment from biological and chemical data. *Expert Opinion on Drug Metabolism & Toxicology*, **7**, 1497–1511.

Predictive safety assessment is incorporated at various stages of drug development in a number of ways: *in silico* methods are used in early discovery to prioritize compounds or to flag potential liabilities; *in vitro* assays are performed to filter out compounds with toxic potential; following lead selection, animal experiments are performed in various species to evaluate pharmacokinetics, pharmacodynamics, potential biomarkers toxicology, gene expression, etc. Authors suggest that the role of computational toxicology is to identify potential issues needing to be followed up by more conventional safety assessment techniques. This article describes different categories of computational toxicology tools: expert- or rule-based systems, statistical models, quantum mechanical calculations, structure-based approaches, and the use of safety panels. Computational approaches may be able to help uncover associations of AEs with chemical structure and activity. Bayesian models have been used to identify relationships between *in vivo* binding profiles and AEs.

[17] Ioannidis, J.P.A. and Lau, J. (2002) Improving safety reporting from randomized trials. *Drug Safety*, **25**, 77–84.

Empirical evidence across diverse medical fields suggests that the reporting of safety information in clinical trials is largely neglected and receives less attention compared with efficacy outcomes. Safety data need to be collected and analyzed in a systematic fashion and active surveillance for toxicity during the conduct of a randomized trial is preferable to passive surveillance. Common errors include (1) not reporting safety data at all; (2) making only vague statements; (3) reporting events without a breakdown by study arm; (4) lumping different kinds of AEs under broad categories; (5) combining severity levels; (6) giving $p$-values but no event counts; (7) providing information on only a few or the most common AEs; (8) not providing information on AEs leading to withdrawal from the trial; (9) over-interpreting and over-analyzing safety data; (10) over-interpreting the absence of AEs; (11) failing to define scales used to categorize AE severity; (12) reporting data without relevant information about the experimental unit, such as duration of exposure. Some recommendations from the article are as follows: (1) specify the number of patients withdrawn because of AEs per study arm and AE; (2) use widely known, standardized scales for AEs; (3) specify the schedule for safety information collection, specific tests performed, questionnaires used, and whether surveillance was active or passive; (4) provide the number of specific AEs per study arm and per type of AE; (5) tabulate safety information per study arm and severity grade for each AE.

[18] Ioannidis, J.P.A., Evans, S.J.W., Gotzsche, P.C. *et al.* (2004) Better reporting of harms in randomized trials: an extension of the CONSORT statement. *Annals of Internal Medicine*, **141**, 781–788.

This article describes an extension of 10 new recommendations to the standard CONSORT checklist about reporting harms-related issues. The recommendations are as follows: (1) State in title or abstract if the study collected data on harms and benefits. (2) The introduction should state if the trial addresses both harms and benefits. (3) Define the recorded AEs in the Methods section, clarifying whether all AEs or only a selected sample are included, whether only expected or also unexpected AEs are included, etc. (4) Clarify how harms-related information was collected. (5) Describe statistical methods planned for presenting and analyzing harms information. (6) Describe the participant withdrawals due to harms from each study arm, and the experience with the allocated treatment. (7) Provide the denominators for analyses of harms. (8) Present the absolute risk of each AE (type, grade, severity) per arm, and present appropriate metrics for recurrent events. (9) Describe any subgroup analyses and exploratory harms analyses. (10) Provide in the Discussion section a balanced discussion of benefits and harms, with emphasis on study limitations, generalizability, etc.

[19] Ioannidis, J.P.A., Mulrow, C.D. and Goodman, S.N. (2006) Adverse events: the more you search, the more you find. *Annals of Internal Medicine*, **144**, 298–300.

Medication-related harms can be identified from many sources, typically case reports, observational studies, and randomized trials. How one defines and looks for problems affects the numbers of AEs that patients report. Patients' judgments about tolerable harm can depend on whether they felt they had effective therapeutic alternatives. it is important to follow appropriate guidelines specifying how and when harms-related information was collected. It is almost always inappropriate to make statements about no difference in AE rates based on non-significant $p$-values.

[20] Balakrishnan, N., Read, C.B., Vidakovic, B. *et al.* (2010) *Methods and Applications of Statistics in the Life and Health Sciences*, John Wiley & Sons, Inc., Hoboken, NJ.

[21] Chow, S.C. and Liu, J.P. (2013) *Design and Analysis of Clinical Trials: Concepts and Methodologies*, 3rd edn, John Wiley & Sons, Inc., Hoboken, NJ.

[22] Everitt, B.S. and Palmer, C.R. (2009) *The Encyclopaedic Companion to Medical Statistics*, John Wiley & Sons, Inc., Hoboken, NJ.

[23] Gad, S.C. (2009) *Drug Safety Evaluation*, John Wiley & Sons, Inc., Hoboken, NJ.

[24] Lachin, J.M. (2000) *Biostatistical Methods: The Assessment of Relative Risks*, John Wiley & Sons, Inc., New York.

[25] Moyé, L.A. (2006) *Statistical Monitoring of Clinical Trials: Fundamentals for Investigators*, Springer, New York.

[26] Proschan, M.A., Lan, K.K.G. and Wittes, J. (2006) *Statistical Monitoring of Clinical Trials*, Springer, New York.

[27] Rao, C.R., Miller, J. and Rao, D.C. (2007) *Epidemiology and Medical Statistics*, Handbook of Statistics, vol. **27**, Elsevier, New York.

[28] Senn, S. (2008) *Statistical Issues in Drug Development*, 2nd ed., John Wiley & Sons, Ltd, Hoboken, New Jersey.

[29] Popper, K.R. (1963) Science as falsification, in *Conjectures and Refutations*, Routledge & Kegan Paul, London.

   This is a short, elegant, and clear explanation of what it takes for a theory to be "scientific." Some points: (1) Confirmations or verifications can be found for any theory if they are sought. (2) Confirmations should count only if they result from "risky predictions", i.e., if there are possible outcomes that could not be explained by the theory. (3) The more a theory forbids, the better it is. (4) A theory which is not refutable is not scientific. (5) Every genuine test of a theory is an attempt to falsify or refute it. (6) Confirming evidence should count only when it can be presented as a serious but unsuccessful attempt to falsify the theory. In short, the scientific status of a theory is determined by its falsifiability, refutability, or testability. The criteria for refutation have to be laid down before obtaining observations to test a theory, i.e., the hypothesis must be stated before the data are obtained.

[30] Altman, D.G. and Bland, J.M. (1991) Improving doctors' understanding of statistics. *Journal of the Royal Statistical Society, Series A*, **154**, 223–267.

   This article discusses the need for statistical knowledge in medicine, what doctors need to know about statistics and whether the state of statistical knowledge among doctors is adequate. The article considers a number of ways in which doctors acquire statistical knowledge, such as undergraduate and postgraduate education, the quality of many textbooks, and the examples given by papers in medical journals. A number of recommendations are offered, including the following: (1) greater emphasis on statistical principles in undergraduate medical education and more postgraduate statistics courses for doctors, taught by experienced medical statisticians; (2) greater attention to the scientific and statistical correctness of papers published by medical journals; (3) more involvement of statisticians in medicine, at all levels of teaching, refereeing medical papers, membership on ethical committees, and more collaboration with doctors and statistical consultancy. The article is accompanied by extensive commentary by many statisticians.

[31] Windish, D.M., Huot, S.J. and Green, M.L. (2007) Medicine residents' understanding of the biostatistics and results in the medical literature. *Journal of the American Medical Association*, **298**, 1010–1022.

   This article describes the result of a survey completed by 277 internal medicine residents in 11 residency programs aimed at evaluating their understanding of biostatistics and research result interpretation. The instrument used for the evaluation was a biostatistics/study design multiple-choice knowledge test. The overall mean percentage correct on statistical knowledge and interpretation of results for the residents was 41% vs 72% for fellows and general medicine faculty with research training. Higher scores were associated with additional advanced degrees (50% vs 41%), prior biostatistics training (45% vs 38%), enrollment in a university-based training program (43% vs 36%), or being male (44% vs 39%). Although most (82%) correctly interpreted a relative risk, the residents were less likely to know how to interpret an adjusted odds ratio from a multivariate regression analysis (37%) or the results of a Kaplan–Meier analysis (10%). Most (75%) did not believe that they understood all of the statistics they encountered in journal articles, but almost all (95%) felt it was important to understand these concepts to be an intelligent reader of the literature. The authors conclude that most residents in this study lacked the knowledge in biostatistics needed to interpret many of the results in published clinical research and that residency programs should include more effective biostatistics training in their curricula.

[32] Wulff, H.R., Andersen, B., Brandenhoff, P. and Guttler, F. (1987) What do doctors know about statistics? *Statistics in Medicine*, **6**, 3–10.

A 10-item multiple-choice test to evaluate statistical knowledge was sent to 250 Danish doctors selected at random from a registry of Danish physicians, who were asked to complete the test without consulting a textbook of statistics; 140 of the doctors completed the questionnaire, as did an additional 97 participants in postgraduate courses in research methods. The median number of correct answers was 2.4 among the random sample and 4 among the additional cohort. The conclusion was that the statistical knowledge of most doctors was so limited that they could not be expected to interpret statistical findings in medical journals correctly.

[33] Food and Drug Administration (2010) The Sentinel Initiative, http://www.fda.gov/Safety/FDASSentinelInitiative/default.htm (accessed 22 July 2014).

An update on FDA progress in building a national electronic system for monitoring post-marketing safety of FDA-approved drugs and other medical products.

[34] ICH Expert Working Group (1996) Guideline for Good Clinical Practice E6(R1), http://www.ich.org/fileadmin/Public_Web_Site/ICH_Products/Guidelines/Efficacy/E6_R1/Step4/E6_R1__Guideline.pdf (accessed 22 July 2014).

A comprehensive international ethical and scientific quality standard for designing, conducting, recording, and reporting trials that involve the participation of human subjects. The objective of the guideline is to provide a unified standard for the EU, Japan and the USA to facilitate the mutual acceptance of clinical data by the various regulatory agencies.

[35] *ICH Expert Working Group* (2014) ICH Safety Guidelines, http://www.ich.org/products/guidelines/safety/article/safety-guidelines.html (accessed 22 July 2014).

[36] Aboelsoud, N.H. (2010) Herbal medicine in ancient Egypt. *Journal of Medicinal Plants Research*, **4**, 82–86.

This paper summarizes documentary evidence that therapeutic herbs and foods were used extensively in ancient Egypt. Medicines also were made from mineral substances. Medications were age-specific. Prescriptions were written with high skill. Most of the medical knowledge was set by 2000 BCE.

[37] Anon. Bald's Leechbook, http://en.wikipedia.org/wiki/Bald's_Leechbook (accessed 13 September 2011).

This Old English medical text in two volumes was probably compiled in the ninth century CE. The first book deals with external disorders, the second with internal problems.

[38] Anon. Authentic Mayan Medicine, http://www.authenticmayan.com/maya_medicine.html (accessed 12 September 2011).

This provides an overview of principles of Mayan medicine. Mayan medicine was holistic by nature, incorporating a medico-religious tradition that took account of the emotional as well as the physical state of the patient. There was an extensive, largely herbal-based, pharmacopoeia.

[39] Jia, W., Gao, W.-Y., Yan, Y.-Q. *et al.* (2011) The rediscovery of ancient Chinese herbal formulas. *Phytotherapeutic Research*, **18**, 681–686.

This review of ancient Chinese herbal medicine principles describes the organization of formulas containing combinations of herbs with specific roles (monarch, minister, adjuvant, guide). It gives examples where the properties/effects of a particular herbal component can be modified, sometimes dramatically, by the inclusion of other herbal components. The mechanism of action of most combination formulas is still unknown. It discourages use of herbal medicines chronically or in high dosages without the involvement of a skilled practitioner diagnosis and the determination of a holistic treatment approach.

[40] Lev, E. (2002) Traditional healing with animals (zootherapy): medieval to present-day Levantine practice. *Journal of Ethnopharmacology*, **85**, 107–118.

This paper reviews the history of the use of medicines derived from animal bodies and organs in the Levant. It provides a detailed summary of names and references to documents from various periods of 99 substances of animal origin identified as being used in traditional medicine from early medieval to present times. Main animal sources include honey, wax, adder, beaver testicles, musk oil, coral, and ambergris. It also provides a detailed list of some 77 animal products currently used.

[41] Nissenbaum, A. (1993) The Dead Sea – an economic resource for 10,000 years. *Hydrobiologia*, **267**, 127–141.

This paper describes various products of the Dead Sea since ancient times. Medicinal use was made of distilled asphalt for treating skin diseases. Dead Sea waters may have been useful for treating eye disease, and are still used for treating psoriasis.

[42] Rahman, S.Z., Khan, R.A. and Latif, A. (2008) Importance of pharmacovigilance in Unani system of medicine. *Indian Journal of Pharmacology*, **40**, 17–20.

This paper provides a historical account of pharmacology over 1000 years ago, when more than 2000 drugs were known and studied. It includes a description of the encyclopedic work of Ibn Sinâ (980–1037 CE) who wrote treatises on cardiac drugs, pharmacologic and pharmacotherapeutic characteristics and methods of preparation of many compounds, and many aspects of toxicology. The notion of patient-tailored therapy also appears in the writings of Ibn Sinâ. The paper also discusses early pharmacovigilance and its relation to Unani (Greco-Arabic) medicine. It reecognizes the present-day need for systematic data on the incidence of adverse events associated with the use of traditional medicines.

[43] Saad, B., Azaizeh, H. and Said, O. (2005) Tradition and perspectives of Arab herbal medicine: a review. *Evidence Based Complementary and Alternative Medicine*, **2**, 475–479.

This is an overview of the history of Arab medicine. Major innovations include the discovery of the immune system and introduction of microbiological science; the separation of medicine from pharmacological science (Avicenna, tenth and eleventh centuries CE); and advances in herbal medicine including extraction of anesthetic compounds from local herbs and the introduction of 350 new plant species to medicinal herbs.

[44] Voultsiadou, E. (2010) Therapeutic properties and uses of marine invertebrates in the ancient Greek world and early Byzantium. *Journal of Ethnopharmacology*, **130**, 237–247.

Review of ancient Greek, Roman, and Byzantine texts regarding the therapeutic properties of marine invertebrates. For over 30 species, provides the scientific, classical, and common names, summarizes their therapeutic properties and uses, and provides references to original texts.

[45] Merchant, B. (1998) Gold, the noble metal and the paradoxes of its toxicology. *Biologicals*, **26**, 49–59.

This paper describes therapeutic uses of metallic gold and gold salts, and some related toxicity issues.

[46] Sarkar, P.K. and Chaudhary, A.K. (2010) Ayurvedic bhasma: the most ancient application of nanomedicine. *Journal of Scientific and Industrial Research*, **69**, 901–905.

Sarkar and Chaudhary describe the preparation of nanoparticle formulations of various metals for therapeutic use.

[47] Griffin, J.P. (2004) Venetian treacle and the foundation of medicines regulation. *British Journal of Clinical Pharmacology*, **58**, 317–325.

This paper describes the history of legislation from the fifteenth century onward regarding oversight of the preparation and assurance of quality of a "universal panacea" known as Venetian treacle. This early legislation stimulated concerns about the quality of all medicines and was the earliest implementation of medicine regulation.

[48] Chan, T.Y.K. (1994) The prevalence, use, and harmful potential of some Chinese herbal medicines in babies and children. *Veterinary and Human Toxicology*, **36**, 238–240.

This article reviews the prevalence use of Chinese herbal medicines (CHM) in Chinese pregnant women, babies and children living in Hong Kong and the harmful potential of some CHM and Chinese proprietary medicines (CPM) in babies and children. The use of CHM appears to be common amongst Chinese pregnant women. The possible effects of these herbs on the fetus and baby and their overall safety are not known. This practice should be discouraged since there is a suggestion that maternal consumption of CHM might increase the risk of neonatal jaundice. Both *chuen-lin* and *yin-chen* can displace bilirubin from their serum protein binding and increase the risk of hyperbilirubinemia. These herbs should not be given to the neonates. The use of CPM containing undeclared drugs of high toxicity or lead, arsenic and mercurial compounds should be banned. The medical profession and the general public should be alerted to the harmful potential of some CHM and CPM. There should be continuing efforts to collect information on the safety of these compounds.

[49] Chitturi, S. and Farrell, G.C. (2008) Herbal hepatotoxicity: an expanding but poorly defined problem. *Journal of Gastroenterology and Hepatology*, **15**, 1093–1099.

Many herbal remedies are hepatotoxic, and many more may be hepatotoxic to an unknown degree. This article provides a list of hepatotoxic herbal compounds and provides several examples of how the hepatotoxicity is manifested.

[50] Ernst, E. (2003) Serious psychiatric and neurological adverse effects of herbal medicines – a systematic review. *Acta Psychiatrica Scandinavica*, **108**, 83–91.

This is a survey of literature, mostly case reports, of adverse events associated with the use of alternative (mostly herbal) medicines. The reports suggest that herbal medicines have often been associated with potentially severe psychiatric and neurological adverse events. The article summarizes reports of herb–drug interactions and adverse events associated with contamination or adultery of the herbal products. The findings are suggestive because many of the reports lack the level of detail necessary to establish clear causal or even associative relationships. However, the reports do suggest that the possibility of herb–drug pharmacokinetic or pharmacodynamic interactions needs to be taken into account in patient management. Since herbal medicines (at least those mentioned in the article) have not been rigorously evaluated for efficacy, informed risk–benefit assessments rarely can be made.

[51] Hu, Z., Yang, X., Ho, P.C.L. *et al.* (2005) Herb–drug interactions. A literature review. *Drugs*, **65**, 1239–1282.

Herb–drug interactions probably are significantly under-reported and underestimated for various reasons. For example, patients do not tell their physicians about the herbal remedies they are using; there is a lack of regulations requiring rigorous preclinical/clinical assessment of herbal remedies; most clinical trials of herbal remedies are poorly designed and executed; there is no comprehensive AE surveillance system in many countries (especially those where herbal remedies are popular); and any herbal compound may contain multiple bioactive constituents whose individual actions are difficult to separate. This article is a substantial survey of literature (with more than 500 references) on interactions between herbal preparations and a wide range of conventional pharmaceutical products.

[52] Niggemann, B. and Grüber, C. (2003) Side-effects of complementary and alternative medicine. *Allergy*, **58**, 707–716.

This article is an extensive literature review of mostly anecdotal reports of various kinds of adverse events associated with herbal medicines and mechanical procedures such as acupuncture. It states that "[v]irtually all herbal remedies have been reported to cause either allergic sensitization or photosensitization." Organ toxicity, especially hepatotoxicity and nephrotoxicity, of herbal medicines can be due to the chemical constituents of the product, or to contamination, adulteration, or misidentification of ingredients. Chronic use of high doses of some herbal preparations has been associated with increased cancer risk.

[53] Saad, B., Azaizeh, H., Abu Hijleh, G. and Said, O. (2006) Safety of traditional Arab herbal medicine. *Evidence Based Complementary and Alternative Medicine*, **3**, 433–439.

This is a systematic review of the safety of traditional Arab medicine and contributions of Arab scholars to toxicology. Ancient Arab sources on toxicology go back to the eighth to tenth centuries

CE. The article summarizes toxicologic findings for commonly used traditional herbal medicines. It provides recommendations for processes to assure safety and consistency of herbal medicines.

[54] Skoulidis, F., Alexander, G.J.M. and Davies, S.M. (2005) Ma huang associated acute liver failure requiring liver transplantation. *European Journal of Gastroenterology and Hepatology*, **17**, 581–584.

This is a case report of hepatotoxicity requiring liver transplant induced by ma huang, which contains ephedrine-type alkaloids. It also reviews literature about potential ma huang induced hepatotoxicity.

[55] Wojcikowski, K., Johnson, D.W. and Gobé, G. (2004) Medicinal herbal extracts – renal friend or foe? Part one: the toxicities of medicinal herbs. *Nephrology*, **9**, 313–318.

Literature review of articles describing cases of renal toxicity.

[56] Lee, P.R. and Herzstein, J. (1986) International drug regulation. *Annual Review of Public Health*, **7**, 217–235.

Drug regulation has a long history, dating back 3000 years. Apothecaries were regulated in Europe and Muslim countries in the Middle Ages, with focus shifting to regulations of drugs from the sixteenth century CE on. The institution of patent laws in the USA and Europe and the isolation of pure morphine in 1805 set the stage for the evolution of the pharmaceutical industry and subsequent development of international drug regulation.

[57] Levey, M. (1963) Fourteenth century Muslim medicine and the *hisba*. *Medical History*, **7**, 176–182.

The article describes the office of the *hisba*, established in the ninth century CE to enforce regulations regarding public safety (among other things). It quotes extensively from a fourteenth-century text regarding regulations concerning physicians, ophthalmologists, surgeons, and bonesetters, and extensive discussion of preparation of various therapeutic agents, typically herbal

[58] Swann, J. P. (2014) About FDA: FDA's Origin, http://www.fda.gov/AboutFDA /WhatWeDo/ History/Origin/ucm124403.htm (accessed 22 July 2014).

This describes the history of the FDA from 1862 through 2001, including the various legislative acts that defined and subsequently expanded its role and responsibility.

[59] Lee, P.R., Lurie, P., Silverman, M.M. and Lydecker, M. (1991) Drug promotion and labeling in developing countries: an update. *Journal of Clinical Epidemiology*, **44** (*Suppl. II*), 49S–55S.

This paper provides a description of changes in promotional practices by multinational and domestic pharmaceutical companies as of late 1980s. Legislation to control drugs was enacted in England in the late nineteenth century, in Switzerland in 1900, in the USA in 1906. Regulations relevant to safety and efficacy were enacted in Norway and Sweden in the 1920s, in the USA in 1938, and in virtually all European countries by early 1960s. The paper points to the double standard of basing promotion in developed countries on scientifically based evidence. It says that the practice of expanding indications in developing nations persists, and unjustified claims of efficacy or safety continue(d) to proliferate.

[60] Food and Drug Administration. About FDA: Significant Dates in US Food and Drug Law History, http://www.fda.gov/AboutFDA/WhatWeDo/History/Milestones/ucm128305.htm (accessed 1 September 2011).

Annotated calendar of dates of significant events in FDA history, especially key court cases and legislation.

[61] Wax, P.M. (1995) Elixirs, diluents, and the passage of the 1938 federal food, drug and cosmetic act. *Annals of Internal Medicine*, **122**, 456–461.

This paper gives a history of the events associated with the Elixir Sulfanilamide disaster of 1937 in which 105 patients died from the use of a preparation of sulfanilamide that used diethyl glycol as a diluent. The events and the subsequent public attention led to the 1938 Federal Food, Drug, and Cosmetic Act that required for the first time testing of new drug products for toxicity.

[62] Council for International Organizations of Medical Sciences, www.cioms.ch (accessed 8 September 2011).

Website for CIOMS, World Health Organization.

[63] International Conference on Harmonisation, http://www.ich.org/ (accessed 8 September 2011).

ICH website.

[64] Safety Guidelines, http://www.ICH.org/fileadmin/Public_Web_Site/ICH_Products/Guidelines/Safety/Safety_Guidelines.zip (accessed 1 June 2010).

Archive file containing the latest version of the ICH safety guidelines.

[65] Efficacy Guidelines, http://www.ICH.org/fileadmin/Public_Web_Site/ICH_Products/Guidelines/Efficacy/Efficacy_Guidelines.zip (accessed 1 June 2010).

Archive file containing the latest version of the ICH efficacy guidelines.

# 2

# Safety graphics

## A. Lawrence Gould

*Merck Research Laboratories, 770 Sumneytown Pike, West Point, PA 19486, USA*

## 2.1 Introduction

### 2.1.1 Example and general objectives

Graphical displays provide an opportunity to convey insight about patterns, trends, or anomalies that may signal potential safety issues in ways that would be difficult to apprehend from tabular or textual presentations. Table 2.1 and Figure 2.1 provide a simple, but effective, example using the incidence of dermatologic adverse events that were reported in a trial comparing Aldara® and its vehicle [1]. Aldara® is a formulation of topical imiquimod that is used to treat certain types of actinic keratoses caused by excess sun exposure. While Table 2.1 actually displays more immediately accessible information than Figure 2.1 does because the incidences are immediately available from Table 2.1 but must be interpolated from Figure 2.1, Figure 2.1 conveys the clearer picture of the dermatologic adverse event profile. It is immediately evident from Figure 2.1, but requires study of Table 2.1, that the incidence of dermatologic events of any grade was noticeably greater following treatment with Aldara® than with its vehicle, but that this was true only for severe grades of erythema, scabbing/crusting, or erosion. Table 2.1 provides the basis of analyses that would determine what conclusions about the potential dermatologic toxicity of Aldara® could legitimately be drawn, but Figure 2.1 provides the visual insight into the clinical meaning of those conclusions.

Graphical displays need to be used thoughtfully. "Like good writing, good graphical displays of data communicate ideas with clarity, precision, and efficiency. Like poor writing, bad graphical displays distort or obscure the data, make it harder to understand or compare, or otherwise thwart the communicative effect which the graph should convey" [2]. Wainer provides examples of graphics demonstrating practices that should be avoided [3].

*Statistical Methods for Evaluating Safety in Medical Product Development*, First Edition.
Edited by A. Lawrence Gould.
© 2015 John Wiley & Sons, Ltd. Published 2015 by John Wiley & Sons, Ltd.

**Table 2.1**  Adverse events from a trial of Aldara® cream versus vehicle [1].

|  | Aldara Cream | | Vehicle | |
|---|---|---|---|---|
|  | n = 184 | | n = 178 | |
|  | Overall[a] | Severe | Overall[a] | Severe |
| Erythema | 184 (100%) | 57 (31%) | 173 (97%) | 4 (2%) |
| Flaking/scaling | 167 (91%) | 7 (4%) | 135 (76%) | 0 (0%) |
| Induration | 154 (84%) | 11 (6%) | 94 (53%) | 0 (0%) |
| Scabbing/crusting | 152 (83%) | 35 (19%) | 61 (34%) | 0 (0%) |
| Edema | 143 (78%) | 13 (7%) | 64 (36%) | 0 (0%) |
| Erosion | 122 (66%) | 23 (13%) | 25 (14%) | 0 (0%) |
| Ulceration | 73 (40%) | 11 (6%) | 6 (3%) | 0 (0%) |
| Vesicles | 57 (31%) | 3 (2%) | 4 (2%) | 0 (0%) |

[a] Mild, moderate, or severe.

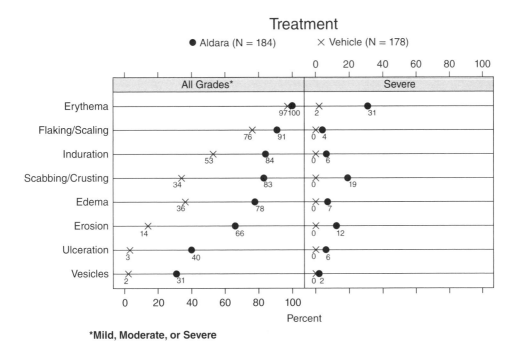

**Figure 2.1**  Dot plots of the information provided in Table 2.1 [1]. There appear to be clear differences between Aldara® and its vehicle with respect to the incidence of any grade of most of the adverse events, but only with respect to erythema, scabbing/crusting, or erosion when just the severe manifestations are considered.

A comprehensive treatment of graphical display construction and software for constructing graphical displays is beyond the scope of this brief chapter. Fortunately, detailed guidance on the construction of effective graphical displays can be found in many books [4–14]. The books by Cleveland [5] and Tufte [13] are seminal resources that provide extensive discussions of the principles underlying effective graphical displays and many examples of effective and ineffective displays. Imaginative and effective graphical displays have been described for conveying insights based on complex data, especially multivariate data and relationships or longitudinal trends such as trends in liver function tests over time [15–17]. These are described further below. Additional general information about the construction of graphical displays, including intriguing and possibly inspiring examples, is readily available on the internet (e.g., [2, 18]), and software packages that can be used to construct effective graphics are readily available [19–25]. Recommendations for graphical displays useful for presenting findings at various stages of medical product development also are described in a recently published book [26]. Table 2.2 provides links to a number of sites providing code and examples.

This chapter has three main objectives: to describe the principles, and provide some practical rules, for constructing effective graphical displays; to provide guidance on how graphical displays can and should be related to their primary purpose of answering specific questions or addressing specific issues related to medical product safety; and to provide examples of the use of effective graphical displays for addressing specific safety issues. The focus in this chapter is on the graphical displays. Details about the design and analysis considerations are not discussed in any detail, nor is there much discussion about specific safety issues such as QT prolongation or hepatotoxicity because these topics are considered in other chapters. The displays described here are based on real data from a number of sources. They are intended

**Table 2.2**    Internet sites providing graphical examples and code for constructing graphical displays.

| Description | URL |
| --- | --- |
| FDA/Industry/Academic Safety Graphics Working Group | https://www.ctspedia.org/StatGraphHome |
| Hmisc R package – contains many functions useful for data analysis, high-level graphics, etc. | http://biostat.mc.vanderbilt.edu/wiki/Main/Hmisc<br>http://cran.r-project.org/web/packages/Hmisc/ |
| HH R package – graphical displays for exploring data and for displaying the analysis | http://cran.r-project.org/web/packages/HH/ |
| SAS® code for producing various graphical displays | http://robslink.com/SAS/democd18/trellis_info.htm<br>http://support.sas.com/kb/43/773.html |
| R packages used to construct graphics | http://cran.r-project.org/web/packages/lattice/<br>http://cran.r-project.org/web/packages/latticeExtra/<br>http://cran.r-project.org/web/packages/ggplot2/<br>http://cran.r-project.org/web/packages/gridExtra/<br>http://cran.r-project.org/web/packages/rms/<br>http://cran.r-project.org/web/packages/prodlim/<br>http://cran.r-project.org/web/packages/rainbow/ |

to be illustrative, and by no means should be regarded as comprehensive. The displays can be produced by a variety of software packages. The code for some of the graphics may not be conveniently available, so is provided here, but only as a point of departure. The reader is invited, in fact encouraged, to make modifications and refinements as needed for specific circumstances.

As a practical matter, while it may be desirable to do all processing using a single software platform (e.g., SAS®, R), the production of graphical displays can be uncoupled from data processing. For example, the data needed to generate a display in R can be exported from (say) SAS® data files, so that the display can be produced using R code without having to do significant programming in SAS®. Consequently, although the displays described in this chapter are produced using code written in R, and sometimes in SAS®, there should be little difficulty in generating the displays even when the data processing occurs in other systems.

It is important to keep in mind that the purpose of all of the displays presented here is to convey a message whose validity is established by appropriate statistical analysis. The analysis establishes the conclusions that the data justify. Effective graphics satisfy three key criteria: immediacy, meaning that the reader grasps the message quickly; "interlocularity," meaning that the message hits the reader between the eyes; and inescapability, meaning that the message cannot be avoided [27]. Most of the graphical displays described here are fairly simple even though software to construct elaborate graphical displays is readily available (see Table 2.2). This represents a deliberate choice driven by three practical considerations: the need to communicate the message to a general audience in line with the criteria just mentioned; the ability to generate the display easily and quickly, without requiring elaborate programming; and general applicability, so that the code used to generate a display in one application can be used in many others. Much of what this chapter covers is based on work carried out over the past few years by the FDA, Industry, and Academia Working Group on Visualizing Safety Data. The reader is encouraged to explore the website containing guidance, examples, and software provided by this working group (Table 2.2).

## 2.1.2    What is the graphic trying to say?

Graphical displays can have a variety of purposes. For example, they are useful, if not essential, for exploratory data analyses to help to find potentially interesting relationships in a set of data. They can be used for descriptive purposes to help make sense of the data, that is, what the findings might mean in, say, a clinical setting. Graphical displays also can be used narratively, to communicate specific aspects of the data, or predictively, as a way to communicate potential scenarios as functions of assumptions about the processes generating the observed data [28].

The most effective graphics are those that clearly communicate a message or the answers to specific questions that specific analyses provide. The role of the graphics is to convey the insight provided by the analyses and to aid the reader in understanding the implications of the findings. Sometimes a graphic display can suggest additional questions that should be addressed or may indicate where alternative analyses should be applied to clarify an issue that became apparent only when displayed graphically.

Evaluating product safety requires addressing specific issues, particularly:

1. Frequency of adverse event reports or occurrences

2. Timing of adverse event reports or occurrences

3. Temporal variation of vital sign and laboratory measurements

4. Association patterns for combinations of vital sign and laboratory measurements

5. Identification of individuals with aberrant values for further evaluation

6. Relationship between baseline and on-treatment values

7. Effect of test medication dosage on occurrence of adverse events or laboratory values.

## 2.2    Principles and guidance for constructing effective graphics

There is no dearth of guidance for constructing effective graphical displays. The brief discussion of some key principles that follows provides touchstones for evaluating the effectiveness of the specific graphical displays that are described later in this chapter.

### 2.2.1    General principles

Table 2.3 provides a list of general criteria for graphical displays given by Tufte [13, p. 14]. These criteria are not restrictive, and allow for a wide variety of graphical displays depending on their intended usage. Since many safety analyses will be part of regulatory submissions, regulatory agencies such as the Food and Drug Administration have provided recommendations for graphics principles and specific graphical displays. Table 2.4 summarizes the principles and key general recommendations provided by the FDA [29]. The FDA recommendations reflect Tufte's criteria and, in addition, provide details about certain aspects of graphics for regulatory submissions. These are useful points to keep in mind when constructing graphical displays to include in regulatory submissions.

## 2.3    Graphical displays for addressing specific issues

### 2.3.1    Frequency of adverse event reports or occurrences

The analyses and graphical displays that address adverse event frequency seek to determine which adverse events occur more frequently on the test agent than on the control and how much more frequently, and which adverse events could be indicators of potential toxicity by

**Table 2.3**    What graphical displays generally should do [13, p. 14].

Show the data
Induce the viewer to think about the substance rather than [the technique or design]
Avoid distorting what the data have to say
Present many numbers in a small space
Make large data sets coherent
Encourage the eye to compare different pieces of data
Reveal the data at several levels of detail, from a broad overview to the fine structure
Serve a reasonably clear purpose: description, exploration, tabulation, or decoration
Be closely integrated with the statistical and verbal descriptions of a data set

**Table 2.4**   Uses of graphical displays and selected attributes of "good" graphics as expressed in a regulatory guidance [29].

A. Common uses of graphs

To present a large amount of data, such as individual subject data points (e.g., distribution of responses)

To show effects of treatment on major events or survival over time

To illustrate changes over time

To illustrate differences in magnitude of response, particularly where more than two treatment groups are being compared

To convey dose–response information

B. Recommendations for constructing good graphics

Label each axis and include units of measurement

Label selected ticks for each axis; face ticks away from the graph and eliminate (or at least reduce the prominence of) grids to reduce clutter

Ensure that the axis scale of measurement (generally the $y$-axis) does not exaggerate the treatment effect or any other variable being measured (e.g., by interruptions). Use consistent scales for similar graphs

Distinguish symbols by size, shape, or fill (do this consistently in a submission)

Represent variability or uncertainty by error bars or shading, and make it clear on the graphic what measure of variability is being used. Include confidence intervals on displays of treatment differences or ratios

Ensure that the legend does not overpower the graph. Labels directly on the graph often are preferable to a legend

Generally not necessary or desirable to include $p$-values in a graph, except possibly for plots of survival curve

Include reference lines for no change or no difference and, where useful, descriptors that denote change, such as an arrow labeled "Improvement"

---

virtue of their frequency of occurrence or severity. The corresponding questions can be made more specific, and addressed by specific graphical displays, in a number of ways, for example:

1. What is the difference, expressed using a metric such as the arithmetic difference, ratio, or odds ratio, between the proportions of patients who experience an adverse event at any time during treatment with the test agent and with the control?

2. What is the difference between the treatment groups with respect to the report frequency of the adverse event? That is, do events recur to individual patients more frequently on the test agent than on the control?

3. What differences are there between the treatment groups with respect to the maximum reported severity of an adverse event? The frequency of recurrence or reporting of the adverse event may be similar among the treatment groups, but the severity of its occurrence may differ.

4. As for 1–3, except broken down by specific strata such as gender, adverse event severity, or body system chosen in advance to minimize spurious findings arising by chance.

**Table 2.5**   Adverse events reported in each treatment group of a trial, with corresponding organ systems. (Organ system codes: GenUr = genital/urinary, GI = gastrointestinal, Misc = miscellaneous, Neur = neurologic/psychriatic, Resp = respiratory.)

| Adverse event | Organ system | Test (431) events | Control (216) events | Adverse event | Organ system | Test (431) events | Control (216) events |
|---|---|---|---|---|---|---|---|
| Dyspnea | Resp | 9 | 15 | Rhinitis | Resp | 17 | 11 |
| Hyperkalemia | Misc | 9 | 4 | Flatulence | GI | 20 | 6 |
| Rash | Misc | 9 | 4 | Back pain | Pain | 23 | 10 |
| Weight decrease | Misc | 9 | 2 | Coughing | Resp | 26 | 13 |
| Bronchitis | Resp | 11 | 8 | Infection viral | Misc | 26 | 12 |
| Respiratory | Resp | 11 | 4 | Insomnia | Neur | 26 | 4 |
| Disorder | – | – | – | Sinusitis | Misc | 28 | 13 |
| Chest pain | Pain | 12 | 9 | Dizziness | Neur | 29 | 9 |
| Gastroesophageal | GI | 12 | 5 | Injury | Misc | 30 | 12 |
| Reflux | – | – | – | Headache | Neur | 36 | 14 |
| Melena | GI | 12 | 7 | Vomiting | GI | 37 | 6 |
| Myalgia | Pain | 12 | 6 | Dyspepsia | GI | 42 | 8 |
| Urinary tract | GenUr | 12 | 6 | Abdominal pain | GI | 61 | 20 |
| Infection | – | – | – | Upper respiratory tract | Resp | 68 | 33 |
| Hematuria | GenUr | 14 | 2 | Infection | – | – | – |
| Anorexia | GI | 15 | 2 | Nausea | GI | 82 | 10 |
| Arthralgia | Pain | 15 | 1 | Diarrhea | GI | 90 | 23 |
| Fatigue | Neur | 16 | 4 | Chronic obstructive | Resp | 95 | 76 |
| Pain | Pain | 17 | 4 | Airway | – | – | – |

Let us take these one at a time, starting with Question 1. Table 2.5 contains observations of the numbers of patients reporting various adverse events during a trial, along with a characterization of the adverse events according to body system [30]. Table 2.6 provides statistics that summarize differences between the test and the control treatments. Interpreting the findings in Table 2.6 requires care, especially when there are many adverse events, because the extreme values actually may represent the order statistics corresponding to a uniform distribution that would be expected even if there were no difference between the treatments [31]. The goal of the graphical displays presented here is to provide a message that the reader can apprehend at a glance, with little or no processing needed to interpret the meaning of the display.

Figure 2.2, obtained using the AEdotplot function from the HH package in R (see Table 2.2) provides overall summaries of the adverse event incidences. Figure 2.2 has three parts: the left-hand panel summarizes the rates of each adverse event in each treatment group; the center panel summarizes the relative risks along with confidence intervals; and the right-hand panel provides the numbers and rates of events in each group, and the relative risks (ratio of event rates). Relative risks (event rate ratios) are the metric used to compare the event rates graphically, and are plotted on an arithmetic scale. The adverse events are ordered by the relative risks, highest to lowest regardless of the organ system. This simple picture clearly identifies the adverse events occurring more frequently in the test than in the

**Table 2.6**  Summary statistics for the adverse event findings in Table 2.3. (Organ system codes: GenUr = genital/urinary, GI = gastrointestinal, Misc = miscellaneous, Neur = neurologic/psychriatic, Resp = respiratory.)

| Adverse event | Organ system | Test event (%) | Cntl event (%) | Relative risk | RRLB | RRUB |
|---|---|---|---|---|---|---|
| Hematuria | GenUr | 3.2 | 0.9 | 3.5 | 0.8 | 15.3 |
| Urinary tract infection | GenUr | 2.8 | 2.8 | 1 | 0.4 | 2.6 |
| Nausea | GI | 19 | 4.6 | 4.1 | 2.2 | 7.8 |
| Anorexia | GI | 3.5 | 0.9 | 3.8 | 0.9 | 16.3 |
| Vomiting | GI | 8.6 | 2.8 | 3.1 | 1.3 | 7.2 |
| Dyspepsia | GI | 9.7 | 3.7 | 2.6 | 1.3 | 5.5 |
| Diarrhea | GI | 20.9 | 10.6 | 2 | 1.3 | 3 |
| Flatulence | GI | 4.6 | 2.8 | 1.7 | 0.7 | 4.1 |
| Abdominal pain | GI | 14.2 | 9.3 | 1.5 | 0.9 | 2.5 |
| Gastroesophageal reflux | GI | 2.8 | 2.3 | 1.2 | 0.4 | 3.4 |
| Melena | GI | 2.8 | 3.2 | 0.9 | 0.3 | 2.2 |
| Weight decrease | Misc | 2.1 | 0.9 | 2.3 | 0.5 | 10.3 |
| Injury | Misc | 7 | 5.6 | 1.3 | 0.7 | 2.4 |
| Hyperkalemia | Misc | 2.1 | 1.9 | 1.1 | 0.4 | 3.6 |
| Infection viral | Misc | 6 | 5.6 | 1.1 | 0.6 | 2.1 |
| Rash | Misc | 2.1 | 1.9 | 1.1 | 0.4 | 3.6 |
| Sinusitis | Misc | 6.5 | 6 | 1.1 | 0.6 | 2 |
| Insomnia | Neur | 6 | 1.9 | 3.3 | 1.2 | 9.2 |
| Fatigue | Neur | 3.7 | 1.9 | 2 | 0.7 | 5.9 |
| Dizziness | Neur | 6.7 | 4.2 | 1.6 | 0.8 | 3.4 |
| Headache | Neur | 8.4 | 6.5 | 1.3 | 0.7 | 2.3 |
| Arthralgia | Pain | 3.5 | 0.5 | 7.5 | 1 | 56.5 |
| Pain | Pain | 3.9 | 1.9 | 2.1 | 0.7 | 6.3 |
| Back pain | Pain | 5.3 | 4.6 | 1.2 | 0.6 | 2.4 |
| Myalgia | Pain | 2.8 | 2.8 | 1 | 0.4 | 2.6 |
| Chest pain | Pain | 2.8 | 4.2 | 0.7 | 0.3 | 1.6 |
| Respiratory disorder | Resp | 2.6 | 1.9 | 1.4 | 0.4 | 4.3 |
| Coughing | Resp | 6 | 6 | 1 | 0.5 | 1.9 |
| Upper respiratory tract infection | Resp | 15.8 | 15.3 | 1 | 0.7 | 1.5 |
| Rhinitis | Resp | 3.9 | 5.1 | 0.8 | 0.4 | 1.6 |
| Bronchitis | Resp | 2.6 | 3.7 | 0.7 | 0.3 | 1.7 |
| Chronic obstructive airway | Resp | 22 | 35.2 | 0.6 | 0.5 | 0.8 |
| Dyspnea | Resp | 2.1 | 6.9 | 0.3 | 0.1 | 0.7 |

Treatment-specific event rates, relative risks, and 95% confidence bounds for each relative risk (uncorrected for multiplicity), sorted by relative risk in descending order within each organ system category.

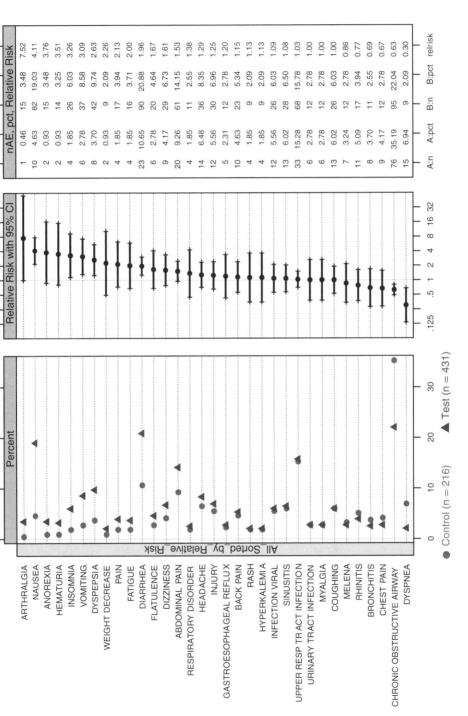

**Figure 2.2** Frequencies of adverse events, sorted by decreasing relative risk, including relative risks with confidence intervals and explicit summary statistics.

control group. Displays similar to Figure 2.2 can be produced from the Hmisc package and using SAS® [20, 32].

Just knowing which adverse events have high associated relative risks does not necessarily provide insight into potential mechanisms of action that may be the cause of the elevated risk. There may be a substantial chance of false positives, especially if events are isolated findings [31]. Figure 2.3 provides a graphical summary similar to Figure 2.2, but with the adverse events grouped by organ system, to provide an additional element of clinical insight by indicating whether the relative risks for adverse events were elevated consistently within an organ system, or whether they were isolated events. This graphic is a way of addressing Question 4 when the grouping is by organ system. The pattern of risk elevation within an organ system category may be useful for understanding potential mechanisms of action for toxicity of the test treatment.

The displays in Figures 2.2 and 2.3 are informative, but must be interpreted carefully because of the potential effect of multiplicity due to the number of different adverse events. This effect can be illustrated using order statistics for the collection of test results. The cumulative distribution function (cdf) of the $k$th-order statistic among $n$ observations $x_1, \ldots, x_n$ drawn from a distribution with density $f(x)$ and cdf $F(x)$ evaluated at $x^*$ is an incomplete beta function with parameters $(k, n + 1 - k)$ evaluated at $F(x^*)$. If, for example, $n = 10$, that is, there are 10 adverse events, and $x^*$, corresponding to a test of a null hypothesis of equal risk of the adverse event in each treatment group, is defined by $F(x^*) = 0.05$, then the cdf of the first-order statistic $X_{1:10}$ evaluated at $x^*$ is 0.4, which is much larger than 0.05 and therefore certainly not "rare." In other words, if there are 10 adverse events, and there is no association between adverse event risk and assigned treatment, then the probability of finding at least one "significant" test result is 0.4. This is why multiplicity adjustments are important, and why the effect of multiplicity needs to be kept in mind when interpreting Figures 2.2 and 2.3.

Figures 2.2 and 2.3 address the issue of overall frequency of adverse event reports, but do not distinguish between reports that occur once or recur often, nor do they address directly differences in severity of adverse events or the frequency or timing of adverse event reports. Insight about treatment differences with respect to timing, recurrence frequency, or maximum severity of reported adverse events can be obtained in various ways, especially from stacked bar charts. These are the issues addressed by Questions 2, 3, 5, and 6. A variety of graphical displays can be used, but stacked bar charts appear to be particularly well suited for conveying relevant insights. Figure 2.4 illustrates their use for summarizing the distribution of maximum intensity. Similar charts can be used to compare treatments with respect to emergence of adverse effects by appropriately categorizing the time scale, for example, week 1, weeks 2–4, after week 4, and so on. The categories then would correspond to patients who never reported the adverse event, or to the patients who initially reported the event during the first week, and so on. The charts can be used to compare observed recurrence frequency, so that, for example, the categories could correspond to patients who never reported the event, who reported the event once, or twice, or three times, or more than three times. These charts provide more detail than Figures 2.2 and 2.3, and so ordinarily would be used only for a subset of the reported adverse events. They provide less detail than charts such as Figure 2.5, so information about collections of adverse events, such as events corresponding to an organ system, can be presented together. The charts can be produced for subsets of patients (e.g., by gender or by age group), and for subsets of adverse events (e.g., "severe" events), to address Questions 5 and 6. The purpose of these charts is to provide immediate insight about potentially important differences in patterns of adverse event timing, recurrence, or severity between two treatment groups in a compact, easily apprehended form in the spirit of Tukey's recommendations [27].

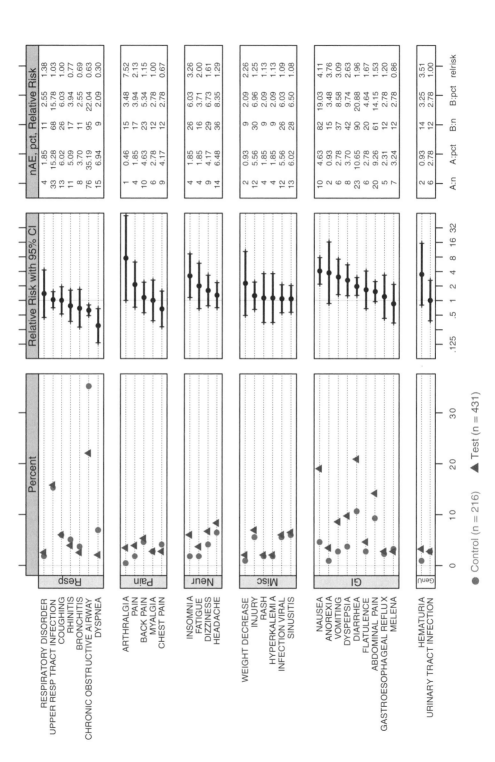

**Figure 2.3** Frequencies of adverse events, grouped by organ system class, including relative risks with confidence intervals and explicit summary statistics.

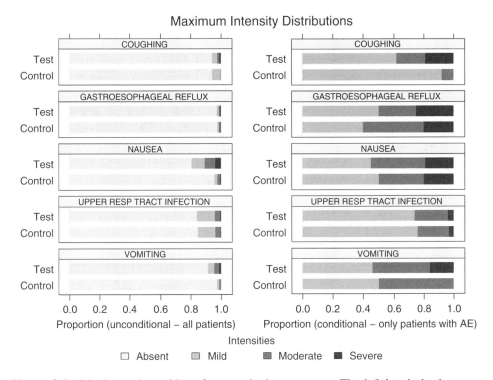

**Figure 2.4**    Maximum intensities of reported adverse events. The left-hand plot is unconditional, including all patients. The right-hand plot is conditional, including only patients reporting the adverse event. This figure also can be used to display event recurrence frequency or times to onset of events.

Definitive inferences about differences in patterns would be determined by formal statistical analyses.

Figure 2.4 provides two variations. One variation consists of an unconditional distribution that includes all patients and so partially reproduces some of the information provided in Figures 2.2 and 2.3. The other variation consists of a conditional distribution that includes only the patients reporting at least one occurrence of the adverse event, to better emphasize differences in patterns of occurrence or severity. The examples presented in Figure 2.4 are univariate, like Figure 2.2. Code for producing these figures is provided in Appendix 2.A.

## 2.3.2    Timing of adverse event reports or occurrences

It often will be useful, and sometimes essential, to know when adverse events occur, not just how often they occur. Toxicities can arise shortly after initiating treatment with a drug, reflecting an acute response, or may require weeks or months of exposure to become evident, or in fact may not become evident until years have passed when toxicities become evident only because of the effects on children. The specific questions usually are of the form:

1. What is the trend in risk over time (or with exposure to treatment) of a specific adverse event?

2. Do the treatment groups differ in the time to first occurrence of an adverse event?

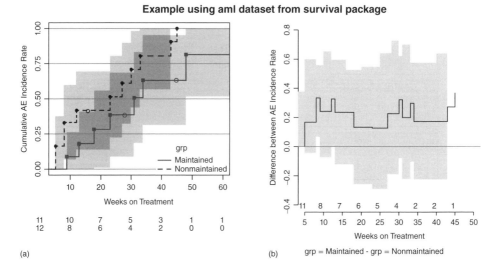

**Figure 2.5**   (a) Cumulative adverse event incidences with 95% confidence bounds for each group, and (b) cumulative between-group differences between the adverse event rates, with simultaneous 95% confidence bounds. Open circles identify censored observations. Data from aml dataset provided in R survival package (see Table 2.2).

These questions refer to time to event, which is conventionally (and, usually, best) handled by plots of cumulative survival or incidence or, depending on the application, cumulative hazard. Many software packages provide programs for producing graphical displays useful for addressing these questions. Figure 2.5 provides two ways of displaying incidence information that can be useful for comparisons between treatment groups. Appendix 2.A includes R code for generating either or both of the displays in Figure 2.5. The left-hand panel displays cumulative incidence curves for each treatment, along with shaded simultaneous 95% confidence regions. The right-hand panel displays the difference between the two cumulative incidence curves with a 95% confidence region. These two panels clearly describe the time course of first occurrences of a particular adverse event. Separate graphical displays can be constructed easily for important subsets of the data and of the adverse events. For example, one might wish to provide displays like Figure 2.5 separately for men and women, or for just serious occurrences of the adverse event. These displays can be produced for individual adverse events, or for collections of adverse events such as organ system events.

The confidence bands are important features of these displays, since they provide a context in which to interpret differences between incidence curves. Thus, for example, even though the average difference between incidence rates in the two groups displayed in the right-hand panel of Figure 2.5 is of the order of 20 percentage points for all times on treatment, the confidence intervals generally include zero, so that what seems to be a fairly definitive difference between the incidence rates in the two groups in fact may not be. There seems to be a tendency for the rate to be higher in the "maintained" group, but there does not seem to be a clear difference between the rates for the two groups. This also would be the conclusion reached from examining the left-hand panel of Figure 2.5, since the confidence bands for the two incidence trajectories overlap sufficiently that the bands for the trajectory corresponding to either group largely include the trajectory for the other.

Various software packages can be used to obtain displays similar to the left-hand panel of Figure 2.5 when there are more than two treatment groups. It may be preferable to omit the confidence bounds to make the display easier to read as, for example, in Figure 2.6. These curves have less detail than the left-hand panel of Figure 2.5, but they also have the different objective of highlighting possible differences between the curves, that is, between the pattern of occurrence of the adverse event(s) in question. Figure 2.6 provides two alternative displays (code in Appendix 2.A).

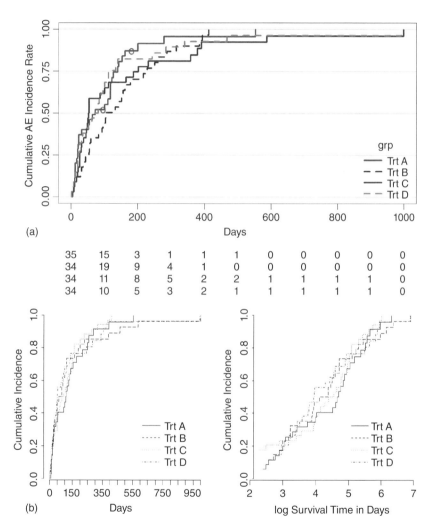

**Figure 2.6**  Cumulative adverse event incidences for each of four treatment groups: (a) linear time scale only (note that censored points are identified); (b) linear and logarithmic time scales.

### 2.3.3   Temporal variation of vital sign and laboratory measurements

The displays in this section use data from the CDISC Pilot Project [33]. An archived data file can be downloaded from https://www.ctspedia.org/do/view/CTSpedia/DataSetPageCDISC. All of the figures described here are designed to illustrate clearly estimated trends with a measure of uncertainty about the true trends. Most of the examples that follow use liver function metric values for illustration. The individual liver function metrics are identified by acronyms: albumin (ALB), alkaline phosphatase (ALP), alanine aminotransferase (ALT), aspartate aminotransferase (AST), bilirubin (BIL), and gamma-glutamyl transferase (GGT). Chapter 9 contains a comprehensive discussion of liver function metrics and their interpretation.

Figure 2.7 illustrates variations on a straightforward boxplot display of values that can be used to display distributions of vital sign and laboratory measurements as a function of an appropriate covariate such as time. Trend lines are omitted for clarity of presentation; they are unnecessary for these plots. Four variations are shown in Figure 2.7 using observations on ALT from the CDISC dataset. Two variations are based on the ALT and log-transformed ALT values, and two are based on the values of ALT divided by the upper limit of the normal range (ALT/ULN) and log(ALT/ULN). In both of these latter plots, a horizontal line is added at the value of 2 (absolute scale) or log(2) (log scale) to identify observations exceeding twice the upper limit of the normal range All four of the displays in Figure 2.7 are produced by the same concise code (Fig7.fn in Appendix 2.A) that uses functions in the ggplot2 package in the R system. Note that the $x$ variable "Week" in Figure 2.7 is treated as a category and not as a continuous variable. This can be rectified by additional programming, but in fact is not necessarily a defect. Not using a continuous scale makes for a more concise figure because empty gaps are omitted, and outliers and potential toxicity issues can be identified easily. The disadvantage is that it is not possible to plot a sensible trend line with this graphic. That can be resolved with a different graphic (see Figure 2.9).

Figure 2.8 illustrates a version of Figure 2.7 that can be produced in SAS®. Figure 2.8 also provides considerable detail without clutter, and additionally includes useful summary information such as the numbers of patients/subjects in each treatment group providing measurements at each time point and the numbers of patients whose values exceed twice the upper limit of the normal range, which is especially useful for monitoring laboratory safety measurements such as liver or renal function tests. Figures 2.7 and 2.8 are likely to be especially useful when there are many individual data points and it would be more informative simply to summarize the distributions at each time point by, for example, boxplots. More elaborate versions of the boxplots could be used, including notched boxplots and violin plots, and the reader is encouraged to try constructing them.

Sometimes, it may be useful and informative to include trend lines. Figure 2.9, corresponding to the log-transformed examples in Figure 2.7, plots the actual data points and includes local regression (loess) curves with shaded 95% confidence regions around each curve to illustrate the temporal trends in each treatment group. Including individual data points provides a sense of the distributions of the values in each treatment group at each time point. Plotting the values divided by the upper limit of the normal range simplifies the identification of observations corresponding to potential toxicity. The R code that produced Figure 2.9 (Fig9.fn) also is quite concise, and is given in Appendix 2.A.

Figures 2.7–2.9 convey a number of messages. Firstly, there does not appear to be a noticeable change in ALT values over time in any of the treatment groups. Secondly, the values in

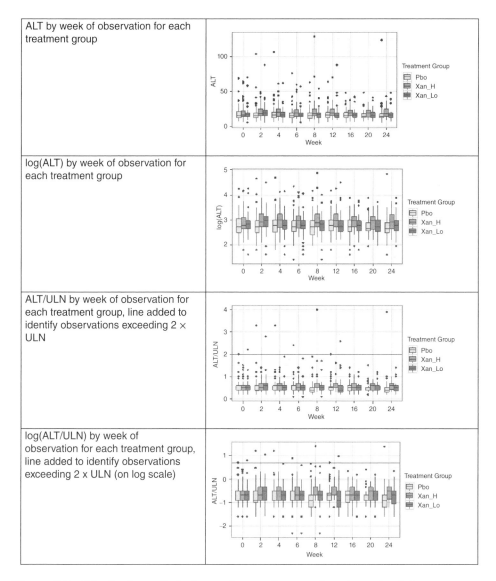

| ALT by week of observation for each treatment group | |
| log(ALT) by week of observation for each treatment group | |
| ALT/ULN by week of observation for each treatment group, line added to identify observations exceeding 2 × ULN | |
| log(ALT/ULN) by week of observation for each treatment group, line added to identify observations exceeding 2 x ULN (on log scale) | |

**Figure 2.7** Distributions of alanine aminotransferase values in each of three treatment groups over time.

the placebo and low-dose groups appear to be about the same at all time points, while the values in the high-dose group appear to be somewhat elevated relative to the other two treatment groups. Finally, the values in any treatment group at any time point do not appear to be symmetrically distributed, suggesting that a transformation of the data would be advisable before applying conventional analysis methods. Figures 2.7 and 2.9 suggest that a logarithmic transformation of the data would diminish the asymmetry of the observations.

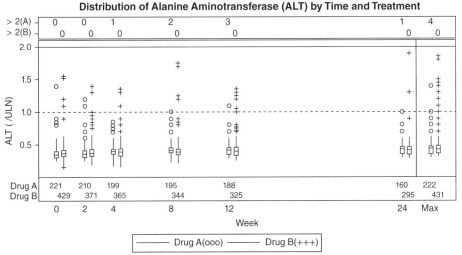

**Figure 2.8**  Distributions of alanine aminotransferase values in each of two treatment groups over time, including counts of patients providing values at each time point, and counts of patients whose values exceeded twice the upper limit of the normal range. From https://www.ctspedia.org/do/view/CTSpedia/ClinLFTGraph007, based on [32]. See also http://support.sas.com/kb/43/912.html.

It often will be of interest to display trends in differences among treatment groups with respect to changes from baseline, such as in Figure 2.10, which displays changes in serum albumin from baseline over time. The two panels of Figure 2.10 plot the same data, namely percentage changes from baseline, but with one important difference. The left-hand panel, following almost universal practice, includes a line connecting the constructed zero difference from baseline at baseline to the first time point. The right-hand panel does not include these lines, nor does it include a point at (0,0). There are three reasons why the right-hand panel may be a better choice. Firstly, and most obviously, the point at (0,0) is not a datum – the difference from baseline at baseline is zero *by construction*, and therefore adds no information. Secondly, drawing a line from (0,0) to the first time point assumes that the change from baseline to the first time point really is linear, even though there is no evidence to support such an assumption. Finally, the extraneous line can be misleading because it diverts attention from the pattern that does exist in the data. In fact, the trends in values during treatment in each treatment group are nearly the same. However, the left-hand display suggests an initial drop in serum albumin over the first couple of weeks followed by a gradual increase to essentially a zero mean change, which seems clinically implausible, and is an artifact arising from the inclusion of a point that is not a datum. The right-hand display suggests that there was a very slight increase in serum albumin over the first 8 weeks. Only actual data contribute to the trend line in the right-hand display. The difference between the two displays is not large, but may be enough to be misleading about the trend in serum albumin values over time. These differences may not be so subtle in other circumstances.

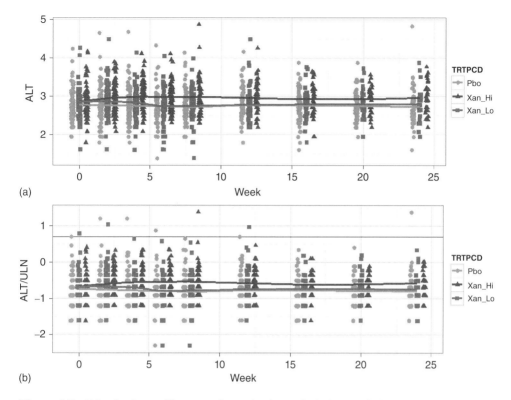

**Figure 2.9**    Distributions of log-transformed values of (a) ALT and (b) ALT/ULN values in each of three treatment groups over time, with loess trend lines and simultaneous confidence bands added.

### 2.3.4    Temporal variation of combinations of vital sign and laboratory measurements

Figures 2.7–2.10 are especially useful for evaluating one laboratory or vital sign metric at a time. Often, however, the evaluation of safety requires considering variation in two or more related observations. Bivariate scatterplots are particularly useful for this purpose, and can be constructed in various ways. Figure 2.11 illustrates one possibility, in which maximum values of four liver function tests on treatment are plotted against their baseline values. The metrics are plotted separately, and not against each other, but the plots are arranged in such a way that the eye can perceive potential toxicity, or lack thereof, by the consistency of the patterns of points. Figure 2.11 contains two variations. The variation on the left-hand panel corresponds to conventional scatterplots, including the values for all patients. However, since most patients do not experience potentially toxic changes in laboratory values, the greatest density of points will lie in the regions corresponding to unremarkable values, which is not where the viewer's attention should focus.

The right-hand panel of Figure 2.11 blanks out the portion of the graphic corresponding to measurements that are below the ULN for that measurement. The viewer's attention now

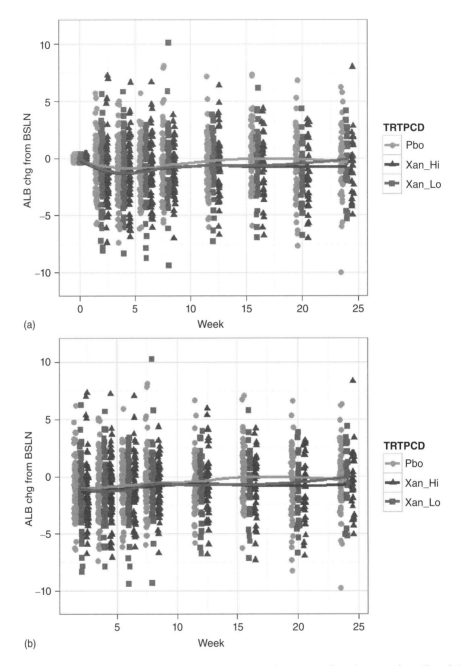

**Figure 2.10**   Two displays of changes from baseline in serum albumin over time. Panel (a) includes an artificial zero point that panel (b) excludes.

focuses on the values that are above the ULN at baseline and/or on treatment. Examination of Figure 2.11 suggests that the maximum on-treatment values exceeding the ULN appeared for the most part to do so modestly regardless of what the baseline values were. On the other hand, some patients experienced appreciable elevations on treatment in both groups.

Figure 2.12 provides two views of a true bivariate relationship. As with Figure 2.11, the scatterplots in the left-hand panel include all patients. Ordinarily, as is evident from the left-hand panel of Figure 2.12, the greatest density of points will lie in the regions corresponding to unremarkable values because most patients do not exhibit potentially toxic organ function measurements. This potential misdirection of attention, and possible obscuring of important differences between treatments, can be corrected simply by blanking out the region of unremarkable values, as shown on the right-hand panel. The result is to remove the distraction of the unimportant findings and focus the viewer's attention on the findings that may be important for evaluating potential toxicity.

Many variations of these generic displays would be useful for evaluating safety as expressed by laboratory tests such as liver function or kidney function tests, or for changes

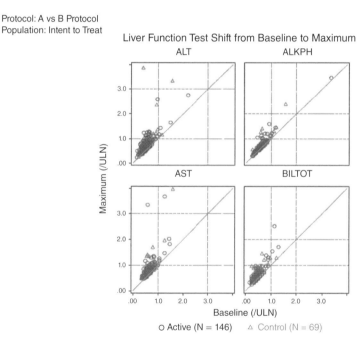

**Figure 2.11**    Bivariate scatterplots of laboratory values (liver function tests in this example) with indications of upper limits of normal (ULN). The left-hand panel includes points corresponding to patients whose value did not exceed ULN, the right-hand panel omits these points and focuses only on the patients whose values were above ULN at baseline or at some time during treatment. AST = aspartate aminotransferase, ALKPH = alkaline phosphatase, BILTOT = total bilirubin. Areas of clinical concern are $2 \times$ ULN (upper limit of normal) for BILTOT and ALKPH, 3 or $5 \times$ ULN for AST and ALT. 10 and $20 \times$ ULN identify toxicity grades. From https://www.ctspedia.org/do/view/CTSpedia/ClinLFTGraph002.

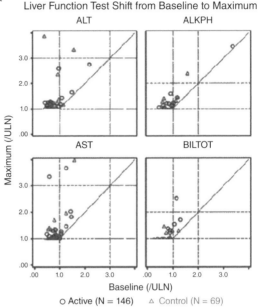

Protocol: A vs B Protocol
Population: Intent to Treat

**Figure 2.11**    (*continued*)

in vital signs. These include plots of the maximum value/ULN for pairs of liver or renal function tests to identify patients with possibly severe toxicity, plots of values on treatment versus baseline values for a single laboratory value over time, to evaluate the progression of toxicity over time, and, for the same reason, plots of the values of pairs of laboratory values at various time points. These plots can be made interactive, so that clicking on any point brings up the record for the corresponding patient.

Examining trends over time for combinations of related measurements can provide useful clinical insights, essentially as a combination of the objectives of the preceding figures. Figure 2.13 illustrates one application of this idea, to a collection of electrocardiogram (ECG) component values over time for a set of treatment groups. This display omits information about variability or precision to minimize clutter, so should not be regarded as definitive. However, the clarity of insight about the patterns of variation of the various components compensates for the lack of detail. Definitive conclusions can rest on formal statistical analyses; the advantage of Figure 2.13 is that it suggests what the conclusions might be, or at least what specific hypotheses to address by the formal analyses.

There are other ways to visualize the progress of combinations (vectors) of measurements over time. For example, Trost and Freston [34, Figure 2], provide three-dimensional plots of values of triplets of liver function test values at baseline and at various follow-up times relative to the positions of regions of normal variation for an active drug group and a placebo group. The divergences in three dimensions between the two groups became increasingly evident over time, suggesting that possible liver toxicity could be detected sooner than by conventional means.

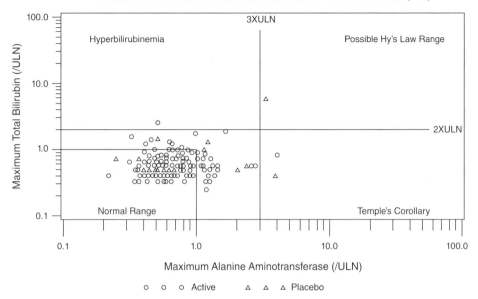

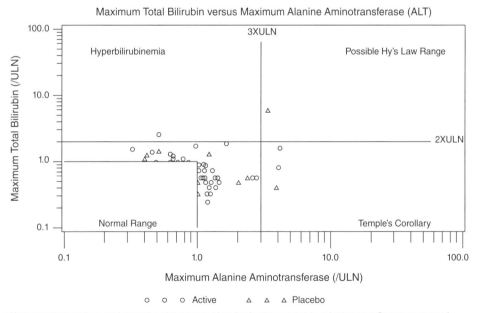

**Figure 2.12**   Bivariate scatterplots especially suited to liver function laboratory values by virtue of identification and labeling of specific areas in the plane of laboratory values. The right-hand panel omits the points that fall within both normal ranges, to focus attention on the points that fall outside either normal range.   From https://www.ctspedia.org/do/view/ CTSpedia/ClinLFTGraph000.

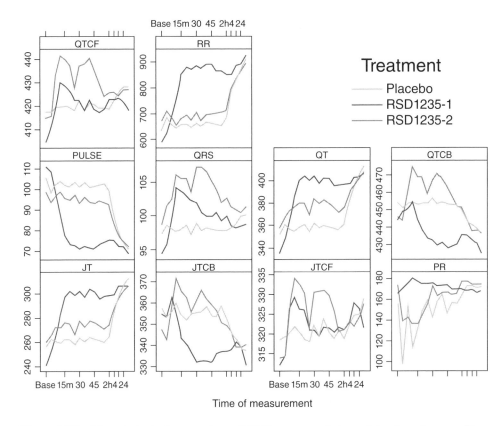

**Figure 2.13**   Mean trajectories over time of ECG components in each treatment group. From https://www.ctspedia.org/do/view/CTSpedia/StatGraphTopic015.

## 2.3.5   Functional/multidimensional data

The displays illustrated so far take scalars or pairs of observations as the basis for analysis, usually at single time points. However, the advent and increasing use of more sophisticated measuring equipment and tools can be anticipated to generate more complex data collections, for example, time series such as ECGs, electroencephalograms (EEGs), or hypnograms (for sleep studies), or highly multidimensional data such as obtained by imaging or gene expression, for which simple methods of analysis may be inadequate. Insightful analyses and informative visualizations based on these measurements often require explicit or implicit data reduction that collectively can be categorized under the rubric of functional data analysis, in which the objects of analysis are curves or reductions of multidimensional observations by, for example, principal components analysis. The objective of safety analyses employing functional data analysis techniques is to identify possibly toxicity-related pattern variations. There is a considerable literature on functional data analysis (see the books by Ramsay and Silverman [35, 36] and bibliographies in [15, 37–39]).

Hyndman and Shang [15] describe, and provide software for computing, displays appropriate for functional data, of which two, the "functional depth" and the "functional highest density region (HDR) boxplot", appear to have especially attractive properties. To illustrate the calculations, suppose that the data can be viewed as a matrix whose columns are $p$-element observation vectors, say $\mathbf{y}_1, \ldots, \mathbf{y}_n$. Suppose also that a $p$-element index vector $\mathbf{x}$ orders the rows of the data matrix. The observation vectors could be sequences of observations of individual laboratory, vital signs, or other essentially continuous safety-related values, in which case the elements of $\mathbf{x}$ would index the time points. The observations also could be collections of values of measurements of various components of a body system such as a collection of values from liver function tests or collections of values from ECG or EEG readings at specific points in time, in which case the elements of $\mathbf{x}$ would identify the specific tests or components of the ECG or EEG.

The method assumes that the essential features of the observation vectors can be captured by the first two principal components, which are calculated for each column using a robust method [40]; call the corresponding vectors of components $(z_{11}, \ldots, z_{n1})$ and $(z_{12}, \ldots, z_{n2})$, and let $\mathbf{z}_i = (z_{i1}, z_{i2})$. The data columns could be ordered in a meaningful way or not, which usually would be the case if the observations corresponded to individual patients. If the data columns are ordered, then the trajectories of individual observation vectors can be plotted using the elements of the vector specifying the ordering of the rows as the independent variable. If the data columns are not ordered (and even if they are), then the $\mathbf{z}_i$ values can be ordered in terms of a bivariate score density or a depth measure. Hyndman and Shang discuss a number alternative ordering strategies, and the rainbow package in R provides software to carry out the calculations required for these strategies. The functional depth plot assigns colors or shades of gray to reflect the ordering of the $\mathbf{z}_i$ values (and, therefore, the observation vectors), and plots each column of the data matrix against the values in the index vector $\mathbf{x}$. The individual data trajectories can be plotted, but it should be more useful in practice to identify regions containing, say, 50% or 95% of the trajectories and plot only those individual trajectories that the depth algorithm identifies as possible outliers. A separate function (foutlier) provides a way to identify outliers using various algorithms and a tuning parameter to adjust the sensitivity of the detection procedure. This provides a way to interpret patterns of apparent outliers. An example given below illustrates the process.

The functional HDR boxplot is based on the bivariate HDR boxplot [41] that uses the first two principal components of each observation vector to calculate a bivariate kernel density estimate for each observation vector. The inner (more darkly shaded) region of the functional HDR boxplot (in the plane of values for the two principal components) corresponds to the boundary in the plane of principal component values encompassing the points where the probability content under the bivariate kernel density is 0.5. The outer, more lightly shaded, region corresponds to the boundary encompassing points where the bivariate kernel density probability content is 0.95. The HDR region is one way to express bivariate variation; bagplots [42] provide an alternative (and can be generated by the software provided in the rainbow package). There are a number of differences between the regions that these two approaches produce, the most notable of which is that the bagplot regions are convex and unimodal, while the HDR regions do not need to be convex, unimodal, or even connected. Consequently, they do not necessarily identify the same outlying observations.

The graphical displays can be constructed using the data from all of the patients and, separately, for the data from each of the treatment groups. This is useful because the principal components calculated for any subset of the patients do not have to correspond to the components calculated for any other subset. Constructing a graph based on all of the patients identifies those patients who could be detected during monitoring of an ongoing trial without breaking the blinding of the trial. Graphs based on patients within a treatment group would

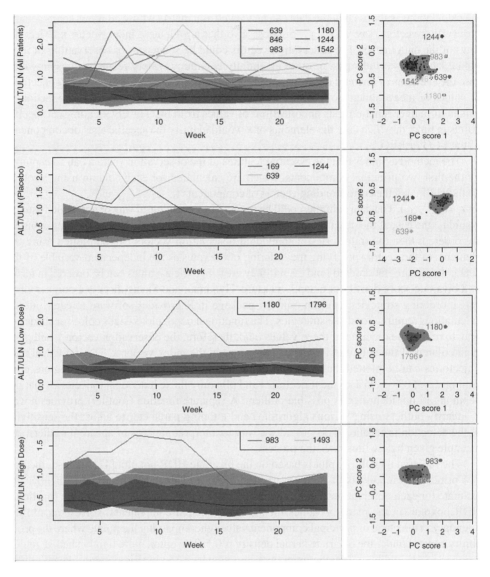

**Figure 2.14** Functional depth plots (left-hand side) and functional HDR boxplots (right-hand side) corresponding to ALT values measured at weeks 2, 4, 6, 8, 12, 16, 20, and 24 relative to the upper limit of normal overall and separately for each treatment group.

identify patients whose pattern of values differed markedly from the patterns of the remaining patients in the treatment group.

Figure 2.14 provides examples of functional depth plots and functional HDR plots based on a robust principal components decomposition of a multinomial outcome which, in this case, is the 24-week observation period. The fboxplot function was used for both displays. The values plotted in the functional depth graphic (left-hand side) are directly interpretable. The HDR plots (right-hand side) are in terms of the principal components, provide a more concise summary of the multivariate observations and simplify identification of potential outliers. The outliers identified by the plotting program are:

| All patients | Placebo | Low dose | High dose |
|---|---|---|---|
| 639, 846, 983, 1180, 1244, 1542 | 169, 639, 1244 | 1180, 1796 | 983, 1493 |

The outlier detection method described by Hyndman and Ullah [43] was used, with the tuning parameter set to 2, except for the high-dose group where a value of 1.65 was used. Examination of the graphics in Figure 2.14 suggests that the separate calculation of outliers can help the interpretation of the graphical findings. The patterns for the patients detected separately using the foutlier function clearly differ substantially from the patterns for the remaining patients. The graphical display for all patients identified two additional possible outliers, patients 1542 and 846. However, examination of the trajectories for these two patients suggests that their trajectories did not differ substantially from the trajectories of the remaining patients.

Table 2.7 displays the actual ALT/ULN values for patients identified as outliers in Figure 2.14.

**Table 2.7**  Mean of weekly ALT/ULN values for patients on placebo, low dose, and high dose identified as outliers in the bivariate boxplots displayed in Figure 2.14.

| | | Week | | | | | | | |
|---|---|---|---|---|---|---|---|---|---|
| | | 2 | 4 | 6 | 8 | 12 | 16 | 20 | 24 |
| Placebo | Mean | 0.5 | 0.5 | 0.5 | 0.5 | 0.5 | 0.5 | 0.5 | 0.5 |
| Obs. no. | 169 | 0.9 | 1.2 | 1.1 | 1.1 | 1.1 | 1.1 | 0.9 | 0.9 |
| | 639 | 0.8 | 0.8 | 2.4 | 1.4 | 2 | 0.8 | 1.5 | 0.9 |
| | 1244 | 1.6 | 1.3 | 1.2 | 1.9 | 1 | 0.6 | 0.6 | 0.8 |
| | | Week | | | | | | | |
| | | 2 | 4 | 6 | 8 | 12 | 16 | 20 | 24 |
| Low dose | Mean | 0.6 | 0.5 | 0.4 | 0.5 | 0.5 | 0.5 | 0.5 | 0.5 |
| Obs. no. | 846 | 0.8 | 1 | 0.7 | 0.8 | 0.9 | 1 | 1.1 | 1.1 |
| | 1180 | 0.9 | 1 | 0.8 | 0.7 | 2.6 | 1.2 | 1.2 | 1.4 |
| | 1796 | 1.3 | 0.6 | 0.6 | 0.6 | 0.6 | 0.6 | 0.7 | 0.6 |
| | | Week | | | | | | | |
| | | 2 | 4 | 6 | 8 | 12 | 16 | 20 | 24 |
| High dose | Mean | 0.7 | 0.7 | 0.6 | 0.6 | 0.7 | 0.6 | 0.6 | 0.6 |
| Obs. no. | 983 | 1.1 | 1.4 | 1.4 | 1.7 | 1.6 | 0.8 | 0.8 | 1 |
| | 1493 | 0.9 | 0.9 | 1 | 1 | 0.9 | 1.1 | 0.9 | 1 |

The values of a collection of (say) liver function test values at a point in time may provide useful information about potential toxicity beyond what sequences of values over time of individual tests may provide. Figure 2.15 plots the first two principal components corresponding to a collection of values (divided by the upper limit of normal) of six liver function tests at week 4. Since there is no natural ordering of the individual liver function tests, nor are the relative elevations above the upper limit of the corresponding normal ranges necessarily equally meaningful clinically, a functional depth plot is unlikely to be of great value. The following patients were identified as having a potentially outlying suite of liver function values at week 4 on the basis of a separate calculation carried out to identify outliers using the foutlier function:

| All patients | Placebo | Low dose | High dose |
| --- | --- | --- | --- |
| 668, 811, 877, 1198, 1282, 1298, 1470 | 560, 811, 1470 | 466, 668, 1182, 1298 | 134, 985, 1198 |

Table 2.8 displays the mean values of the week 4 liver values (/ULN) for patients identified as outliers using the foutlier function corresponding to Figure 2.15. It is intriguing that the suites of potential outliers are not entirely coincident. This may be due to different algorithms being used to identify outliers, or may be due to the fact that the algorithms are sensitive to different patterns of deviation from the general run of liver function values.

## 2.3.6 Multivariate outlier detection with multiplicity adjustment based on robust estimates of mean and covariance matrix

Suppose as before that the data consist of $n$ observation vectors, each of length $p$, presumably arising from a distribution with mean vector $\boldsymbol{\mu}$ and covariance matrix $\boldsymbol{\Sigma}$. As an alternative to the functional data analysis approach, one may test a set of null hypotheses, $H_{0i}$: $E(\mathbf{y}_i) = \boldsymbol{\mu}$, at a significance level $\alpha$, and label as outliers those values of $\mathbf{y}_i$ for which $H_{0i}$ is rejected. An approach using this strategy was described by Cerioli [44, 45] based on multiplicity-adjusted multivariate comparisons using robust estimators of the mean and covariance matrix when the observations are (nearly) normal. The robust estimate is a reweighted version of the minimum covariance determinant (MCD) estimator [46, 47] that can be computed using available software, for example, the covMcd procedure in [48]. $p$-values for rejecting the hypotheses $H_{0i}$ are obtained using an accurate approximation to the exact distribution of the robust distances, and the ranks of these $p$-values are determined from lowest to highest. Three approaches for identifying outliers are described. The first, based on the Benjamini–Hochberg approach [49] for controlling the false discovery rate (FDR), rejects the $i$th null hypothesis, that is, declares the $i$th observation an outlier, if the $i$th $p$-value is less than the product rank$(p_i)\alpha/n$. The second, seeking to control the false discovery exceedence (FDX) [50, 51] rejects $H_{0i}$ if the $i$th $p$-value is less than $(\eta_i + 1)\alpha/(n + \eta_i - \text{rank}(p_i))$, where $\eta_i$ is equal to the integer part of the product $c \times \text{rank}(p_i)$, with $c$ usually set to 0.1. The Benjamini–Hochberg (BH in Tables 2.9 and 2.10) procedure seeks to control the expected false discovery fraction, while the FDX procedure (LR in Tables 2.9 and 2.10) seeks to control the probability that the false discovery fraction exceeds a defined threshold. The third procedure, based on the iterative reweighted minimum covariance determinant (IRMCD) estimator, accepts all observations as not outliers

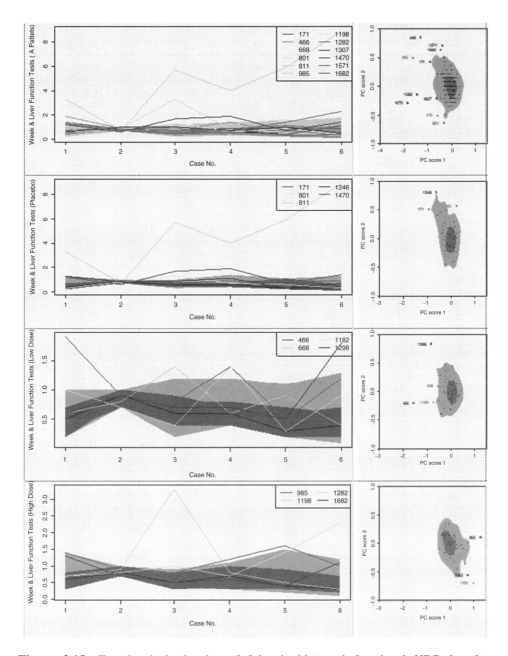

**Figure 2.15** Functional depth plots (left-hand side) and functional HDR boxplots (right-hand side) corresponding to liver function values measured at week 4 relative to the upper limit of normal overall and separately for each treatment group. The liver function tests corresponding to the case number label on the *x*-axis of the functional depth plot are: 1, ALT; 2, ALB; 3, ALP; 4, AST; 5, BIL; 6, GGT.

**Table 2.8**  Mean of various liver function metric values divided by the upper limit of the normal range at week 4 for patients on placebo, low dose, and high dose identified as outliers using the foutlier function corresponding to the bivariate boxplots displayed in Figure 2.15.

| | | Liver function metric | | | | | |
|---|---|---|---|---|---|---|---|
| | | ALT | ALB | ALP | AST | BIL | GGT |
| Placebo | Mean | 0.5 | 0.8 | 0.7 | 0.7 | 0.5 | 0.5 |
| Obs. no. | 171 | 1.2 | 0.9 | 0.7 | 0.9 | 0.9 | 0.9 |
| | 801 | 0.3 | 0.8 | 1.3 | 0.7 | 0.6 | 0.3 |
| | 1246 | 1.3 | 0.8 | 0.9 | 1.1 | 0.3 | 0.7 |
| | | Liver function metric | | | | | |
| | | ALT | ALB | ALP | AST | BIL | GGT |
| Low dose | Mean | 0.5 | 0.8 | 0.6 | 0.6 | 0.4 | 0.4 |
| Obs. no. | 668 | 0.6 | 0.8 | 1.4 | 0.6 | 0.9 | 0.4 |
| | 1182 | 1 | 0.7 | 0.4 | 1.4 | 0.3 | 0.9 |
| | 1298 | 0.6 | 0.9 | 0.7 | 0.7 | 0.5 | 1.8 |
| | | Liver function metric | | | | | |
| | | ALT | ALB | ALP | AST | BIL | GGT |
| High dose | Mean | 0.6 | 0.8 | 0.6 | 0.7 | 0.5 | 0.5 |
| Obs. no. | 985 | 1.4 | 0.9 | 0.8 | 1.2 | 1.6 | 1 |
| | 1282 | 0.7 | 0.8 | 1 | 0.7 | 1.4 | 2.3 |
| | 1682 | 1.3 | 0.7 | 0.5 | 0.6 | 0.4 | 1.1 |

if the smallest $p$-value exceeds $\alpha$; if this is not true, then observations whose $p$-values are less than $\alpha$ are labeled as outliers. R code for carrying out the calculations (Cerioli.fn) is provided in Appendix 2.A. Simulation studies suggest that the IRMCD procedure may be particularly useful [44, 45].

Figure 2.16 illustrates how outliers can be identified, with the treatment group membership of each potential outlier identified after the identification. That is, the outliers were identified without using information about their treatment group membership. Figure 2.16 also illustrates the effect of choice of coverage ratio, with versions using a ratio of 0.6 and a ratio of 0.75. In this example, the considerable variability of the original observations was tempered appreciably by an initial logarithmic transformation, leading to the detection of substantially fewer outliers regardless of how they were identified.

Tables 2.9 and 2.10 provide counts of the number of outliers in each treatment group as a function of the metameter/transformation of the individual liver function measurement values and the criterion used to identify outliers. The number of outliers clearly depended on the

**Table 2.9** Numbers of "outliers" detected in each treatment group using robust multiple comparison approaches [44, 45] based on week 4 values of six liver function measurements as a function of the metameter/transformation of the observed values and the criterion used to identify outliers. (LR = FDX = false discovery exceedance, BH = Benjamini–Hochberg, IRMCD = iterative reweighted minimum covariance determinant.)

| | | Liver function test metameter/transformation | | | | | |
|---|---|---|---|---|---|---|---|
| Criterion | Treatment | Value | Value change from baseline | Value/ ULN | Value/ULN change from baseline | log (value) | log (value/ ULN) |
| LR | Placebo | 4 | 6 | 4 | 5 | 2 | 2 |
| | Low | 5 | 5 | 5 | 2 | 0 | 0 |
| | High | 7 | 6 | 8 | 6 | 1 | 1 |
| BH | Placebo | 11 | 9 | 7 | 6 | 2 | 2 |
| | Low | 7 | 7 | 6 | 4 | 0 | 0 |
| | High | 9 | 7 | 10 | 6 | 1 | 1 |
| IRMCD | Placebo | 11 | 9 | 7 | 8 | 2 | 2 |
| | Low | 7 | 7 | 7 | 4 | 0 | 1 |
| | High | 9 | 8 | 10 | 6 | 3 | 2 |

The breakdown factor was set at 0.6 and the significance level ($\alpha$) was set at 0.025.

**Table 2.10** Numbers of "outliers" detected in each treatment group using robust multiple comparison approaches [44, 45] based on week 4 values of six liver function measurements as a function of the metameter/transformation of the observed values and the criterion used to identify outliers. (LR = FDX = false discovery exceedance, BH = Benjamini–Hochberg, IRMCD = iterative reweighted minimum covariance determinant.)

| | | Liver function test metameter/transformation | | | | | |
|---|---|---|---|---|---|---|---|
| Criterion | Treatment | Value | Value change from baseline | Value/ ULN | Value/ULN change from baseline | log (value) | log (value/ ULN) |
| LR | Placebo | 7 | 8 | 5 | 6 | 2 | 2 |
| | Low | 5 | 6 | 6 | 3 | 0 | 0 |
| | High | 9 | 6 | 9 | 6 | 1 | 1 |
| BH | Placebo | 12 | 10 | 11 | 9 | 2 | 2 |
| | Low | 8 | 10 | 7 | 7 | 0 | 0 |
| | High | 10 | 9 | 11 | 7 | 3 | 1 |
| IRMCD | Placebo | 2 | 2 | 2 | 2 | 1 | 1 |
| | Low | 1 | 1 | 0 | 1 | 0 | 0 |
| | High | 3 | 2 | 2 | 1 | 0 | 1 |

The breakdown factor was set at 0.75 and the significance level ($\alpha$) was set at 0.1.

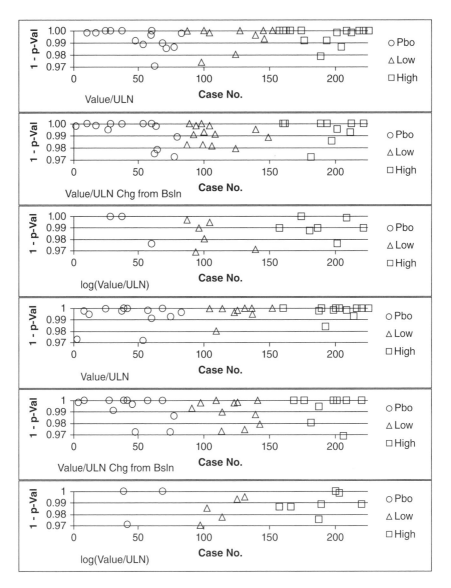

**Figure 2.16** Potential outliers identified by application of the Cerioli [44, 45] method to various transformations of the values of six liver function test measurements at week 4. The coverages are $0.6n$ for the top three plots and $0.75n$ for the bottom three.

criterion and on the metameter used, at least for this example and choice of tuning parameters for the method.

This approach should be regarded as complementary to the functional data analysis approach described in Section 3.5. The sets of outliers identified with these two approaches when applied to the same data overlapped considerably but were not identical and, indeed, depended on the criteria used to identify outliers.

### 2.3.7    Monitoring individual patient trends

It will often be useful to evaluate patterns of sequences of safety (e.g., liver function) tests over time for individual patients in order to get an idea of the occurrence and/or persistence of abnormal values. Since an individual may have transiently elevated values that do not persist with treatment, maximum values over a period of treatment may not be providing a true indication of potential toxicity. Values may be elevated shortly after initiating treatment or may slowly increase with accumulated exposure. Chapter 7, on recurrent adverse events, addresses this issue in more detail.

Two methods that can be useful for visualizing trends of this sort over time are event charts [52–54] for discrete events such as the occurrence of an elevated test value, and spaghetti or lasagna plots [55] for visualizing trends in the values of frequently measured ordered categories or discretized continuous variables. Software for carrying out the calculations is readily available. The Hmisc R package (see Table 2.2) contains a function called event.chart that can produce a variety of event charts. Supplementary material corresponding to the description of lasagna plots by Swihart *et al.* [55] includes code for producing different flavors of these plots.

## 2.4    Discussion

The key objective of this chapter is the description of graphical displays that directly address questions and issues arising in the evaluation of medical product safety. A number of graphical examples that address specific questions are provided, illustrated with real data, along with code for generating the display when the code needed to produce that specific display is not readily available. The displays are intended to be clear about the message the graphic seeks to convey, to provide insight and perspective about the conclusions from formal analyses, to illustrate key features of the data so that they can be grasped easily, and to help identify specific cases of potential toxicity. The collection certainly is not exhaustive. The chapter provides a bibliography on principles for constructing effective graphics and on published sources of code for producing various graphics that may be useful for individuals wishing to extend the graphical displays provided here.

The graphical displays described here are driven by, and organized in terms of, very specific issues. These include the incidence of adverse events globally and by stratum or organ system, the characterization of patterns of AE occurrence by, for example, frequency of recurrence or distribution of severity, how laboratory and vital signs measurements vary over time, and how insight about potential toxicity can be obtained by considering an entire sequence of measurements over time or by considering how potential toxicity might be manifested in terms of the values of a collection of related measurements such as liver function measurements. The latter displays constitute an attempt to understand, and clearly convey, the effect of different treatments on the overall picture of potential organ system toxicity. Clarity about the message a graphic is intended to convey is essential to producing an effective graphic.

The aim of the chapter is to present practical ways to construct graphical displays reflecting good practice and principles that help readers, especially those with limited statistical backgrounds, to interpret findings from clinical trials and other sources that bear on medical product safety. These are not the only displays that can be used for this purpose, and they very well may benefit from further refinement. The reader is invited, in fact encouraged, to make modifications and refinements as needed for specific circumstances [56–68].

# Appendix 2.A  R code for selected graphics

The following R code can be used to produce graphics like Figure 2.4.

```
Fig4.fn <- function(dta,pAE2=pAE2,pAE1=pAE1,
        title="Maximum Intensity Distributions",Intens=Intens,
        aspect=0.2, ygrob=.98, stripbg="grey96",
        leg.title="Intensities", leg.cex=1.15, title.cex=1.3,
        leg.text=c("Absent","Mild","Moderate","Severe"),
        leg.inset=-0.125, x.cex=1, strip.cex=0.8)
#
#  This program produces two sets of stacked bar charts giving
#  distributions of adverse events among ordered categories that can
#  be defined in various ways, e.g., maximum intensity ("Absent",
#  "Mild", "Moderate", "Severe").  One set provides unconditional
#  distributions, so that "Absent" is one of the possible categories.
#  The other set provides conditional (on having reported the AE)
#  distributions.  Separate plots are provided for each adverse event
#  in the dataset.
#
#  INPUT:
#       dta = dataset containing for each Adverse Event the numbers
#             and proportions of patients in the test and control
#             groups demonstrating each AE category.
#      pAE1 = variable in dta providing the proportion of all patients
#             demonstrating the corresponding category of the AE.
#      pAE2 = variable dta providing the conditional proportion of
#             patients reporting the corresponding category of the AE
#             given that the patient reported the AE.
#     title = title for plot(s)
#    Intens = name of variable in dta providing the category values
#             (usually maximum intensity)
# leg.title = title of legend
#  leg.text = names of AE categories
#
#             plus additional parameters governing text size, etc.
#  The program uses routines from the HH, gridBase, and lattice
#  packages.
#                 A. L. Gould   November 2012
{
  tempdta <- dta
  nn <- length(unique(tempdta$AEname))
  nr <- nrow(tempdta)
  j <- 0
  xx <- NULL
  tempdta$Intens <- as.character(tempdta$Intens)
  for (i in 1:(nr/3))
  {
    x <- rbind(tempdta[j+1,],tempdta[j+1:3,])
    x$pAE2[1] <- 1-sum(x$pAE2[2:4])
    x$pAE1[1] <- 0
    x$Intens[1] <- "Absnt"
    xx <- rbind(xx,x)
    j <- j + 3
  }
  grid.newpage()
```

```
pushViewport(viewport(x=0,y=.6,height=.8,width=.5,just="left"))
w2 <- tapply(xx$pAE2,list(xx$TRT,xx$AEname,xx$Intens),FUN=mean)
bc1 <- barchart(w2,stack=T,
              xlab="Proportion (unconditional - all patients)",
              layout=c(1,nn),aspect=aspect, col=gray(c(.93,.8,.5,.1)),
              between=list(y=0.5),par.strip.text=list (cex=strip.cex),
              scales=list(cex=x.cex),border="transparent",
   par.settings=list(strip.background=list (col=c(stripbg,rep(0,6)))))
bc1 <- update(bc1,index.cond=list(nn:1))
print(bc1,newpage=F)
popViewport()
pushViewport(viewport(x=0.5,y=.6,height=.8,width=0.5,just="left"))
w1 <- tapply(dta$pAE1,list(dta$TRT,dta$AEname,dta$Intens), FUN=mean)
bc2 <- barchart(w1,stack=T, xlab=
              "Proportion (conditional - only patients with AE)",
              layout=c(1,nn),aspect=aspect,col=gray(c(.8,.5,.1)),
              between=list(y=0.5),  par.strip.text=list (cex=strip.cex),
              scales=list(cex=x.cex), border="transparent",
   par.settings=list(strip.background=list (col=c(stripbg,rep(0,6)))))
bc2 <- update(bc2,index.cond=list(nn:1))
print(bc2,newpage=F)
popViewport()
legend("bottom",leg.text,fill=gray(c(.93,.8,.5,.1)),horiz=T,
       bty="n",inset=leg.inset,title=leg.title,cex=leg.cex)
title.grob(main=title,y=ygrob,gp=gpar(cex=title.cex))
return(list(call=sys.call(),date=date(),dta.aug=xx,w1=w1,w2=w2))
}
```

The following R code can be used to produce graphics like Figures 2.5 and 2.6(a).

```
Fig5and6a.fn <- function(option, dta, time, AE, grp, linetype=c(1,2),
                    linecol=c("red","black"), plotevpts=FALSE,
                    pch=c(15,16), censmark="o", xmax1=0,
                    xmax2=0, lwid=3, xlab="Weeks on Treatment",
                    ylab1="Cumulative AE Incidence Rate",
                    ylab2="Difference between AE Incidence Rates",
                    cnfint = T, ylim1=c(0,1),ylim2=c(-.4,.4),
                    title=NULL, time.inc=NULL,
                    atRiskline=c(-2,-1), atrisk=F,
                    atRiskTimes=seq(0,xlim1[2],by=10),
                    atRisklabels="",n.risk.diff=T)
#
#  This program produces a simple Kaplan-Meier plot of cumulative
#  incidences of first occurrences of adverse events with allowance
#  for right censoring.  It uses processing and plotting programs from
#  the 'prodlim' and 'rms' packages.
#
#  INPUT:
#   option = 1 for plot of separate curves for each treatment
#            2 for plot of difference between the two survival curves
#            3 for both plots side by side
#            4 for plot on actual and log time scales side by side
#      dta = dataset containing times of AE events and censoring for
#            each subject
#     time = variable in 'dataset' containing event & censoring times
```

```
#       AE = variable in 'dataset' indicating for each subject whether
#            an event occurred at that time (AE = 1) or the individual
#            was censored at that time (AE = 0).
#      grp = variable in 'dataset' that identifies the treatment group
#            or stratum (this version of the program assumes 2 groups)
# linetype = line texture used to plot each survival curve
#  linecol = color of each survival curve
#      pch = specification of character plotted at each event time
#            for each survival curve.  These characters will have the
#            same colors as their corresponding curves.
#    xlab = x axis label; default is "Weeks on Treatment"
#   ylab1 = y axis label for separate curves
#   ylab2 = y axis label for difference between curves
#   title = title for graph; default is NULL (no title)
#
#  A. L. Gould  October, December 2012
{
  attach(dta)
  if (option < 4)                         # Survival calculations:
  {
    if (xmax1==0) max.x <- max(time)      # Fix upper time limit
    else max.x <- min(xmax1,max(time))    #  for separate survival
    xlim1 <- c(min(time),max.x)           #  curves
    if (xmax2==0) max.x <- max(time)      # Fix upper time limit
    else max.x <- min(xmax2,max(time))    #  for difference between
    xlim2 <- c(0,max.x)                   #  survival curves
    srv.fit <- prodlim(Hist(time,AE) ~ grp, data=dta)   # Fit KM model
    srvd <- Surv(time,AE)                 # Get Surv object
    srvd.fit <- npsurv(srvd ~ grp, data=dta) # Fit KM survival model
    srv.sum <- summary(srv.fit)
    ngps <- length(srv.sum$table)
    evpts <- vector(mode="list",length=ngps)    # Get distinct event
    cenpts <- vector(mode="list",length=ngps)   # & censoring points
    ne <- 0
    nc <- 0
    for (i in 1:ngps)
    {
      xx <- as.data.frame(srv.sum$table[i])
      xx[,5] <- 1 - xx[,5]
      if (length(xx[,3]) > 0)
        { ne <- ne + 1; evpts[[ne]] <- xx[xx[,3]>0,c(1,5)] }
      if (length(xx[,4]) > 0)
        { nc <- nc + 1; cenpts[[nc]] <- xx[xx[,4]>0,c(1,5)] }
    }
                                    # Plot both curves if just 2 gps
    if ((option==3) & (ngps==2)) oldpar <- par(mfrow=c(1,2))
    if (option %in% c(1,3))               # Plot the incidence curves
    {
      aRlabs <- as.character(srv.fit$X$grp)
      if (atrisk)
      srv.plot <- plot(srv.fit, type="cuminc",xlim=xlim1, ylim=ylim1,
                       confint=cnfint, lty=linetype, col=linecol,
                       xlab=xlab, ylab=ylab1, lwd=lwid,
                       percent=F, atRisk.times=atRiskTimes,
                       atRisk.labels=atRisklabels,
                       atRisk.line=atRiskline,legend.x="bottomright",
```

```
                    legend.bty="n",legend.cex=1)
     else srv.plot <- plot(srv.fit, type="cuminc",xlim=xlim1,
                       ylim=ylim1, confint=cnfint, lty=linetype,
                       col=linecol, xlab=xlab, ylab=ylab1,
                       percent=F, lwd=lwid, legend.x="bottomright",
                       legend.bty="n",legend.cex=1)
            # Plot distinct event and censored points
     if (plotevpts & (ne > 0))
       for (i in 1:ne)
         points(evpts[[i]],pch=pch[i],col=linecol[i],cex=1.2)
     if (nc > 0)
       for (i in 1:nc)
         points(cenpts[[i]],pch=censmark,col=linecol[i],cex=1.2)
   }
                         # Plot difference between incidence curves
   if ((option %in% 2:3) & (ngps==2))
     srv.diff <- survdiffplot(srvd.fit, order=1:2,
                   fun=function(y) 1-y, xlim=xlim2, ylim2, xlab=xlab,
                   ylab=ylab2, time.inc=time.inc, conf.int=.95,
                   conf="shaded", add=FALSE, lty=1, lwd=lwid,
                   col=1, n.risk=T, adj.n.risk=1, cex.n.risk=.9)
   if (option==3) oldpar <- par(mfrow=c(1,1))
   title(title)
   detach(dta)
   return(list(call=sys.call(),date=date(),srv.fit=srv.fit,
               srvd.fit=srvd.fit))
 }
```

The following R code can be used to produce graphics like Figure 2.6(b).

```
Fig6b.fn <- function()
{
#  This program produces Figure 2.6b. Needs the 'rms' package.
#
  Trt <- c(sample(c(rep("Trt A",35),rep("Trt B",34))),
           sample(c(rep("Trt C",34),rep("Trt D",34))))
  dta <- survival::veteran
  dta <- cbind(dta,Trt)
  srv.fit <- survfit(Surv(time,status)~Trt,data=dta)
  par(mfrow=c(1,2))
  survplot(srv.fit,fun=function(y){1-y},conf="none",label.curves=F,
           ylab="Cumulative Incidence",time.inc=50)
  legend(x=600,y=.4,c("Trt A","Trt B","Trt C","Trt D"),
         lty=1:4,merge=T,bty="n")
  survplot(srv.fit,fun=function(y){1-y},conf="none",label.curves=F,
           ylab="Cumulative Incidence",logt=T)
  legend(x=5,y=.4,c("Trt A","Trt B","Trt C","Trt D"),lty=1:4,
          merge=T,bty="n")
  par(mfrow=c(1,1))
}
```

The following R code can be used to produce graphics like Figure 2.7.

```
Fig7.fn <- function(dta="adlbc.lflst",varname="ALT",hline=F,
                    logtrans=F)
```

```
#   INPUT:
#      dta = character string giving name of file containing the data
#  varname = name of variable to plot (as character string)
#    hline = T to include a horizontal line at y = 2 (or log 2 if
#            logtrans = T)
# logtrans = T to plot log-transformed variable values, F to plot
#            actual values
#                                    A. L. Gould   January 2013
{
  xy <- Set.gg2plot.fn(dta=dta,var=varname)
  if (logtrans) eval(parse(text=paste0("xy$",varname, "=log(xy$",
                                        varname,")")))
  eval(parse(text=paste0("pb <- ggplot(xy,aes(x=factor(WEEK), y=",
                                        varname,"))")))
  pb <- pb + theme_bw()+xlab("Week")+ylab(varname)
  ppb <- pb + geom_boxplot(aes(fill=xy$TRTPCD))
  if (hline)
    if (logtrans)  ppb <- ppb + geom_hline(yintercept=log(2))
    else ppb <- ppb + geom_hline(yintercept=2)
  ppb + scale_fill_manual("Treatment Group",
                          values=c(gray(.9),gray(.7),gray(.5)))
}


Set.gg2plot.fn <- function(dta="adlbc.lflst",var="ALT")
{
#  Set up data file for plots using Fig7.fn and Fig9.fn
  wks <- c(0,2,4,6,8,12,16,20,24)
  x <- eval(parse(text=paste0("cbind(",dta,"[,c(1,5,10)],",dta,"$",
                              var,")")))
  dimnames(x)[[2]][4] <- var
  x<-x[x$VISIT_mod<10,]
  WEEK <- wks[x$VISIT_mod]
  x <- cbind(x,WEEK)
  return(x)
}
```

The following R code can be used to produce graphics like Figure 2.9.

```
Fig9.fn <- function(dta="adlbc.lflst",varname="ALT",hline=F,
                    logtrans=F)
#   INPUT:
#      dta = character string giving name of file containing the data
#  varname = name of variable to plot (as character string)
#    hline = T to include a horizontal line at y = 2 (or log 2 if
#            logtrans = T)
# logtrans = T to plot log-transformed variable values, F to plot
#            actual values
#                                    A. L. Gould   January 2013
{
  xy <- Set.gg2plot.fn(dta=dta,var=varname)
  if (logtrans) eval(parse(text=paste0("xy$",varname,"=log(xy$",
                                        varname,")")))
  xx <- paste0("p <- ggplot(xy,aes(x=(WEEK+.5*(TRTPCD==\"Xan_Hi\")
                         -.5*(TRTPCD==\"Pbo\")),y=",varname,"))")
  eval(parse(text=xx))
  pp <- p + theme_bw() + xlab("Week") + ylab(varname)
```

```
  if (hline)
    if (logtrans)  pp <- pp + geom_hline(yintercept=log(2))
    else pp <- pp + geom_hline(yintercept=2)
  pp <- pp + geom_jitter(aes(shape=TRTPCD,color=TRTPCD),
                         position=position_jitter(w=0.1),size=2.5)
  pp <-  pp + scale_color_manual(values=c(Pbo=gray(.7),
                                  Xan_Lo=gray(.5), Xan_Hi=gray(.3)))
  xx <- paste0("pp + geom_smooth(aes(x=WEEK,y=",varname,",
               group=TRTPCD, color=TRTPCD), lwd=1.25)")
  eval(parse(text=xx))
}
```

Figure 2.16 can be produced using the following functions:

```
Cerioli.fn <- function(X,trt,alpha=0.5,siglev=0.025,c.LR=0.1)
{
  i0 <- apply(!apply(X,1,is.na),2,"all")
  XX <- X[i0,]
  trts <- trt[i0]
  nX <- dim(XX)[1]
  vX <- dim(XX)[2]
  d2.rob <- array(0,nX)
  pvals <- array(0,nX)
  rob <- covMcd(XX,alpha=alpha)
  d.rob <- XX - t(array(rob$center,rev(dim(XX))))
  for (i in 1:nX) d2.rob[i] <- d.rob[i,]%*%solve(rob$cov)%*%d.rob[i,]
  mX <- sum(rob$raw.weights)
  i0 <- (1:nX)[rob$raw.weights == 0]
  i1 <- (1:nX)[rob$raw.weights == 1]
  c0 <- mX*(mX-vX)/(vX*(mX^2-1))
  c1 <- mX/(mX-1)^2
  if (length(i0) > 0)
    pvals[i0] <- pf(c0*d2.rob[i0],vX,mX-vX,lower.tail=F)
  if (length(i1) > 0)
    pvals[i1] <- pbeta(c1*d2.rob[i1],vX/2,(mX-vX)/2,lower.tail=F)
  rank.pvals <- rank(pvals)
  BH.crit <- rank.pvals*siglev/nX
  BH.rej <- (1:nX)[pvals < BH.crit]
  w <- floor(rank.pvals*c.LR)
  LR.crit <- (w + 1)*siglev/(nX + w + 1 - rank.pvals)
  LR.rej <- (1:nX)[pvals < LR.crit]
  if (min(pvals) > siglev) IRMCD.rej <- NULL
  else IRMCD.rej <- (1:nX)[pvals < (1 - siglev)^nX]
  pvals <- cbind(pvals,trts)
  return(list(call=sys.call(),date=date(),data=XX,center.
         rob=rob$center,cov.rob=rob$cov,pvals=round(pvals,3),
         trts=trts,BH.rej=BH.rej,LR.rej=LR.rej,IRMCD.rej=IRMCD.rej))

CerioliFig.fn <- function(alpha=0.5,siglev=0.025)
# Essentially a driver routine for Cerioli.fn.  Figure 2.16 can be
# produced from the output of this function using the graphing
# capabilities of a spreadsheet.
{
  WK4 <- adlbc.lflst[adlbc.lflst$VISIT=="WK4",]
  trt <- WK4$TRTPCD
  n <- dim(WK4)[1]
```

```
vals <- array(0,c(n,6))
vals0 <- array(0,c(n,6))
vals.uln <- array(0,c(n,6))
x0 <- array(0,c(n,6))
for (i in 1:6)
{
  vals[,i] <- as.numeric(WK4[,10+i])
  vals0[,i] <- as.numeric(WK4[,16+i])
  vals.uln[,i] <- as.numeric(WK4[,28+i])
  x0[,i] <- as.numeric(WK4[,34+i])
}
chgs <- vals - vals0
chgs.uln <- vals.uln - x0
lvals <- log(vals)
lvals.uln <- log(vals.uln)
lchgs <- lvals - log(vals0)
lchgs.uln <- lvals.uln - log(x0)
z.vals <- Cerioli.fn(vals,trt,alpha=alpha,siglev=siglev)
z.chgs <- Cerioli.fn(chgs,trt,alpha=alpha,siglev=siglev)
z.ulns <- Cerioli.fn(vals.uln,trt,alpha=alpha,siglev=siglev)
z.chgsuln <- Cerioli.fn(chgs.uln,trt,alpha=alpha,siglev=siglev)
z.lvals <- Cerioli.fn(lvals,trt,alpha=alpha,siglev=siglev)
z.lchgs <- Cerioli.fn(lchgs,trt,alpha=alpha,siglev=siglev)
z.lulns <- Cerioli.fn(lvals.uln,trt,alpha=alpha,siglev=siglev)
z.lchgsuln <- Cerioli.fn(lchgs.uln,trt,alpha=alpha,siglev=siglev)
return(list(call=sys.call(),date=date(),vals=z.vals,chgs=z.chgs,
            ulns=z.ulns,chgsuln=z.chgsuln,lvals=z.lvals,
            lchgs=z.lchgs,lulns=z.lulns,lchgsuln=z.lchgsuln))
}
```

# References

[1] Brueckner, A. The Forest for the Trees: Visualizing Adverse Events, www.ctspedia.org/do/view/CTSpedia/GraphicsPresentationArchive#The_Forest_for_the_Trees_Visuali (accessed 17 October 2012).

[2] Friendly, M. (2012) Gallery of Data Visualization, http://www.datavis.ca/gallery/index.php (accessed 24 June 2014).
    A collection of some excellent, effective graphics, including unusual graphics such as the table plot, with extensive descriptions of their interpretations and, in many cases, code to produce them. Also includes some examples that deliberately or inadvertently mislead the viewer, as instructive lessons in what not to do graphically.

[3] Wainer, H. (1984) How to display data badly. *American Statistician*, **38**, 137–147.
    This article provides 12 rules for displaying data badly in various ways or, even worse, for misleading the reader, whether deliberately or inadvertently. The description is useful for understanding why the examples are so bad, and the paper provides guidance on how to avoid committing the same sins. Statisticians are not immune from making these errors: two of the examples are from the *Journal of the American Statistical Association*.

[4] Bertin, J. (2001) *Semiology of Graphics*, Esri Press, Redlands, CA.

[5] Cleveland, W.S. (1993) *Visualizing Data*, Hobart Press, Summit, NJ.
    A fundamental treatment of the effective use of graphical displays that focuses on their use for visualizing the structure of data. A number of displays are described, some new such as multiway dot plots, and some previously described such as boxplots, quantile plots, and quantile–quantile

plots. Illuminates how simple individual graphical displays can be stacked and otherwise arranged to provide insight into relationships that otherwise would be difficult if not impossible to discern.

[6] Cleveland, W.S. (1994) *Elements of Graphing Data*, Hobart Press, Summit, NJ.

[7] Few, S. (2012) *Show Me the Numbers: Designing Tables and Graphs to Enlighten*, 2nd edn, Analytics Press, Burlingame, CA.

[8] Nicol, A.A.M. and Pexman, P.M. (2010) *Displaying Your Findings: A Practical Guide for Creating Figures, Posters, and Presentations*, 6th edn, American Psychological Association, Washington, DC.

[9] Robbins, N.B. (2005) *Creating More Effective Graphs*, Wiley Interscience, Hoboken, NJ.

[10] Schmid, C.F. (1954) *Handbook of Graphic Presentation*, Ronald Press, New York.

[11] Tufte, E.R. (1990) *Envisioning Information*, Graphics Press, Cheshire, CT.

[12] Tufte, E.R. (1997) *Visual Explanations: Images and Quantiles, Evidence and Narrative*, Graphics Press, Cheshire, CT.

[13] Tufte, E.R. (2001) *The Visual Display of Qualitative Information*, 2nd edn, Graphics Press, Cheshire, CT.
    A fundamental reference for constructing effective graphical displays in general. It discusses in detail graphical design principles that maximize the effectiveness of graphical displays in communicting messages with as little superfluous detail as possible to interfere with the message of the display.

[14] Wainer, H. (2009) *Picturing the Uncertain World*, Princeton University Press, Princeton, NJ.

[15] Hyndman, R.J. and Shang, H.L. (2010) Rainbow plots, bagplots, and boxpolots for functional data. *Journal of Computational and Graphical Statistics*, **19**, 29–45.
    This paper describes ways to visualize, and graphically detect, outliers when the observations are functional data, that is, smooth curves or trends in time such as with organ function tests or possible EEGs or ECGs. The sequences of observations are reduced to the first two (or possibly more) principal components or by other appropriate dimension-reducing techniques. The results are displays either of functional densities of individual trajectories with outliers identified, or of highest bivariate density regions of pairs of principal components based on a bivariate kernel density estimate that provides the analogs of boxplots.

[16] Polzehl, J. and Tabelow, K. (2007) fmri: a package for analyzing fmri data. *R News*, **7**, 13–17.

[17] Rossling, H. and Johansson, C. (2009) Gapminder: Liberating the x-axis from the burden of time. *Statistical Computing and Graphics Newsletter*, **20**, 4–10.

[18] Harrell, F.E. Statistical Graphics, http://biostat.mc.vanderbilt.edu/twiki/pub/Main/StatGraph Course/graphscourse.pdf (accessed 14 September 2012).

[19] Heiberger, R. and Holland, B. (2004) *Statistical Analysis and Data Display*, Springer, New York.

[20] Matange, S. Tips and Tricks for Clinical Graphics Using ODS Graphics, http://support.sas.com/ resources/papers/proceedings11/281-2011.pdf (accessed 11 July 2014).

[21] Murrell, P. (2011) *R Graphics*, 2nd edn, CRC Press, Boca Raton, FL.
    This book describes, and provides the code for, a very extensive collection of graphical displays. Also describes in detail various display-producing packages, including lattice, ggplot2, and grid graphics. Each of these packages comprises a suite of functions for producing a variety of graphical displays.

[22] Rodriguez, R.N. *An Overview of ODS Statistical Graphics in SAS© 9.3*, http://support.sas.com/ resources/papers/76822_ODSGraph2011.pdf (accessed 16 October 2012).

[23] Sarkar, D. (2008) *Lattice: Multivariate Data Visualization with R*, Springer, New York.
    The reference manual for the use of the lattice graphical display system implemented in R.

[24] SAS Institute (2011) *SAS 9.3 ODS Graphics: Getting Started with Business and Statistical Graphics*, SAS Institute, Cary, NC.

[25] Wickham, H. (2009) *ggplot2: Elegant Graphics for Data Analysis*, Springer, New York.

[26] Krause, A. and O'Connell, M. (2013) *A Picture is Worth a Thousand Tables*, Springer-Verlag/AAPS, New York.

[27] Tukey, J.W. (1990) Data-based graphics: visual display in the decades to come. *Statistical Science*, **5**, 327–339.

[28] Few, S. Criteria for Evaluating Visual EDA Tools, Visual Business Intelligence Newsletter, http://www.perceptualedge.com/articles/visual_business_intelligence/evaluating_visual_eda_tools.pdf (accessed 25 September 2012).

[29] FDA Guidance for Industry: Clinical Studies Section of Labeling for Human Prescription Drug and Biological Products – Content and Format, Food and Drug Administration, http://www.fda.gov/RegulatoryInformation/Guidances/ucm127509.htm (acceesed 4 July 2014).

[30] Amit, O., Heiberger, R.M. and Lane, P.W. (2008) Graphical approaches to the analysis of safety data from clinical trials. *Pharmaceutical Statistics*, **7**, 20–35.
    This paper describes some graphical displays for three categories of safety data evaluation: ECGs, clinical laboratory tests, and spontaneous patient-reported adverse events. The displays have two aims: confirmation and further evaluation of known safety signals and identifying emerging safety issues. Three QTc interval displays are described: an empirical cdf for maximum change from baseline in QTc with indicator lines at changes of 30 and 60 milliseconds to provide an overall picture of QTc change during the entire period of observation; boxplots of QTc changes in each treatment group at each week, also with indicator lines; and a line plot of mean QTc changes from baseline at each time point with confidence intervals (plus means and confidence intervals for LOCF values). For liver function tests, the current value, often divided by the upper limit of normal, usually is more important than the change from baseline. Boxplots of the test values at each week are proposed, with extreme outliers counted above the corresponding boxplot rather than plotted, along with a marginal plot of the maximum value over the observation period. One also can include boxplots of the maximum (relative to ULN) values of various test measurements over the observation period in the same graphic, although this requires recognizing that the maxima for the various tests may not occur at the same time point. Scatterplots of test values for individual patients also are presented, both on-treatment versus baseline values, and (as trellis plots) on-treatment values for pairs of tests. Profiles of test values at the various time points during the study can be compiled for individual patients, and profiles for several patients arranged as a series of panels. Care needs to be taken in order to assure that the individual plots are readable. Three displays for summarizing the incidence of spontaneously reported adverse events are described. A two-panel graphic provides on the left panel a dot plot relating adverse event (*y*-axis) to frequency (*x*-axis) for each treatment; the right panel provides for each adverse event an estimate of the relative risk of the test treatment to the control along with a 95% confidence interval. The adverse experience names are sorted so that the estimated relative risks increase monotonically from the bottom to the top. Variations on this graphic also are briefly described. The second graphic consists of time-to-event plots for adverse events. The third graphic, complementary to the second, is a plot of the hazard functions for specific adverse events, along with their standard errors.

[31] Schweder, T. and Spjøtvoll, E. (1982) Plots of P-values to evaluate many tests simultaneously. *Biometrika*, **69**, 493–502.

[32] Matange, S. *Clincal Graphics Using ODS Graphics*, http://support.sas.com/resources/papers/wusspaper.pdf (accessed 28 January 2013).

[33] CDISC CDISC SDTM/ADaM Pilot Project Report, Cerebrovascular Diseases (accessed 27 November 2012).

[34] Trost, D.C. and Freston, J.W. (2008) Vector analysis to detect hepatotoxicity signals in drug development. *Drug Information Journal*, **42**, 27–34.

[35] Ramsay, J.O. and Silverman, B.W. (2002) *Applied Functional Data Analysis: Methods and Case Studies*, Springer, New York.

[36] Ramsay, J.O. and Silverman, B.W. (2005) *Functional Data Analysis*, Springer, New York.

[37] Epifanio, I. and Ventura-Campos, N. (2011) Functional data analysis in shape analysis. *Computational Statistics and Data Analysis*, **55**, 2578–2773.

[38] González Manteiga, W. and Vieu, P. (2007) Statistics for functional data. *Computational Statistics and Data Analysis*, **51**, 4788–4792.

[39] Martínez-Camblor, P. and Corral, N. (2011) Repeated measures analysis for functional data. *Computational Statistics and Data Analysis*, **55**, 3244–3256.

[40] Croux, C. and Ruiz-Gazen, A. (2005) High breakdown estimators for principal components: the projection-pursuit approach revisited. *Journal of Multivariate Analysis*, **95**, 206–226.

[41] Hyndman, R.J. (1996) Computing and graphing highest density regions. *American Statistician*, **50**, 241–250.

[42] Rousseeuw, P., Ruts, I. and Tukey, J.W. (1999) The bagplot: a bivariate boxplot. *American Statistician*, **53**, 382–387.

[43] Hyndman, R.J. and Ullah, M.S. (2007) Robust forecasting of mortality and fertility rates: a functional data approach. *Computational Statistics and Data Analysis*, **51**, 4942–4956.

[44] Cerioli, A. (2010) Multivariate outlier detection with high-breakdown estimators. *Journal of the American Statistical Association*, **105**, 147–156.

[45] Cerioli, A. and Farcomeni, A. (2011) Error rates for multivariate outlier detection. *Computational Statistics and Data Analysis*, **55**, 544–553.

[46] Hawkins, D.M. and Olive, D.J. (1999) Improved feasible solution algorithms for high breakdown estimation. *Computational Statistics and Data Analysis*, **30**, 1–11.

[47] Rousseeuw, P.J. and Van Driessen, K. (1999) A fast algorithm for the minimum covariance determinant estimator. *Technometrics*, **41**, 212–233.

[48] Maechler, M. robustbase: Basic Robust Statistics, http://cran.r-project.org (accessed 27 June 2014).

[49] Benjamini, Y. and Hochberg, Y. (1995) Controlling the false discovery rate: a practical and powerful approach to multiple testing. *Journal of the Royal Statistical Society, Series B*, **57**, 289–300.

[50] Lehmann, E.L. and Romano, J.P. (2005) Generalizations of the familywise error rate. *Annals of Statistics*, **33**, 1154.

[51] van der Laan, M.J., Dudoit, S. and Pollard, K.S. (2004) Augmentation procedures for control of the generalized faimily-wise error rate and tail probabilities for the proportion of false positives. *Statistical Applications in Genetics and Molecular Biology*, **3** article 15.

[52] Dubin, J.A., Muller, H.-G. and Hess, K.R. (2001) Event history graphs for censored survival data. *Statistics in Medicine*, **20**, 2951–2964.

[53] Goldman, A.I. (1992) EVENTCHARTS: visualizing survival and other timed-events data. *American Statistician*, **46**, 13–18.

[54] Lee, J.J., Hess, K.R. and Dubin, J.A. (2000) Extensions and applications of event charts. *American Statistician*, **54**, 63–70.

[55] Swihart, B.J., Caffo, B., James, B.D. *et al.* (2010) Lasagna plots: a saucy alternative to spaghetti plots. *Epidemiology*, **21**, 621–625.

This paper describes a graphical display similar to a heat map that provides a way to visualize trends in measurements in individual subjects over time. A typical starting display is visualized as a rectangular grid of stacked boxes, with the rows corresponding to subjects and the columns corresponding to time points at which measurements are made. The observation for an individual at a point in time is represented by the color or shading of the box corresponding to that individual at that time. Various shading or color schemes can be used to represent ordered measurement values, and some recommendations are given for effective color/shading schemes. The sequences of values for different individuals are distinct because they correspond to different rows fo the array, as opposed to typical "spaghetti plots" of measurement vs time trajectories of individual patients that can overlap so much that no pattern can be discerned. The rows and/or columns can be sorted or aggregated, e.g., by patient strata, in various ways to highlight interesting data features.

[56]  Cox, D.R. and Wong, M.Y. (2004) A simple procedure for the selection of significant effects. *Journal of the Royal Statistical Society, Series B*, **66**, 395–400.

[57]  Crowe, B.J., Xia, H.A., Berlin, J.A. *et al.* (2009) Recommendations for safety planning, data collection, evaluation and reporting during drug, biologic and vaccine development: a report of the safety planning, evaluation, and reporting team. *Clinical Trials*, **6**, 430–440.

[58]  Gait, J.E., Smith, S. and Brown, S.L. (2000) Evaluation of safety data from controlled clinical trials: the clinical principles explained. *DIA Journal*, **34**, 273–287.

[59]  Haemer, K.W. (1947) The perils of perspective. *American Statistician*, **1**, 19–19.
        Charts drawn in perspective usually are difficult to read even with approximate accuracy. The interpretation of the message of a chart can depend on the perspective used to draw it. If a perspective view really is necessary, then it should be used with restraint and the same perspective should be used for all of the charts. Horizontal rulings should be provided to allow the reader to interpret the figures.

[60]  Haemer, K.W. (1950) Color in chart presentation. *American Statistician*, **4**, 20–20.
        This article recommends not using color just because one can: color has to perform a specific service. Generally, using fewer colors is better than using many, and it is possible for color to make a figure more difficult to understand. A few subtleties: (1) Some colors are not easily visible either by themselves or when used with other colors; red is easy to see, yellow is not, and deep colors can be difficult to distinguish. (2) Colors have suggestion values and connotations: for example, red and green convey different subconscious messages.

[61]  Haemer, K.W. (1951) The pseudo third dimension. *American Statistician*, **5**, 28–28.
        This paper recommends not giving bars in a bar chart a three-dimensional appearance unless it really is needed to tell the story. If a 3D appearance really is necessary then recommends (1) keeping the third dimension thin and avoiding dramatic perspectives; (2) using the same perspective view for all charts in a series; (3) shading the front of the columns (bars) with the strongest tone and, if bottoms or tops must be shown, keeping them light to avoid adding to column length.

[62]  Levine, J.G. Gersonides, www.gersonides.com (accessed 25 September 2011).
        This is a collection of graphical displays along with code (usually in R) and example data sets that can be run in real time that are useful for summarizing data from clinical trials, based on the author's experience as a regulatory reviewer. Unusual, but potentially useful, displays include boxplots with overlaid density plots, dot plots to summarize sample sizes in various study subgroups, and bubble plots to summarize how many patients were exposed to various doses for how long.

[63]  Pocock, S., Travison, T. and Wruck, L. (2008) How to interpret figures in reports of clinical trials. *British Medical Journal*, **336**, 1166–1169.

[64]  Pocock, S.J., Clayton, T.C. and Altman, D.G. (2002) Survival plots of time-to-event outcomes in clinical trials: good practice and pitfalls. *Lancet*, **359**, 1686–1689.

[65]  Pocock, S.J., Traviston, T.G. and Wruck, L.M. (2007) Figures in clinical trial reports: current practice and scope for improvement. *Trials*, **8**, 36–17.
        This paper provides recommendations for improving figures used to communicate results of clinical trials on the basis of a survey of 77 reports of randomized clinical trials published in five general medical journals from November 2006 to January 2007. Key general recommendations include: (i) deciding if a figure really is needed instead of a table; (ii) clear labeling and presentation and a good legend so that the figure can be understood without reference to the text; (iii) clearly identifying treatment groups and using color carefully so that message is not lost in a black and white copy; (iv) indicating numbers of patients in each treatment group; (v) including measures of

uncertainty such as error bars or confidence intervals; (vi) clearly stating the primary inferences to avoid misinterpretation by readers; and (vii) paying careful attention to principles of graphical and visual display.

[66] Squassante, L., Robinson, C.N. and Palmer, R.L. (2006) Simple graphical methods of displaying multiple clinical results. *Pharmaceutical Statistics*, **5**, 51–60.

   This paper provides examples of how complex issues can be summarized graphically to give effective insight. Of particular interest are topographical maps of *p*-values (considered only as descriptive weights) corresponding to between-group comparisons of EEG leads, using shading to indicate relative weight, and star plots to identify patterns of difference among multivariate measurements.

[67] Steele, J. and Ilinsky, N. (2010) *Beautiful Visualization: Looking at Data through the Eyes of Experts*, O'Reilly Media, Sebastopol, CA.

[68] Tufte, E.R. (2003) *The Cognitive Style of PowerPoint 2003*, Graphics Press, Cheshire, CT.

# 3

# QSAR modeling: prediction of biological activity from chemical structure

**Andy Liaw and Vladimir Svetnik**

*Biometrics Research, Merck & Co., Inc, Rahway, NJ 07065, USA*

## 3.1    Introduction

This chapter describes a very important application of statistical methods to drug discovery, namely quantitative structure–activity relationship (QSAR) models. These models are most often used in the lead optimization stage, when a few families of molecules have been iden- tified as active *in vitro* against the biological target of interest. At this stage the medicinal chemists' effort in modifying the molecular structures is focused on: (i) maximizing potency; (ii) improving the absorption, distribution, metabolism, excretion (ADME) properties of the compounds as possible drugs; and (iii) minimizing potential liabilities with respect to toxic- ity. QSAR models can help prioritize a list of candidate compounds for experimental testing, as well as giving hints as to the effects of possible structural modifications on biological activities.

A QSAR model is a regression or classification model that uses variables derived from the structure of molecules (chemical descriptors) to predict their biological activities. The biolog- ical activities are typically obtained experimentally from *in vitro* assays. These models (and indeed, medicinal chemistry) are based on a fundamental assumption that structurally similar molecules usually have similar biological activities, while structurally dissimilar molecules may or may not have similar activities [1]. There are exceptions to this, sometimes referred to as the "activity cliff," where a small change in molecular structure leads to a large change in

*Statistical Methods for Evaluating Safety in Medical Product Development*, First Edition.
Edited by A. Lawrence Gould.
© 2015 John Wiley & Sons, Ltd. Published 2015 by John Wiley & Sons, Ltd.

biological activity [2]. In general, there are two ways QSAR models are utilized. The first is via predictions, when the activities of candidate molecules predicted by the model are used in screening for potential undesirable effects and/or for ranking molecules in terms of their prioritization for the follow-up testing. The second use is to generate hypotheses on how changes in molecular structures affect the biological activity of interest.

The remainder of the chapter is organized as follows. In Section 3.2 we describe the characteristics of data used for building QSAR models. In Section 3.3 we describe two particular methods of building QSAR models: random forests (RFs) and boosting. In Section 3.4, we discuss the model validation process and how the models may provide insight that chemists can use to optimize molecules. In Section 3.5 we show a modeling process on an example data set. Section 3.6 provides a concluding discussion.

## 3.2    Data

### 3.2.1    Chemical descriptors

A bewildering number of chemical descriptors have been proposed in the chemoinformatics literature (see [3] for a survey). Chemical descriptors fall generally into one of several categories: constitutional (e.g., molecular weights), topological, geometrical, and so on. The use of chemical descriptors is not limited to QSAR model building: for example, they are also commonly used in molecular database search and chemical library design.

The two-dimensional descriptors are based on a 2D representation of the molecules. Two of them that commonly are used in QSAR applications are atom pairs (APs) [4] and extended connectivity fingerprints (ECFPs) [5]. There is for either approach a collection or "dictionary" of specific descriptors. The data for any molecule consist of the frequencies of occurrence of the descriptors in the representation of the molecule. Most of these frequencies will be zero (sparse data) because although the dictionaries may contain many possible descriptors, relatively few will apply to any individual molecule. It is not uncommon to see a data matrix with no more than 5% non-zero entries. For example, for the 250 molecules used as the training set in Section 3.5, most molecules have less than 15% non-zero AP descriptors and less than 2% ECFP4 descriptors. This makes some modeling methods unsuitable, especially those that rely on assumptions about the distributions of the descriptors (e.g., linear discriminant analysis). Dimension reduction sometimes is useful for dealing with descriptors that number in the thousands or more.

The three-dimensional descriptors are based on the 3D structures of the molecules. They are computationally more demanding to generate, partly because there usually does not exist a unique rigid three-dimensional conformation of a molecule; that is, a molecule has some flexibility and can change shape somewhat. There are experimental procedures to elucidate the 3D structures. If such information is not available, there are computational methods that can produce a low-energy conformation of a molecule based on the 2D structural information. One of the most commonly used types of 3D descriptors is a 3D pharmacophore fingerprint. A pharmacophore point is a molecular feature that may be involved in molecular interaction. A pharmacophore fingerprint is a set of (either three or four) pharmacophore points and the physical distances (e.g., in angstroms) among them (with distances discretized into discrete bins). This class of descriptors is conceptually more precise than the others. However, in practice, and especially in QSAR applications, the use of these descriptors rarely justifies the additional computational burden required. They rarely provide more precise characterizations than, say, 2D descriptors, even though they can easily number in the millions. Brown and Martin had found that none of the 3D descriptors they studied performed as well as some 2D descriptors in separating biologically active molecules from the inactive ones [6].

When gathering data for building QSAR models, one should consider how the data came about. Available data rarely come from designed experiments with the goal of building predictive QSAR models. Rather, they usually come as a result of chemists' attempts to optimize the properties (potency against the target as well as drug-like properties) for a specific therapeutic target by creating many close analogs based on a handful of core molecular structures. Accumulating such data over time and over many different projects can lead to a very large collection of molecules that lack chemical diversity (for example, the molecules may form just a few large clusters of similars). This characteristic of the data leads to the issue of "local" versus "global" models: should one build QSAR models only from structurally related molecules, in hope of better prediction in the neighborhood of the chemical space being modeled, or should one use all available data and build models that are applicable to a much more diverse chemical space [7]? At the most basic level, this depends on the intended use of the model as well as the method being used for building the model. Methods that do not have the flexibility to handle nonlinear trends or possible interactions among descriptors are most likely not suitable for building global models.

### 3.2.2   Activity data

The characteristics of molecules being predicted in QSAR models are usually biological activities of the molecules measured in *in vitro* assays. These can be activity at a single concentration, or potency determined from multiple concentrations. It is worthwhile to point out that precision of the experimental measurements can be a useful information in determining the quality of a QSAR model: if the magnitude of prediction error of a model is close to that of the experimental measurements, then we know that there is not much to gain from use of the model.

There are a few points about the nature of the data available for building QSAR models that are worth keeping in mind. The first is the potential skewness of the activity data, either due to the nature of the assay, or "by design": chemists usually synthesize molecules for testing in the hope that they give "good" biological activities. It is not common that molecules that are known to be "undesirable" are tested. The second is the information content of the assay data. Some assays are inherently difficult in producing precise numerical results, and as such are more qualitative than quantitative. With such data, it may be more appropriate to build a classification model that predicts the probability that a molecule falls in certain range, rather than a regression model that provides a numerical prediction of expected assay results. For some assays, especially for ADME or toxicology-related endpoints, there may be a significant proportion of the molecules with qualified results, meaning the values are only known to be above (or below) certain constants (e.g., detection limit of the assay, or concentration range tested). Such data also pose significant challenges to most commonly used methods. The qualified data in reality consist of the censored values. However, very few methods for building QSAR models can adequately handle such data. On the other hand, very few statistical methods for handling censored data are adequate for building QSAR models.

## 3.3   Model building

A QSAR model is a regression (or classification) model that predicts the biological activity of a molecule based on some representation of its structure,

$$Y = f(\mathbf{x}) + \varepsilon,$$

where $Y$ denotes the biological activity (perhaps suitably transformed), $\mathbf{x}$ is the vector of chemical descriptors, and $\varepsilon$ is the error. Any statistical or machine learning method that produces such a model can be (and most likely has been) brought to bear. Among several methods that have been popular in the QSAR literature are the naïve Bayes classifier, partial least squares, recursive partitioning, artificial neural networks, support vector machines (SVMs), Gaussian processes, and ensemble methods such as boosting and random forests [8]. We describe below two ensemble methods, RFs [9] and stochastic gradient boosting models (GBMs) [10,11] in more detail.

### 3.3.1   Random forests

RF is an ensemble method that builds a "forest" of classification or regression trees, and forms predictions by either voting (for classification) or averaging (for regression). We first describe the "base learner" in the ensemble: the individual classification and regression trees.

A classification and regression tree is a data partitioning method [12]. The algorithm starts with all of the data in the "root" node. Each predictor variable is evaluated to see how well it can separate the data into two descendent ("daughter") nodes. For classification, the criterion is the decrease in the Gini index, whereas for regression it is the reduction in mean squared errors. The best splitting point for the best variable is used to form the binary split. The process is then repeated on each of the descendant nodes until no further split is possible. For regression the process is stopped when the number of data points in a node falls below a minimum (e.g., 5). In the usual tree-based method there is a pruning process to cut the tree down to a size that is less likely to overfit the data. This is usually accomplished via cross-validation [12].

In RF [9], the ensemble is formed by injecting randomness into the tree-growing process (hence the name). Firstly, a random sample, usually a bootstrap sample, is drawn from the data to grow each tree. This corresponds to bagging (bootstrap aggregating). Within each tree, a random subset of variables is evaluated for splitting at each node. The trees are grown to maximum size and not pruned back. After all trees are grown, prediction of a new data point is done by aggregating the predictions from all trees for that data point. For classification, the fraction of trees predicting a particular class is taken as the estimated probability of that class, and the class with the largest probability is the predicted class. For regression, the prediction of a tree is formed by averaging the training data points that fall into the same terminal node as the data point being predicted. Then the predicted values from all trees are averaged.

The rationale for the deliberately added randomness is as follows. Predictions from a tree grown to its maximum size have low bias but high variance. By averaging over many such trees, low bias is retained while the variance is reduced. This would only work if the quantities being averaged have low correlation. The random split selection at each node was designed to reduce the correlation among trees.

The random sampling of the training set to grow each tree also produces a side benefit. One can view the sampling as partitioning of the training set into "training" (the "in-bag" portion) and "test" (the "out-of-bag" (OOB) portion) sets for the particular tree to be grown. The predictions of the OOB data by that tree are legitimate out-of-sample predictions. Thus by aggregating these OOB predictions we can get an "honest" out-of-sample estimate of error rate (or mean squared errors) of the model. The OOB prediction of each data point is based on about 36% of the trees (since each data point has about a 36% chance of being OOB, if the sampling is the regular $n$-out-of-$n$ with replacement bootstrap). The mean squared error decreases initially quickly and then slowly as a function of the number of trees. Consequently, the OOB estimate of error is reasonably accurate and can be obtained at little additional computational cost as long as there are sufficient trees in the ensemble.

The RF approach has some appealing attributes. First, it can handle many different data types, and has very few tuning parameters. Breiman considered "mtry," the number of variables tested for splitting at each node, as the only tuning parameter [9]. Second, it is robust against overfitting, so one can grow as many trees in the ensemble as is practical without having to worry about overfitting. Third, it often performs quite well compared to other algorithms, and rarely performs poorly, so it is a "safe" algorithm to use. The potential drawbacks of the algorithm are that it generates very large and complex models, which also makes it nearly impossible to discern how the model relates predictor variables to the response. The variable importance measures described in the next section should help in this respect.

There have been many extensions and modifications of the RF algorithm since its introduction, though Breiman's work remains the reference to which others are compared. We will only mention a few developments that readers may want to explore further. The first is the cforest implementation in the party package for R [13–15]. The principal differences between this package and Breiman's original implementation are in how the trees are grown and predictions are aggregated. The base learners in cforest use conditional inference, and predictions are formed by averaging weights produced by the trees. The variable importance measure from cforest attempts to correct for the bias in RFs that tends to favor variables with more possible splitting points [16]. Another interesting tree ensemble method is bart in the BayesTree package for R [17]. This method uses a Markov chain Monte Carlo backfitting algorithm to produce a posterior distribution of trees, so one can obtain not only point estimates for prediction (either by median or mean of the posterior distribution) but also the uncertainty intervals.

### 3.3.2  Stochastic gradient boosting

Boosting has some similarities to RFs, yet in some respects they are almost polar opposites. Both are ensembles of trees (although other "base learners" are possible as well in both). However, RF is "embarrassingly parallel" in nature (every tree is grown independently of any other tree), while boosting grows trees sequentially. In RFs, trees are grown to their maximum size. In boosting, usually very small trees (as small as a single split or a "decision stump") are grown. Yet the two algorithms frequently perform similarly well on a wide variety of data sets. Comparisons of RFs, stochastic gradient boosting, SVMs, and a few other methods popular in the QSAR literature found RFs and stochastic gradient boosting to be the best performers across several QSAR data sets [10, 18].

Stochastic gradient boosting is a general framework that can give rise to several different boosting algorithms [10, 11]. The algorithm proceeds as follows:

---

**Algorithm**

1. $F_0 = \left\{ \sum_{i=1}^{n} Y_i \right\} / n.$

2. For $m = 1, \dots, M$ DO:

3. Compute the residuals $r_i = Y_i - F_{m-1}(\mathbf{X}_i)$, $i = 1, \dots, n$.

4. Draw a random sample of size $s$ from the indices $1, \dots, n$: $\{i_1, \dots, i_s\}$.

5. Grow a regression tree $T_m$ with up to $n_{node}$ terminal nodes from the sampled residuals and data $\{(r_{i1}, \mathbf{X}_{i1}), \dots, (r_{is}, \mathbf{X}_{is})\}$.

6. Update the model: $F_m(\mathbf{X}) = F_{m-1}(\mathbf{X}) + \gamma T_m(\mathbf{X})$, where $\gamma \in (0, 1)$ is the shrinkage factor.

7. End the for loop.

---

This process can be seen as a stagewise, greedy optimization of a loss function [10]. The residuals in step 3 above can be thought of as the derivatives of the loss function evaluated at the estimate of the function at the $(m - 1)$th iteration. The form of the algorithm above is least squares regression (using regression trees as the base learner). Other boosting algorithms, such as least absolute deviation regression or logistic regression, can be obtained by suitable modification of steps 1 and 3.

The algorithm as presented has three tuning parameters: the number of iterations, $M$; the size of the trees (i.e., the number of terminal nodes), $n_{node}$; and the shrinkage parameter, $\gamma$. These parameters usually are interdependent. Increasing the size of the trees amounts to allowing higher-order interactions among the descriptors. (Using decision stumps yields additive models.) As the base learner gets more complex, more regularization (by using a smaller value of $\gamma$) tends to work better, and as regularization gets stronger, more iterations usually are needed to achieve better performance.

Boosting has proved to be such a popular algorithm that many other extensions and variations have been produced since its introduction by Freund and Shapire [19, 20]. Several R packages implement various boosting methods. Friedman's method as described above is available in the gbm package [21], with some minor differences from Friedman's own implementation. The Machine Learning Task View for R (http://cran.r-project.org/web/views/MachineLearning.html) is a valuable resource for methods available in R, and has a list of available packages that contain various flavors of boosting.

## 3.4    Model validation and interpretation

One of the most important tasks in building predictive models such as QSAR is assessing and tuning the prediction performance of models. To discuss model tuning and performance assessment, we first need to have a measure of performance as a basis. The various performance metrics usually are related to the residuals: the differences between the observed and predicted values. Before we go on to discuss the performance metrics, it is important to discuss the metrics computed on the training set versus the test set. We would like to emphasize that performance metrics computed on the training data are usually not useful, and for some methods they are not informative at all. As an example, the boosting and RF algorithms are basically designed to drive the errors on the training data as low as possible, and frequently will give zero training error in classification data. Some people take this as an indication of overfitting, but we would argue that overfitting should be reserved strictly for when the prediction performance on test data degrades as the model becomes more complex [22, p. 220]. Low training data error does not have to coincide with high test data error, which is what really matters.

For regression data, the most commonly used performance metric would be either the mean squared error or its square root. More often a dimensionless metric is desired, and the prediction squared correlation coefficient,

$$Q^2 = 1 - \frac{\sum_{\text{test}}(Y - \hat{Y})^2}{\sum_{\text{test}}(Y - \overline{Y})^2}.$$

where the summations are over data in the test set. $Y$ denotes the observed activities, $\hat{Y}$ denotes the predicted activities, and $\overline{Y}$ is the mean activity of the test set.

There is a larger variety of performance metrics for classification data. The most commonly used is the misclassification rate, or equivalently, percent accuracy. These make use only of the predicted class labels. An alternative measure that is also used is Cohen's $\kappa$ index, originally intended to measure agreement between two raters. For methods that can produce estimated class probabilities or some numerical measures that indicate likelihood of belonging to a class, there may be more informative metrics such as area under the receiver operating characteristic curve (AUROC). If the task at hand is akin to screening, so that the number of molecules belonging to one class is much smaller than that of the second class, then the costs of misclassification should not be symmetric; that is, the cost of predicting an inactive molecule as active is not the same as predicting an active molecule as inactive. In such cases the error rate may be weighted accordingly. In such a situation the AUROC can also be modified for "early recognition" (ranking the rare class as high as possible) [23].

With the appropriate performance metric in hand, we can move on to model tuning and performance assessment. There are two commonly used methods: $k$-fold cross-validation and bootstrap [24]. These methods can become computationally costly when the data set is large. In such cases repeated random data splitting (into training and test sets) can be done instead.

Because the dimension of some descriptor types (AP, ECFP, 3D pharmacophores, etc.) can be very high, even though the number of informative descriptors can be relatively low, some feature selection or dimension reduction step can be taken as part of the model building process. The importance of including any feature selection or dimension reduction as part of the model building process cannot be overemphasized, and any validation and performance assessment must be done external to that. In other words, any data used in feature selection or dimension reduction must be considered as part of the training data, and not used to assess performance. If this is not done carefully, one may end up with an overly optimistic estimate of prediction performance due to selection bias [25]. One way to ensure that such selection bias does not happen is to employ nested cross-validation or bootstrapping, where the "outer" loop is used for performance assessment, and any feature selection, dimension reduction, and model tuning is done in the "inner" loop. Svetnik gives an example procedure for feature selection with the RF algorithm, where the feature selection is done within the cross-validation loop [26].

Due to the fact that most data available for building QSAR models came from past experiments that were not designed for building predictive models, the models often can be used to predict data that are on the boundary, or even outside the domain, of the training data. This can be addressed in two ways. The first is in the performance assessment or model selection step. Sheridan proposed "time-split" cross-validation, which splits the training data into two parts by the time the experimental data were generated [27]. This is meant to simulate how a model would be used "in the field." A model that gives better performance under the time-split cross-validation will likely do well in predicting molecules in the (near) future. The other way of addressing the issue is to estimate how well a molecule not in the training data can be predicted by the model. This is called domain of applicability in the QSAR literature [28, 29]. This approach is usually implemented by modeling the prediction error of a molecule using information from its "neighbors," such as similarities to the neighbors, the prediction errors of the neighbors, and/or other model-derived metrics (e.g., standard deviation of predictions from the individual trees in an RF).

In addition to predictions, QSAR models can be used to generate hypotheses about structural changes in molecules that are influential to biological activity. Such knowledge can aid chemists in synthesizing new molecules with better properties. Even for "black box" methods such as RFs and boosting, we can get some hints from the models through variable importance measures and partial dependence functions [10]. Tree-based methods (including ensembles) using single variable split at each node can measure the importance of a variable by summing the decrease in the node impurity index due to splitting on that variable [12]. For other methods, a bootstrap procedure similar to RFs can be used: in each bootstrap iteration, the cases not included in the bootstrap sample (OOB data) can be treated as test set, and the prediction error (mean squared error, error rate, etc.) computed on them, say $E_i$ for the $i$th bootstrap iteration. Then for each variable in the OOB data, we randomly permute the values of that variable, and compute the prediction error on this modified data, say $\widetilde{E}_{ik}$ for the $k$th variable. Then the importance of the $k$th variable can be computed as

$$I_k = \frac{1}{B} \sum_{i=1}^{B} (\widetilde{E}_{ik} - E_i).$$

Note that $\widetilde{E}_{ik}$ is not necessarily larger than $E_i$, so the importance measures need not be strictly positive. Some authors truncate the values at 0. By randomly permuting the variable in the OOB data, the correlation between that variable and the response or any other variable is removed, while the marginal distribution of the variable is preserved. If the prediction error increases substantially after permuting a variable, then that variable should have an important contribution to the prediction accuracy of the model.

After determining which variables have high importance in the model, one would naturally want to know the nature of the relationship between these variables and the response. For methods that do not directly produce such relations, we can use partial dependence plots, proposed by Friedman [10]. Denote the QSAR model by $g(Y) = \widehat{f}(x)$, where $g$ is a link function, and $\mathbf{x}$ is the vector of descriptors. Let $\mathbf{x}_t$ be the set of descriptors for which we are interested in exploring the relationship with $Y$, and $\mathbf{x}_r$ be all other descriptors, so that $\mathbf{x} = \mathbf{x}_t \cup \mathbf{x}_r$, and we denote $\widehat{f}(\mathbf{x})$ as $\widehat{f}(\mathbf{x}_t, \mathbf{x}_r)$. The partial dependence function is defined as

$$p(\mathbf{x}_t) = \int \widehat{f}(\mathbf{x}_t, \mathbf{x}_r) h(\mathbf{x}_r) d\mathbf{x}_r,$$

where $h$ is the marginal density of $\mathbf{x}_r$. In finite samples, the function can be estimated as

$$\widehat{p}(\mathbf{x}_t) = \frac{1}{n} \sum_{i=1}^{n} \widehat{f}(\mathbf{x}_t, \mathbf{x}_{i, r}).$$

Such functions can be plotted as a graphical summary of the marginal effects of the important variables. If the descriptors can be mapped back onto molecules, then it may be possible to "color" the structures of molecules to see which part of the molecules have positive or negative influence on the biological activity.

## 3.5  Data example

One very important *in vitro* assay that is related to safety of putative therapeutic compounds is the one that measures molecules' interaction with the human ether-à-go-go related gene (hERG). This is important because blockade of hERG is related to the potentially lethal effect of QT interval elongation [30]. Su *et al.* collected data on 356 structurally diverse sets of molecules and their hERG activities from the literature [31]. Based on this (and other publicly available data), they built several QSAR models for predicting hERG activity from the structure of a molecule. In this section we will use this data set to demonstrate the QSAR model building process. A transcript of an R session that demonstrates the whole process from reading in the data to generating the performance output is provided in Appendix 3.A. Parts of the code make use of the caret package for R [32] which provides a unified framework for model building, tuning, and validation with a single interface to a large number of classification and regression methods available in various R packages.

From the molecular structures (provided as mol files in the supplementary material of [31]), we generated three sets of chemical descriptors: AP, ECFP4, and a set of 2D descriptors produced by the MOE software (MOE2D). There are 2488 AP descriptors, 2828 ECFP4 descriptors, and 165 MOE2D descriptors. We follow [31] in dividing the molecules into a set of 250 for training, and 106 for validation. For each descriptor type, we build both a regression model (predicting pIC50 of molecules) as well as a classification model (predicting whether the molecule is likely a hERG blocker, using 40 µM as cutoff). Figure 3.1 shows the distribution of the pIC50 values of the compounds in the two sets.

We build models using the two methods described earlier: RFs and stochastic GBMs. For RF, we also apply the descriptor deduction method described in [26]. For RF, we can use the built-in OOB estimate of prediction errors, while for GBM we use three repeats of fivefold cross-validation to find the optimal combination of tuning parameters. We fixed the interaction depth at 3, and varied the shrinkage factor among 0.01, 0.05, and 0.1, and the number of iterations (trees) among 150, 500, and 1000. Table 3.1 shows the estimated performance of the classification and regression models in the validation set. For RF with reduced descriptors

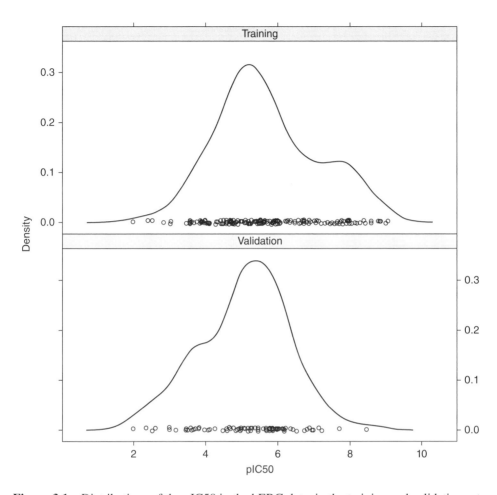

**Figure 3.1**    Distributions of the pIC50 in the hERG data, in the training and validation sets.

**Table 3.1**    Error rates (classification) and $Q^2$ (regression) of various QSAR models (SGB = stochastic gradient boosting).

| Method | Descriptor | Classification | Regression |
|--------|-----------|----------------|------------|
| RF | AP | 0.330 | 0.272 |
| RF | ECFP | 0.330 | 0.134 |
| RF | MOE2D | 0.208 | 0.258 |
| RF_sub | AP | 0.358 | 0.277 |
| RF_sub | ECFP | 0.302 | 0.163 |
| RF_sub | MOE2D | 0.198 | 0.279 |
| SGB | AP | 0.330 | 0.279 |
| SGB | ECFP | 0.311 | 0.000 |
| SGB | MOE2D | 0.198 | 0.295 |

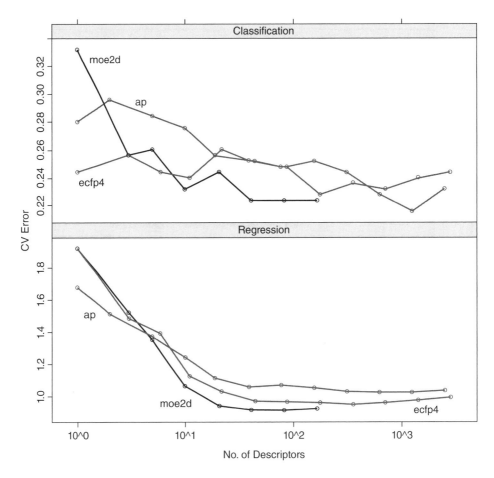

**Figure 3.2**  Cross-validated errors of random forests as the number of descriptors is reduced.

(AP and ECFP4 only), Figure 3.2 shows how the estimated prediction error changes as the number of descriptors is reduced.

Based on the best models, we can examine the most important descriptors responsible for the prediction performance. Chemists might be able to form hypotheses about molecular features that influence hERG activity from these important descriptors.

## 3.6   Discussion

We have described in this chapter how QSAR models are used in the drug discovery process. Such models are used routinely in screening or prioritizing candidate molecules, as well as helping chemists gain insight into how molecular features influence biological activities. We have described some potential challenges that may arise from the data available for building QSAR models. It is worth emphasizing that care must be taken to address these challenges, or else the usefulness of the models can be limited. It is conceivable that the entire model building and prediction process can be fully automated in a system, and it may be very tempting to do so. However, such an automated process rarely accounts for the potential challenges that exist in the data, and it may take some expert knowledge to understand the limitations of such a system.

It is also worth pointing out that one area where statistical principles and methods can have important impact is in improving repeatability and reproducibility of the assays. The smaller the experimental error, the more predictive the QSAR models based on such data can be.

# Appendix 3.A  Transcript of an R Session for the Model Building of the hERG Data

```
R version 3.0.2 (2013-09-25) - "Frisbee Sailing"
Copyright (C) 2013 The R Foundation for Statistical Computing
Platform: i386-w64-mingw32/i386 (32-bit)

[...]

> # Build various models to predict hERG activities, using data from
> # Su et al. JCIM v50, #3, 2010, containing 250 training
> # and 106 validation molecules culled from literature.
> ####################################################################
> setwd("c:/home/safety_chapter_QSAR")
>
> stopifnot(require(lattice))
Loading required package: lattice
> stopifnot(require(caret))
Loading required package: caret
Loading required package: cluster
Loading required package: foreach
Loading required package: plyr
Loading required package: reshape2
> stopifnot(require(gbm))
Loading required package: gbm
Loading required package: survival
Loading required package: splines
Loading required package: parallel
Loaded gbm 2.1
> stopifnot(require(randomForest))
Loading required package: randomForest
randomForest 4.6-7
Type rfNews() to see new features/changes/bug fixes.
>
> makeNewdata <- function (x, desList) {
+   n <- nrow(x)
+   p <- length(desList)
+   newx <- data.frame(matrix(0, n, p, dimnames = list(rownames(x),
+         desList)))
+   if (any(colnames(x) %in% desList)) {
+     des <- colnames(x)
+     des <- des[des %in% desList]
+     newx[, des] <- x[, des]
+   }
+   newx
```

```
+ }
>
> rsq <- function(y, pred) {
+   ssy <- sum((y - mean(y))^2)
+   sse <- sum((y - pred)^2)
+   1 - sse / ssy
+ }
> rmse <- function(y, pred) sqrt(mean((y - pred)^2))
>
> train.act <- read.csv("train.csv", header=TRUE,
  colClasses=c("NULL", "numeric"))
> train.act$blocker <- factor(train.act$pIC50 >= 5)
> valid.act <- read.csv("valid.csv", header=TRUE,
  colClasses=c("NULL", "numeric"))
> valid.act$blocker <- factor(valid.act$pIC50 >= 5)
>
> both.act <- cbind(Set=factor(rep(c("Training", "Validation"),
+     c(nrow(train.act), nrow(valid.act)))),
+   rbind(train.act, valid.act))
> ## Compare the distribution of pIC50 between the two sets.
> print(densityplot(~ pIC50 | Set, data=both.act, layout=c(1, 2),
  as.table=TRUE))
>
> desType <- c("ap", "ecfp4", "moe2d")
> names(desType) <- desType
> sets <- c("train", "valid")
> names(sets) <- sets
> desList <- lapply(desType, function(d) {
+     x <- lapply(sets, function(s) {
+       fn <- paste(s, d, sep=".")
+       dat <- read.table(fn, row=1, header=TRUE)
+       dat <- dat[order(as.numeric(row.names(dat))), ]
+     })
+   if (! all(names(x$train) == names(x$valid))) {
+     x$valid <- makeNewdata(x$valid, names(x$train))
+   }
+   sd0 <- which(apply(x$train, 2, sd) < 1e-7)
+   if (length(sd0) > 0) {
+     x$train <- x$train[-sd0]
+     x$valid <- x$valid[-sd0]
+   }
+   x
+ })
>
> set.seed(6432)
> rfList <- lapply(desList, function(des) {
+     randomForest(des$train, train.act$pIC50,
+       des$valid, valid.act$pIC50, importance=TRUE)
+   })
R> perf.regRF <- t(sapply(rfList, function(d) {
+     c(RMSE=sqrt(d$test$mse[500]), Rsq=d$test$rsq[500])
+   }))
R> print(round(perf.regRF, 3))
      RMSE    Rsq
ap 1.044 0.279
ecfp4 1.139 0.142
```

```
moe2d 1.049 0.272
>
> set.seed(6432)
> crfList <- lapply(desList, function(des) {
+    randomForest(des$train, train.act$blocker,
+      des$valid, valid.act$blocker,
+      importance=TRUE)
+    })
R> perf.clsRF <- sapply(crfList, function(d) d$test$err.rate[500, "Test"])
R> print(round(perf.clsRF, 3))
   ap.Test ecfp4.Test moe2d.Test
     0.311      0.311      0.189
>
> set.seed(6327)
> rfcvList <- lapply(desList, function(des) {
+    rfcv(des$train, train.act$pIC50)
+    })
>
> set.seed(6327)
> crfcvList <- lapply(desList, function(des) {
+    rfcv(des$train, train.act$blocker)
+    })
>
> reg.err <- lapply(rfcvList[1:3], function(x) as.data.frame(x[1:2]))
> nr <- sapply(reg.err, nrow)
> err1 <- cbind(do.call(rbind, reg.err), Descriptor=rep(names(reg.err), nr),
Model=rep("Regression", sum(nr)))
> cls.err <- lapply(crfcvList[1:3], function(x) as.data.frame(x[1:2]))
> nr <- sapply(cls.err, nrow)
> err2 <- cbind(do.call(rbind, cls.err), Descriptor=rep(names(cls.err), nr),
Model=rep("Classification", sum(nr)))
> err <- rbind(err1, err2)
> xyplot(error.cv ~ n.var | Model, groups=Descriptor, data=err, type="o",
+    lwd=2,scale=listlist,(relation="free"), x=list(log=TRUE)),
+    layout=c(1,2),auto.key=list(columns=3), xlab="No. of Descriptonrs",
+    ylab="CV Error")
>
> ## Best number of descriptors to keep for final RF models.
> ndesCls <- list(ap=622, ecfp4=1771, moe2d=41)
> ndesReg <- list(ap=311, ecfp4=354, moe2d=41)
>
> bestClsRF <- bestRegRF <- vector(mode="list", length=3)
> names(bestClsRF) <- names(bestRegRF) <- names(ndesReg)
>
> bestRF <- function(x, y, xtest, ytest, fullRF, nvar, ...) {
+  imp <- importance(fullRF, type=1)[, 1]
+  impord <- order(imp, decreasing=TRUE)[1:nvar]
+  bRF <- randomForest(x[impord], y, xtest[impord], ytest, ...)
+  bRF
+ }
>
> set.seed(1428)
> for (i in seq_along(ndesCls)) {
+  bestClsRF[[i]] <- bestRF(desList[[i]]$train, train.act$blocker,
+    desList[[i]]$valid, valid.act$blocker,
+    crfList[[i]], ndesCls[[i]])
```

```
+   bestRegRF[[i]] <- bestRF(desList[[i]]$train, train.act$pIC50,
+     desList[[i]]$valid, valid.act$pIC50,
+     rfList[[i]], ndesReg[[i]])
+ }
>
R> perf.clsRFCV <- sapply(bestClsRF,
+   function(d)d$test$err.rate[500, "Test"])
R> print(round(perf.clsRFCV, 3))
   ap.Test ecfp4.Test moe2d.Test
     0.340      0.321      0.226


R> perf.regRFCV <- t(sapply(bestRegRF, function(d) {
+       c(RMSE=sqrt(d$test$mse[500]), Rsq=d$test$rsq[500])
+       }))
R> print(round(perf.regRFCV, 3))
       RMSE    Rsq
ap     1.032 0.296
ecfp4  1.120 0.170
moe2d  1.069 0.245
>
> fitControl <- trainControl(method="repeatedcv", number=5, repeats=3)
> set.seed(4581)
> gbm.ap <- train(desList$ap$train, train.act$pIC50, method="gbm",
+   tuneGrid=expand.grid(.interaction.depth=2:4, .n.trees=c(500, 1000, 1500),
+   .shrinkage=c(.005,.01)),
+   trControl = fitControl, n.minobsinnode=3, verbose = FALSE)
There were 50 or more warnings (use warnings() to see the first 50)
>
> set.seed(4581)
> gbm.ecfp <- train(desList$ecfp4$train, train.act$pIC50, method="gbm",
+   tuneGrid=expand.grid(.interaction.depth=2:4, .n.trees=c(500, 1000, 1500),
+   .shrinkage=.01),
+   trControl = fitControl, n.minobsinnode=3, verbose = FALSE)
There were 50 or more warnings (use warnings() to see the first 50)
>
> set.seed(4581)
> gbm.moe <- train(desList$moe2d$train, train.act$pIC50, method="gbm",
+   .shrinkage=c(.005, .01, .05)),
+   tuneGrid=expand.grid(.interaction.depth=3:4, .n.trees=c(200, 500, 1000),
+   trControl = fitControl, n.minobsinnode=3, verbose = FALSE)
There were 24 warnings (use warnings() to see them)
>
> rsq.gbm <- c(AP=rsq(valid.act$pIC50, predict(gbm.ap$finalModel,
+ desList$ap$valid, n.trees=1500)),
+  ECFP4=rsq(valid.act$pIC50, predict(gbm.ecfp$finalModel,
+ desList$ecfp4$valid, n.trees=1500)),
+  MOE2D=rsq(valid.act$pIC50, predict(gbm.moe$finalModel,
+ desList$moe2d$valid, n.trees=1000)))
> rmse.gbm <- c(AP=rmse(valid.act$pIC50, predict(gbm.ap$finalModel,
+ desList$ap$valid, n.trees=1500)),
+  ECFP4=rmse(valid.act$pIC50, predict(gbm.ecfp$finalModel,
+ desList$ecfp4$valid, n.trees=1500)),
+  MOE2D=rmse(valid.act$pIC50, predict(gbm.moe$finalModel,
+ desList$moe2d$valid, n.trees=1000)))
> print(round(rsq.gbm, 3))
    AP   ECFP4   MOE2D
```

```
  0.277 -0.002   0.294
> print(round(rmse.gbm, 3))
   AP ECFP4 MOE2D
1.043 1.228 1.031
>
> set.seed(4581)
> clsgbm.ap <- train(desList$ap$train, train.act$blocker, method="gbm",
+    tuneGrid=expand.grid(.interaction.depth=2:4, .n.trees=c(500, 1000, 1500),
+    .shrinkage=c(.005, .01)),
+    trControl = fitControl, n.minobsinnode=3, verbose = FALSE)
Loading required package: class
There were 50 or more warnings (use warnings() to see the first 50)
>
> set.seed(4581)
> clsgbm.ecfp <- train(desList$ecfp4$train, train.act$blocker, method="gbm",
+    tuneGrid=expand.grid(.interaction.depth=2:4, .n.trees=c(500, 1000, 1500),
+    .shrinkage=c(.005, .01)),
+    trControl = fitControl, n.minobsinnode=3, verbose = FALSE)
>
>
> set.seed(4581)
> clsgbm.moe <- train(desList$moe2d$train, train.act$blocker, method="gbm",
+    tuneGrid=expand.grid(.interaction.depth=2:4, .n.trees=c(200, 500, 1000),
+    .shrinkage=c(.005, .01)),
+    trControl = fitControl, n.minobsinnode=3, verbose = FALSE)
>
> errRate.gbm <- c(AP=mean(valid.act$blocker != predict(clsgbm.ap,
+  desList$ap$valid)),ECFP4=mean(valid.act$blocker != predict(clsgbm.ecfp,
+  desList$ecfp4$valid)),
+  MOE2D=mean(valid.act$blocker != predict(clsgbm.moe, desList$moe2d$valid)))
> print(round(errRate.gbm, 3))
   AP ECFP4 MOE2D
0.321 0.311 0.198
```

# References

[1] Patterson, D.E., Cramer, R.D., Ferguson, A.M. *et al.* (1996) Neighborhood behavior: a useful concept for validation of "molecular diversity" descriptors. *Journal of Medicinal Chemistry*, **39**, 3049–3059.

[2] Dimova, D., Heikamp, K., Stumpfe, D. and Bajorath, J. (2013) Do medicinal chemists learn from activity cliffs? A systematic evaluation of cliff progression in evolving compound data sets. *Journal of Medicinal Chemistry*, **56**, 3339–3345.

[3] Todeschini, R. and Consonni, V. (2009) *Molecular Descriptors for Chemoinformatics*, John Wiley & Sons, Inc., Hoboken, NJ.

[4] Carhart, R.E., Smith, D.H. and Venkataraghavan, R. (1985) Atom pairs as molecular features in structure-activity studies: definition and applications. *Journal of Chemical Information and Computer Sciences*, **25**, 64–73.

[5] Rogers, D. and Hahn, M. (2010) Extended-connectivity fingerprints. *Journal of Chemical Information and Modeling*, **50**, 742–754.

[6] Brown, R.D. and Martin, Y.C. (1997) **The information content** of 2D and 2D structural descriptors relevant to ligand-receptor binding. *Journal of Chemical Information and Computer Sciences*, **37**, 1–9.

[7] Helgee, E.A., Carlsson, L., Boyer, S. and Norinder, U. (2010) Evaluation of quantitative structure-activity relationship modeling strategies: local and global models. *Journal of Chemical Information and Modeling*, **50**, 677–689.

[8] Yee, L.C. and Wei, Y.C. (2012) Current modeling methods used in QSAR/QSPR, in *Statistical Modeling of Molecular Descriptors in QSAR/QSPR* (eds M. Dehmer, K. Varmuza and D. Bonchev), Wiley-VCH Verlag, Weinheim, Germany.

[9] Breiman, L. (2001) Random forests. *Machine Learning*, **45**, 5–32.

[10] Friedman, J. (2001) Greedy function approximation: a gradient boosting machine. *Annals of Statistics*, **29**, 1189–1232.

[11] Friedman, J.H. (2002) Stochastic gradient boosting. *Computational Statistics and Data Analysis*, **38**, 367–378.

[12] Breiman, L., Friedman, J., Stone, C.J. and Olshen, R.A. (1984) *Classification and Regression Trees*, Wadsworth, Belmont, CA.

[13] Hothorn, T., Lausen, B., Benner, A. and Radespiel-Troeger, M. (2004) Bagging survival trees. *Statistics in Medicine*, **23**, 77–91.

[14] Hothorn, T., Hornik, K. and Zeileis, A. (2006) Unbiased recursive partitioning: a conditional inference framework. *Journal of Computational and Graphical Statistics*, **15**, 651–674.

[15] Hothorn, L.A. (2006) Multiple comparisons and multiple contrasts in randomized dose–response trials – confidence interval oriented approaches. *Journal of Biopharmaceutical Statistics*, **16**, 711–731.

[16] Strobl, C., Malley, J. and Tutz, G. (2009) An introduction to recursive partitioning: rationale, application, and characteristics of classification and regression trees, bagging, and random forests. *Psychological Methods*, **14**, 323–348.

[17] Chipman, H., George, E.I. and McCulloch, R.E. (2010) BART: Bayesian additive regression trees. *Annals of Applied Statistics*, **4**, 266–298.

[18] Svetnik, V., Want, T., Tong, C. *et al.* (2005) Boosting: an ensemble learning tool for compound classification and QSAR modeling. *Journal of Chemical Information and Modeling*, **45**, 786–799.

[19] Freund, Y. and Shapire, R. Experiments with a new boosting algorithm, *Machine Learning: Proceedings of the 13th International Conference* (ICML '96), Bari, Italy, 1996, pp. 148–156, Morgan Kaufmann, San Francisco (1996).

[20] Freund, Y. (1995) Boosting a weak learning algorithm by majority. *Information and Computation*, **121**, 256–285.

[21] Ridgeway, G. (2013) gbm: Generalized Boosted Regression Models, http://CRAN.R-project.org/package=gbm (accessed 25 June 2014).

[22] Hastie, T., Tibshirani, R. and Friedman, J.H. (2009) *The Elements of Statistical Learning: Data Mining, Inference, and Prediction*, 2nd edn, Springer, New York.

[23] Truchon, J.-F. and Bayly, C.I. (2007) Evaluating virtual screening methods: good and bad metrics for the "early recognition" problem. *Journal of Chemical Information and Modeling*, **47**, 488–508.

[24] Leisch, F., Zeileis, A. and Hornik, K. (2005) The design and analysis of benchmark experiments. *Journal of Computational and Graphical Statistics*, **14**, 675–699.

[25] Ambroise, C. and McLachlan, G.J. (2002) Selection bias in gene extraction on the basis of microarray gene-expression data. *Proceedings of the National Academy of Sciences of the USA*, **99**, 6562–6566.

[26] Svetnik, V., Liaw, A., Tong, C. and Wang, T. (2004) Application of Breiman's random forest to modeling structure-activity relationships of pharmaceutical molecules, in *Multiple Classifier Systems* (eds F. Roli, J. Kittler and T. Windeatt), Springer-Verlag, Berlin.

[27] Sheridan, R.P. (2013) Time-split cross-validation as a method for estimating the goodness of prospective prediction. *Journal of Chemical Information and Modeling*, **53**, 783–790.

[28] Keefer, C.E., Kauffman, G.W. and Gupta, R.R. (2013) Interpretable, probability-based confidence metric for continuous quantitative structure activity relationship models. *Journal of Chemical Information and Modeling*, **53**, 368–383.

[29] Sheridan, R.P. (2012) Three useful dimensions for domain applicability in QSAR models using random forest. *Journal of Chemical Information and Modeling*, **52**, 814–823.

[30] Jamieson, C., Moir, E.M., Rankovic, Z. and Wishart, G. (2006) Medicinal chemistry of hERG optimizations: highlights and hang-ups. *Journal of Medicinal Chemistry*, **49**, 5029–5046.

[31] Su, B.H., Shen, M.Y., Esposito, E.X. *et al.* (2010) In silico binary classification QSAR models based on 4D-fingerprints and MOE descriptors for prediction of hERG blockage. *Journal of Chemical Information and Modeling*, **50**, 1304–1318.

[32] Kuhn, M. (2013) caret: Classification and Regression Training http://CRAN.R-project.org/package=caret (accessed 25 July 2014).

# 4

# Ethical and practical issues in phase 1 trials in healthy volunteers

## Stephen Senn

*Competence Center for Methodology and Statistics, Strassen, Luxembourg*

## 4.1 Introduction

On 13 March 2006 eight healthy male volunteers entered the first phase of a 'first-in-man' study, TGN1412-HV, designed to test the safety of TGN1412, a monoclonal antibody produced by the company TeGenero. Six were allocated to active treatment and two to placebo. Well before the end of that day all doubt regarding the safety of TGN1412 had been resolved: all six young men who had been given it were showing the symptoms of an acute reaction to the product and were, in fact, suffering from what is sometimes referred to as a *cytokine storm*. By 16 hours after the start of the trial all six were in intensive care and two were close to death [1].

Six years later, Thomas Hünig, one of the founders of TeGenero, published an article with the title 'The storm has cleared: lessons from the CD28 superagonist TGN1412 trial' [2]. The title was unfortunate since at least one of the six young men treated with TGN1412, Ryan Wilson, has been permanently partially disabled as a result of his experiences, having suffered multiple amputations to toes and tips of fingers. For him the storm might have cleared but the effects have not.

---

*Statistical Methods for Evaluating Safety in Medical Product Development*, First Edition.
Edited by A. Lawrence Gould.
© 2015 John Wiley & Sons, Ltd. Published 2015 by John Wiley & Sons, Ltd.

Hünig's paper makes many interesting points regarding biology, specifically immunology and also as regards setting safe doses using animal studies and *in vitro* studies, and suggests that many important lessons have been learned. Nowhere, however, does he discuss the lessons learned or that should have been learned about trial design. It is issues with the design and (since a good design must always have the end in sight) analysis of such trials that form the basis of this chapter. Although this chapter is not just about the TGN1412-HV trial, the trial is a useful one to use to make many points of relevance to first-in-man studies generally. Furthermore, the catastrophic events of March 2006 had such an effect on thinking as regards first-in-man studies (even if all the lessons were not learned) that it marks the beginning of an era. We live in the post-TGN1412 era just as drug regulation from the mid-1960s onwards has been part of the post-thalidomide era. For example, the European Medicines Agency (EMA) introduced regulations in the wake of the TGN1412-HV trial to cover first-in-man studies [3]. Therefore, since it is impossible now to write about first-in-man studies without having the TGN1412-HV trial in mind, the design and other features of that trial will be referred to frequently.

Much of the material in this chapter is not original, being largely based on the report [4] of the Royal Statistical Society (RSS) Working Party (of which this author was the chair) that was set up to consider what advice statistics and statisticians could give regarding the future design of first-in-man studies. (However, some further discussion and analysis is given based on subsequent research.) Although this working party included a clinician and a leading immunologist, it consisted mainly of statisticians and, as might be expected from its remit, it concentrated mainly on statistical issues: probabilistic assessment of risk, communication of risk, design of trials and analysis of results. This emphasis was justified because at the same time an official working party was reporting to the UK government, led by the distinguished pharmacologist Professor Gordon (later Sir Gordon) Duff, but did *not* include any statisticians [5]. Therefore, in the sections that follow, we will consider the lessons from a statistical point of view. Before doing so, however, we turn to consider one issue that cannot be ignored, ethics, although even this, as we shall see, has its statistical aspect.

The details that follow will be clearer and more insightful if the overall message of this chapter is kept in mind: that careful planning is necessary for first-in-man studies and that planning is not possible without calculation. Without calculation risks cannot be assessed, and without assessment of risk there can be no informed consent.

## 4.2   Ethical basics

Unpleasant as it may seem, there is no escaping the fact that first-in-man trials in healthy volunteers involve payment for risk. It seems that there must be some acceptable level of risk both for society and for individuals participating in such trials, since, if an acceptable level did not exist, then in the one case they would always be declared illegal and in the other they would fail to recruit any subjects anyway. As was pointed out in the RSS report, the individual and societal perspectives on risk are not necessarily the same [4]. In fact, one can make the following relevant and useful distinction when talking about risk. On the one hand one can consider the risk to an individual in entering a trial of a given design, and on the other one can consider the expected risk (perhaps in the number of serious side-effects) for a given design [6–8]. A concrete example may make this clear.

Suppose we have a treatment for which, based on our best calculation, we consider that the risk of a serious side-effect is 1 in a 1000 prior to any information gained from actual testing in humans. In other words, this is a risk that we consider would apply to the first person taking the experimental treatment. However, an acceptable risk to anyone taking the medicine was judged to be 1 in 5000. It thus follows that the risk of taking this medicine is unacceptable. Now suppose we run a trial in which we have four subjects allocated to placebo and one to the treatment. The estimated risk of a side-effect from the medicine for any individual entering such a trial is now $\frac{1}{5} \times \frac{1}{1000} = \frac{1}{5000}$ and thus, from one point of view, acceptable given the supposed standards.

However, most will surely consider that such a device for diluting risk is unacceptable. The question then is why. One explanation is that it will not reduce the expected number of side-effects [4, 6–8]. If we assume that the trial is devised in such a way that it can be stopped at no risk to any further individuals if one suffers a side-effect (which was not the case for TGN1412-HV) then the expected number of side-effects for the trial is $5 \times \frac{1}{5000} = \frac{1}{1000}$ and thus unchanged. Hence this device does not reduce the expected number of injuries and hence the societal risk. Of course, if one were to take an extreme market point of view one might say that this does not matter since (presumably) the total amount of money spent in recruiting healthy volunteers would be five times what it would otherwise be and this would mean that the exchange of money for risk was acceptable.

Nevertheless, it suffices to show that consideration from the point of view of various parties (volunteers, insurers, society and so forth) may be necessary, as well as careful calculation. The relevance to the TGN1412 example is that the way the trial was designed meant that simultaneous occurrence of serious side-effects was possible (in fact, single occurrences of serious side-effects were unlikely) and therefore any calculations of consequences needed to take this into account. The fact that the calculations did not take this into account is shown by the fact that insurance cover for the trial was not sufficient to deal with the six claims for compensation that followed. This point will be returned to later. However, the more general issue is that although ethics is not *just* a matter of calculation it is *also* a matter of calculation.

## 4.3   Inferential matters

It is not possible to design a trial reasonably without having some idea of the eventual analysis in mind. However, the case of TGN1412-HV raises an important distinction: that between the analysis envisaged and that actually carried out. Of course, in an ideal world all possible eventualities would be envisaged, however unlikely, each having been assigned a probability of occurrence and each having a possible inference associated with it. Assignment of a value to each inference would then make possible a comparison of all possible designs, and if their costs could be taken into account also, this fully Bayesian approach would lead to a truly optimal design.

In practice this seems to be impossible, and it is perhaps useful for the moment to retain a distinction between normal 'contractual' analysis and *force majeure*: what happens when, as was the case with TGN1412-HV, unforeseen and dramatic events require a revision of all plans. In fact first-in-man studies are *not* designed to observe the effects of life-threatening doses. They would never receive ethical approval if that were the case. The issue of normal

**Table 4.1**  Subjects cross-classified by treatment given and result.

| Treatment | Yes | No | Total |
|-----------|-----|-----|-------|
| TGN1412   | 6   | 0   | 6     |
| Placebo   | 0   | 2   | 2     |
| Total     | 6   | 2   | 8     |

'contractual' design and analysis will be covered later in the chapter. For the moment we consider the issue of the analysis of the serious side-effects observed in TGN1412-HV.

## 4.3.1  Analysis of serious side-effects

The first point to note is that a conventional frequentist analysis is clearly inappropriate. We can represent the results as in Table 4.1. A conventional analysis of these results using Fisher's exact test [9] does not result in a very impressive $P$-value. We have here the most extreme table possible, given the marginal totals of 6 and 2 and 6 and 2, and the probability of this from the hypergeometric distribution is $P = 0.036$ (to two significant figures). Whether or not one chooses to double this (as in a two-tailed test), it is clear that this does not begin to do justice to the evidence provided by the trial, and using alternatives to the Fisher exact test (about whose propriety one might argue), such as Barnard's test [10] (which produces a $P$-value of 0.011), makes only a cosmetic difference to the result.

   If we stop to consider *why*, then it is clear that there are at least two sources of information that any such analysis fails to take into account. First, there is the information on rarity of cytokine storms. It is not impossible for otherwise healthy young men to suffer these, and it has been speculated that the high mortality in the 1918–1919 influenza epidemic was caused by excessive immune reactions resulting in a cytokine storm [11]. Nevertheless it is clear that such events are extremely rare. The sort of analysis conventionally carried out on such tables is appropriate (if at all) in circumstances in which we have little or no information about the rate of side-effects. As already, mentioned, such trials are expected to stop at a dose at which non-serious and at most unpleasant or perhaps only discomforting side-effects such as dry mouth might occur. In such a case we might hesitate to nominate some sort of upper bound for the probability of such an event in particular because we may fear a nocebo effect (a noxious placebo reaction) [12–14]. In other words, it is unsafe to use external information and this, indeed, is the reason why subjects given placebo are treated concurrently.

## 4.3.2  Timing of events

The second sort of information is timing. The side-effects followed swiftly on dose administration and very similar time courses were observed. There has been increased interest in recent years in using data on timing of events to establish causality. For example, Farrington and Whitaker have developed the case-series methodology to use the histories of individuals in terms of both exposure and side-effect as a means of examining the causal role (or otherwise) of treatments [15, 16]. Here again such formal analysis is not needed because the events are so dramatic, but it shows that there is not necessarily a conflict between formal and informal inference.

## 4.4    Design for subject safety

### 4.4.1    Dosing interval

A key recommendation of the RSS report was that a so-called *proper interval* should be established for administering individual treatments [4]. Of course, all such studies are run as dose escalations. That is to say, higher doses are not administered until lower doses have been examined and some interval between doses is observed, partly for administrative necessity (including the need to evaluate results at the lower dose) and sometimes because late consequences of lower doses are considered possible. However, it is also quite common, as was the case with TGN1412-HV, to have doses given by 'cohort'. The protocol for TGN1412-HV mentioned that there would be an interval of at least 14 days before treating the next cohort with a higher dose. The question is, however, what interval is to be observed between dosing members of a given dose cohort. This in fact is a critical question.

In fact, in TGN1412-HV subjects were not dosed simultaneously but at intervals of 10 minutes according to the schedule in Table 4.2. (Note that the reason each subject is not given the same dose of TGN1412 is that the dosing was by body weight at a ratio of 0.1 mg/kg [17].) However, clearly this interval was insufficient to take any action as regards dosing of volunteers to be treated later but as part of the same cohort based on information gained from those treated earlier. The design was vulnerable to what is referred to in the literature on reliability as 'common mode' or 'common cause' failure [18]. In the discussion that follows the minor interval of 10 minutes will be ignored as irrelevant to any consideration of safety, since this is essentially for administrative purposes, and the scheme will be referred to as *contemporary dosing*.

### 4.4.2    Contemporary dosing

In fact the RSS report did not say that contemporary dosing would never be acceptable. Instead the point of view was taken that the issue was one that had to be explicitly addressed in a risk assessment document. There would be some cases, for example where a great deal might be known about the general class of drug to which the new molecule belonged, where first-in-man studies had less uncertainty attached to them. It was, however, the point of view of the RSS report that such contemporary dosing was inappropriate for TGN1412-HV. Of course, hindsight is an exact science. It is one thing to identify a risk once catastrophic events have taken place but quite another to predict it. Nevertheless, it is clear that the trial design fails by other

**Table 4.2**   Dosing schedule for the TGN1412-HV trial.

| A | TGN1412 | 8.4 mg | 08:00 | 16 h |
|---|---|---|---|---|
| B | Placebo | – | 08:10 | – |
| C | TGN1412 | 6.8 mg | 08:20 | 15 h 30 min |
| D | TGN1412 | 8.8 mg | 08:30 | 16 h |
| E | TGN1412 | 8.2 mg | 08:40 | 12 h |
| F | TGN1412 | 7.2 mg | 08:50 | 16 h |
| G | TGN1412 | 8.2 mg | 09:00 | 16 h |
| H | Placebo | – | 09:10 | – |

Based on the table in the RSS report.

features of the protocol. Section 10.2 on p. 52 of the protocol [17] states: 'In accordance with Article 3 of Directive 2001/20/EC (The Protection of Clinical Trials Subjects) [19], a clinical trial may be only undertaken if provision has been made to cover the liability of the investigator and sponsor.'

Furthermore, the informed consent form for the healthy volunteers (Parexel International, unpublished, 2006) also covered compensations, stating: 'Compensation will be paid to you without you having to prove either that the injury arose through negligence or that the product was defective in the sense that it did not fulfil a reasonable expectation of safety', and later 'Payment will be made as soon as is practicable'.

However, one of the problems in the aftermath of the trial was that the sponsoring company, TeGenero, declared bankruptcy but the insurance cover was not enough to cover the claims then being made. (Eventually some of the claims were settled by Parexel.) Thus, one could argue that since the possible risk was not covered by the design, the design and the level of insurance were incompatible. Promises were being made which could not be guaranteed to be kept in view of the design chosen.

## 4.5   Analysis

### 4.5.1   Objectives of first-in-man trials

So far the steps that need to be taken to minimize risk to subject have been stressed. However, as has already been explained, first-in-man trials are not designed to establish toxic doses, or at least are not expected to administer and hence to observe the effects of toxic doses. They are meant to establish *tolerable* doses – doses that can be administered to humans without their suffering inacceptable discomfort. That being so, the design chosen has to be capable of delivering useful information when, as should nearly always be the case, things do *not* go wrong.

Paragraph 2 of Article 3 of the EMA Clinical Trials Directive states quite clearly: 'A clinical trial may be undertaken only if, in particular (a) [t]he foreseeable risks and inconveniences have been weighed against the anticipated benefit for the individual trial subject and other present and future patients' [19].

Obviously, apart from the payment they receive, healthy volunteers do not benefit from the participation in the trial. However, the benefit to *future* patients is clearly something that must be considered, and such benefit is maximized by good design and analysis. In this section appropriate analysis under normal 'contractual' conditions is considered.

### 4.5.2   (In)adequacy of statistical analysis plans

Before proceeding to consider these issues, however, it is useful to consider the statement on analysis in the protocol. In any Phase 3 trial this would be a section that was several pages long or, if not, several paragraphs long, to which, prior to the unblinding of the trial, several pages would be added in the form of a statistical analysis plan. However, here the statement runs to exactly 12 lines, four of which state who will do the analysis using what software. The nearest approximation to a formal analysis of any sort that it is envisaged is covered by two sentences as follows: 'Statistical tests (ANCOVA) will be performed on a purely descriptive level. No adjustment for multiple testing will take place.' This is clearly quite inadequate. It would be a mistake, however, to suppose that the trial protocol for TGN1412-HV was lax by the standards of what was commonly done in first-in-man studies. On the contrary, many such studies contain similarly inadequate statistical statements. Unfortunately a common prejudice in drug development is that if the design is deficient by the standards that would apply in Phase 3, for example by not being randomized in a classic manner or by having few subjects, then formal statistical analysis is inappropriate.

### 4.5.3 'Formal' statistical analyses

This point of view is quite illogical. It would imply that where data are subject to many possible sources of bias and complications, intuition, unaided by formal analysis, would come to a reasonable conclusion. On the other hand, for well-designed large studies, such intuition would be unreliable and only statistical analysis would do. This is simply ridiculous. The price for complexity is complex modelling, and the fact that such clinical trial protocols commonly contain such statements does not mean that this is all that is appropriate. It simply means that the authors do not know what is appropriate and hence that the design as a whole is inadequate, since for a design to be adequate one must know that it is capable of yielding useful information, and this in turn must mean that one knows how the data that arise will be analysed.

Perhaps part of the error being made here is to assume that because a formal conventional statistical analysis is unlikely to produce a significant result, it is irrelevant. However, the fact that conventional statistical significance is inappropriate does not mean that statistical analysis is inappropriate. It may be that the conventional approach of looking for efficient unbiased estimates has to be replaced by one in which mean square error is minimized instead (in other words, where some sort of bias–variance trade-off is considered). However, some sort of rule or procedure for deciding whether the trial may proceed to the next dose step and what the finally established dose is will surely be appropriate.

In the closely related field of dose-finding for cytotoxic drugs in cancer (where, however, it is patients, not healthy volunteers, that are recruited) there is a huge literature on algorithmic approaches to dose-finding with, since the key paper by O'Quigley et al. [20], an increasing emphasis on formal properties of schemes chosen. It is surely the case that healthy volunteer studies also would benefit if protocols established firm rules as to how data will be analysed and what decisions are foreseen even if cases of force majeure have to be allowed for.

## 4.6   Design for analysis

In this section some issues regarding design will be considered. The coverage is not comprehensive, but it is simply meant to give an example of the sort of issues that could be addressed in constructing a design and therefore also in making statements about eventual analysis.

### 4.6.1   Treatment assignments and the role of placebo

A key feature of designs such as that chosen for TGN1412-HV is that placebo is used as a control but that the randomization per dose-escalation is unequal, with more subjects being given the active treatment. The trial protocol envisaged up to four doses, namely 0.1, 0.5, 2 and 5 mg per kilogram of body weight, with eight subjects per dose group in an unequal randomization of six given TGN1412 and two given placebo.

An argument that is often given in favour of the unequal randomization is that by the end of the trial one will have more patients under placebo than under any given dose. For example, if all four doses had completed in TGN141-HV there would have been eight subjects under placebo but only six for each dose. There are, however, at least three objections to this. The first is that the trial may, in fact, not proceed to study all doses. This was, indeed, the case for TGN1412-HV. One could reply that under the circumstances this is irrelevant since, given the results seen, one is in no need of the placebo subjects to come to a conclusion. However, the trial could have reached a situation where (say) one or two subjects given TGN1412 had had very mild possible side-effects of the sort that could easily be seen under placebo. In that case it might have been useful to have more subjects treated under placebo.

The second problem is related to the first. The trial has to serve the objective of providing not only useful information if it completes but also useful information at each stage as to whether it should complete. Potential placebo subjects in future cohorts are of no use in making such decisions.

The third problem is that pooling placebo subjects in this way breaks concurrent control. Some secular trend might be operating and, even if not, comparisons across groups would not be completely blind. For example, if the trial runs to completion, although subjects will *not* know whether they are on the highest dose or placebo they *will* know that they are not on any of the lower doses. Such trials, in which partial knowledge as to the identity of some of the treatments being compared is available, have been referred to as *veiled* [21] and have particular problems of analysis [8]. The efficient analysis, which would pool all subjects given placebo, would not be unbiased, and the unbiased analysis, which would only compare a given dose to the truly concurrent placebo subjects, would not be efficient.

## 4.6.2   Dose-escalation trial design issues

The RSS report specifically considers possible designs for efficiently comparing different doses with each other and placebo where a dose-escalation approach is necessary. Rosemary Bailey, a member of the working party and a co-author of the report, later returned to the particular issues of design in some detail in a paper in *Statistics in Medicine* [22], which will now be considered.

Bailey considers a linear model, such as might be appropriate for analysing effects on some continuous tolerability indicator (perhaps suitably transformed) such as QT interval, liver-enzyme levels or blood pressure, and two possible approaches to analysis, one in which a cohort effect *is not* eliminated and one in which it *is*. Such a distinction was also discussed by Senn in Chapter 20, 'Dose Finding', of *Statistical Issues in Drug Development* [23, 24].

Bailey proposes a set of designs for dose-finding and considers their efficiency for these two cases (cohort effect not eliminated and cohort effect eliminated). The designs are indexed by the number of doses to be compared and the number of cohorts. If the number of cohorts equals the number of doses, the designs are called *standard*. If there is one more cohort than the number of doses, the design is called *extended*. There are very many designs in her paper and the reader is recommended to study the paper for more details. Here, just two designs will be considered, since they serve to make a point. In the discussion that follows, it will be assumed that the cohort effect *is* eliminated.

The first is given in Table 4.3 where the numbers of subjects allocated to placebo and various doses are shown. (It is assumed that the dose 4 is higher than dose 3 which is higher than dose 2 which is higher than dose 1.) This illustrates an ethical freedom that dose-escalation

**Table 4.3**   Dose-escalation design 1e considered by Bailey [22].

| Cohort | Placebo | Dose | | | |
|---|---|---|---|---|---|
| | | 1 | 2 | 3 | 4 |
| 1 | 5 | 5 | 0 | 0 | 0 |
| 2 | 3 | 2 | 5 | 0 | 0 |
| 3 | 1 | 1 | 3 | 5 | 0 |
| 4 | 1 | 1 | 1 | 2 | 5 |
| 5 | 0 | 1 | 1 | 3 | 5 |

This design compares four doses to placebo using either four or five cohorts. The numbers in the table show the numbers of subjects allocated to each treatment in each cohort. The fifth cohort would only be used if a so-called extended design were considered.

**Table 4.4**   A simple dose-escalation design proposed by Senn.

| Cohort | Placebo | Dose | | | |
|---|---|---|---|---|---|
| | | 1 | 2 | 3 | 4 |
| 1 | 5 | 5 | 0 | 0 | 0 |
| 2 | 5 | 0 | 5 | 0 | 0 |
| 3 | 5 | 0 | 0 | 5 | 0 |
| 4 | 5 | 0 | 0 | 0 | 5 |

The numbers in the table show the numbers of subjects allocated to each treatment in each cohort.

designs allow, which Bailey exploits. Although one is *not* permitted to study higher doses until lower ones have been studied, it *is* possible to continue to study lower doses. This is shown in the design in Table 4.3 (design 1e in Bailey's paper) [22]. Here, one continues to study lower doses as one proceeds through the cohorts. If the design is *standard,* only four cohorts are used. If it is extended, a fifth is added. In what follows, only the standard design will be considered.

The standard design will use 10 subjects per cohort in 4 cohorts, and so 40 subjects in total. The design may be compared to one recommended by Senn [23, 24] (although he is very unlikely to have been the first to do so), which is given in Table 4.4.

If the design proposed by Senn proceeds to completion, then each dose contrast comparing the dose to placebo will have a variance proportional to $\frac{1}{5} + \frac{1}{5} = \frac{2}{5} = 0.4$, which (trivially) has an average of 0.4. However, for Bailey's design it can be calculated that the variances for the four dose-contrasts will be (approximately) 0.21, 0.27, 0.38, 0.53, which, with the exception of the last, are lower than the variances for Senn's design. In fact, the average variance for the contrast to placebo for this design is 0.35, and so is lower.

Furthermore, the design will be much better for the purpose of comparing doses to each other. For instance, for the Senn design the variances of contrasts comparing any two doses are simply twice the variances of the contrasts to placebo, since each dose contrast must be

**Table 4.5**   Variances of dose contrasts for Bailey's design 1e.

| Dose | D1 | D2 | D3 | D4 |
|------|------|------|------|------|
| D1 | **0.21** | | | |
| D2 | 0.29 | **0.27** | | |
| D3 | 0.39 | 0.32 | **0.38** | |
| D4 | 0.54 | 0.52 | 0.50 | **0.53** |

The figures in bold on the diagonal are the variances of the contrast to placebo. The off-diagonal figures in light type are the contrasts between doses as indexed by rows and columns.

calculated as the difference of two independent contrasts to placebo. Thus the variances are all equal to $0.4 + 0.4 = 0.8$. However, for Bailey's design 1e the variances are as given in Table 4.5 and it can be seen that these are all appreciably less 0.8. Thus most variances for this design are less than the corresponding variances for Senn's design with the exception of the variance of the contrast for the highest dose compared to placebo.

## 4.6.3   Precision at interim stages

However, as Senn pointed out, there is a practical problem with this design [25] and, indeed, with all others proposed by Bailey. In operating dose-escalation studies, the dose information obtained at the end of each cohort has to be used to guide the decision on whether to continue or not. For this purpose it is *not* the variance of a contrast at the end of a fully completed design that is relevant. It is the variance at the end of each escalation step. The variances of the contrasts to placebo are just the same for the Senn design at the end of the trial as they are once the corresponding stage of escalation has been reached. (See Appendix 4.A.) However, for the design proposed by Bailey, this is not the case. The variances are, in general, higher. The situation is illustrated in Figure 4.1.

Figure 4.1 displays the variances on the *Y*-axis and escalations step (or cohort) on the *X*-axis. Here the variance at the end of each escalation step for the Senn design is always proportional to 0.4 and this is shown as a horizontal line. The dashed lines labelled D1–D4 show the evolution over time of the contrasts for the Bailey design. The points labelled F (for final) are what the variances will be proportional to if the design completes. The point labelled R (for real time) show the variances at the point when a decision has to be made to continue. The solid black line joins the variances for each dose contrast at the point at which the decision has to be made to proceed to the next dose or not. It will be seen that except for the first dose and cohort (for which there is no distinction in numbers between the Bailey and Senn designs) this variance is higher for the Bailey design. So for this purpose, the design is never better and usually worse than the Senn design. Table 4.6 provides the variance multiplier for contrasts of four doses relative to placebo as a function of the dose and when the trial stops.

The main message here is not that any particular given design should be recommended rather than any other, but instead that there are many choices to be made and that this is a matter that should be given serious thought in view of the analysis intended and vice versa. Most trial protocols pre TGN1412-HV were woefully inadequate in this respect, and one fears that the situation has scarcely improved. This is an area in which careful thought on the part of statisticians and their colleagues is called for.

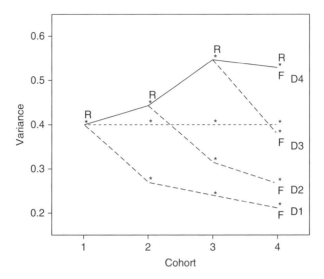

**Figure 4.1** Variance multipliers for contrasts of four doses, D1–D4, compared to placebo Senn and a design of Bailey's (standard case). Dotted line Senn design; dashed lines Bailey design; F, the variances that will be seen if the design runs to completion, and R, the value that will be seen at the point a decision to escalate is taken. The solid black line joins the values of R for Bailey's design.

**Table 4.6**  Variance multipliers for contrasts of four doses, D1–D4 relative to placebo obtained from a design proposed by Senn (Table 4.4) and a design proposed by Bailey (Table 4.3).

|          |       | Stop at cohort | | | Completed trial |
|----------|-------|------|------|------|------|
| Design   | Dose  | 1    | 2    | 3    | 4    |
| Senn     | Any   | 0.4  | 0.4  | 0.4  | 0.4  |
| Bailey   | 1     | 0.4  | 0.27 | 0.24 | 0.21 |
|          | 2     | –    | 0.44 | 0.31 | 0.27 |
|          | 3     | –    | –    | 0.55 | 0.35 |
|          | 4     | –    | –    | –    | 0.53 |

## 4.7  Some final thoughts

### 4.7.1  Sharing information

One of the themes of the RSS report is that risk assessment should be explicit [4]. The point is sometimes made that because risk assessment is difficult and fraught with many uncertainties it cannot be attempted. However, making the attempt can be a useful exercise in clarifying what needs to be known. The RSS report suggested that a risk-assessment document, which could be shared with all interested parties (sponsors, volunteers, insurers and ethics committees) and which covered the issues in Table 4.7 should be produced.

**Table 4.7** Recommendations in the RSS report of matters to be addressed in a formal risk-assessment document (see [4, p. 547]).

| Recommendation no. | Sub-index | Information to be provided |
|---|---|---|
| 4.3.1 | a | A quantitative justification for the starting dose, |
| | b | An estimate of risk for the recommended dose and |
| | c | Estimates of uncertainty regarding these recommendations. |
| 4.3.3 | a | A justification of the proper interval between dosing subjects, |
| | b | A justification of the dose steps the trial will use, |
| | c | A general justification of the design including monitoring and stopping rules and |
| | d | An estimate of the expected number of serious adverse reactions that the trial will produce. |

The three matters addressed as part of recommendation 4.3.1 are those related to the suitability of beginning any trial at all at the proposed starting dose. The four matters addressed in 4.3.3 are very much dependent on other features of the design proposed. These may seem very ambitious, but it is plausible at least that had a simple list like this been addressed, although it might well have been the case that one healthy volunteer would have suffered a serious adverse effect when TGN1412 was first being tried in man, one would not have been faced with the situation where six did.

The information recommended by 4.3.1c may seem rather curious. However, the idea behind this is that it is meant to give some impression as to what further information might be attainable prior to starting the trial. If there was a frank statement that although the estimated risk given under 4.3.1b was low it was not well established, it might be an indication that further *in vitro* or animal studies might be appropriate before proceeding to first-in-man studies.

Another issue addressed in the RSS report is that background information on risks generally would be very useful for the purpose of calibrating risks for given projects. Such information proved to be very hard to get. At the time of the report there were few published studies that could be relied on [26–28]. The Association of Independent Clinical Research Contractors had unpublished data for the years 1991–1998 in which 65 205 health volunteers had been treated to produce 128 serious adverse events, a disturbingly high rate of about 1 in 500 treated subjects.

One of the problems of the field is that drug development does not lead naturally to data-sharing. A recommendation of the RSS report was that this was an area in which regulators, who would get to see the data from many sponsors, should take the lead. Recommendation E.4.18 stated: 'Competent drug regulatory authorities should provide a mechanism for the pharmaceutical industry to collect and share data on adverse reactions in first-in-man studies – to improve a priori risk assessments'. Of course, what such global figures provide are averages, but nevertheless these are part and parcel of the process of calibrating specific forecasts. It is surely an unsatisfactory state of affairs that such figures are not readily available.

## 4.8   Conclusions

The general message of this chapter is that careful planning is necessary for first-in-man studies and that planning is not possible without calculation. Without calculation risks cannot be
assessed, and without assessment of risk there can be no informed consent. It may be objected
that the calculations that are made will be highly speculative, but if the very process of calculation makes it clear how speculative all risk assessments are, this at least is a valuable
contribution to risk communication.

## 4.9   Further reading

The RSS report contains many detailed recommendations [4]. Commentaries are provided by
Senn [6–8] and Julious [29]. The Duff report, whose perspective is more biological but less
statistical, should also be consulted [5]. The book by Julious, Tan and Machin has a chapter
on first-in-man studies [30]. A discussion of the EMA guideline [3] is provided by Milton and
Horvath [31]. More recent discussions of some of these issues will be found in [32–37].

## Acknowledgements

I am grateful to all my colleagues on the RSS working party, Dipti Amin, Rosemary Bailey,
Barbara Bogacka, Peter Coleman, Andrew Garrett, Andrew Grieve and Peter Lachmann, for
their expert help in producing our final report and in understanding many issues. I am also
grateful to Martyn Ward of the MHRA and Martin Lewis of the NHS for helpfully responding
to freedom of information requests at the time of writing the report. The opinions expressed
in this chapter are my responsibility alone.

## Appendix 4.A   Variances for Estimates

Suppose that at any time the design is to be studied we have $k$ cohorts and $l + 1$ doses: 0
(for placebo) and 1, 2, ..., $l$. for the active doses. Let the number of subjects assigned to dose
$j = 0, ..., l$ in cohort $i$ be $n_{ij}$, where in some cases $n_{ij}$ might be 0. Any linear estimator is a linear
combination of the cell means with weights of the form $w_{ij}$. Assuming homoscedasticity, the
variance is now proportional to

$$\sum_{i=1}^{k} \sum_{j=0}^{l} \frac{w_{ij}^2}{n_{ij}} \times (n_{ij} \neq 0) \tag{4.1}$$

This factor (4.1) can be called the *variance multiplier*. Suppose we are interested in estimating the contrast between doses $j = a, a = 0, ..., l$, and $j' = b, b = 0, ..., l, b \neq a$. The
variance function (4.1) now has to be minimized subject to the following constraints:

$$\sum_{j=0}^{l} w_{ij} = 0, \quad i = 1, ..., k, \tag{4.2}$$

$$w_{ij} = 0, \quad \text{if } n_{ij} = 0, \tag{4.3}$$

$$\sum_{i=1}^{k} w_{ia} = 1, \tag{4.4}$$

$$\sum_{i=1}^{k} w_{ib} = -1. \tag{4.5}$$

Minimization of (4.1) subject to the constraints (4.2)–(4.5) yields the solutions for the $w_{ij}$ for any given chosen contrast. These can be plugged into (4.1) to give the variance multiplier for any given contrast.

# References

[1] Suntharalingam, G., Perry, M.R., Ward, S. *et al.* (2006) Cytokine storm in a phase 1 trial of the anti-CD28 monoclonal antibody TGN1412. *New England Journal of Medicine*, **355**, 1018–1028.

[2] Hunig, T. (2012) The storm has cleared: lessons from the CD28 superagonist TGN1412 trial. *Review of Immunology*, **12**, 317–318.

[3] CMPH (2007) Guideline on Strategies to Identify and Mitigate Risks for First-in-Human Clinical Trials with Investigational Medicinal Products. EMEA/CHMP, http://www.ema.europa.eu/docs/en_GB/document_library/Scientific_guideline/2009/09/WC500002988.pdf (accessed 24 June 2014).

[4] Working Party on Statistical Issues in First-in-Man Studies (2007) Statistical issues in first-in-man studies. *Journal of the Royal Statistical Society, Series A*, **170**, 517–579.

[5] ESG (2006) *Expert Scientific Group on Phase One Clinical Trials Final* Report, HM Stationery Office, Norwich, http://webarchive.nationalarchives.gov.uk/+/dh.gov.uk/en/publicationsand statistics/publications/publicationspolicyandguidance/dh_063117.

[6] Senn, S. (2007) Lessons from TGN1412. *Applied Clinical Trials*, **16**, 18–22.

[7] Senn, S. (2007) Safety first. *Significance*, **4**, 79–80.

[8] Senn, S. (2008) Lessons from TGN1412 and TARGET: implications for observational studies and meta-analysis. *Pharmaceutical Statistics*, **7**, 294–301.

[9] Fisher, R.A. (1971) *The Design of Experiments*, Macmillan, New York.

[10] Barnard, G.A. (1945) A new test for 2 × 2 tables. *Nature*, **156**, 177.

[11] Salomon, R. and Webster, R.G. (2009) The influenza virus enigma. *Cell*, **136**, 402–410.

[12] Data-Franco, J. and Berk, M. (2012) The nocebo effect: a clinician's guide. *Australian and New Zealand Journal of Psychiatry*, **47**, 617–623.

[13] Kennedy, W.P. (1961) The nocebo reaction. *Medical World*, **95**, 203–205.

[14] Schweiger, A. and Parducci, A. (1981) Nocebo: the psychologic induction of pain. *Pavlovian Journal of Biological Science*, **16**, 140–143.

[15] Farrington, C.P. and Whitaker, H.J. (2006) Semiparametric analysis of case series data (with discussion). *Applied Statistics*, **55**, 1–28.

[16] Senn, S.J. (2006) Comment on Farrington and Whitaker: semiparametric analysis of case series data. *Applied Statistics*, **55**, 581–583.

[17] Parexel International (2006) *A Phase 1 Single Centre, Double-Blind, Randomized, Placebo-Controlled, Escalating Dose Group Study, to Assess the Safety, Pharmacokinetics, Pharmacodynamics, and Immunogenicity of Single Doses of TGN1412 Administered to Health Volunteers*, Clinical Trial Protocol, Harrow.

[18] Dhillon, B.S. (1978) On common-cause failures – bibliography. *Microelectronics Reliability*, **18**, 533–534.

[19] European Parliament (2001) Directive 2001/20/EC of the European Parliament and of the Council of 4 April 2001, European Parliament, http://www.eortc.be/services/doc/clinical-eu-directive-04-april-01.pdf (accessed 24 June 2014).

[20] O'Quigley, J., Pepe, M.S. and Fisher, L. (1990) Continual reassessment method: a practical design for Phase-1 clinical trials in cancer. *Biometrics*, **46**, 33–48.

[21] Senn, S.J. (1995) A personal view of some controversies in allocating treatment to patients in clinical trials. *Statistics in Medicine*, **14**, 2661–2674.

[22] Bailey, R.A. (2009) Designs for dose-escalation trials with quantitative responses. *Statistics in Medicine*, **28**, 3721–3738; 3759–3760.

[23] Senn, S.J. (1997) *Statistical Issues in Drug Development*, John Wiley & Sons, Ltd, Chichester.

[24] Senn, S.J. (2007) *Statistical Issues in Drug Development*, 2nd edn, John Wiley & Sons, Inc., Hoboken, NJ.

[25] Senn, S.J. (2009) Commentary on designs for dose-escalation trials with quantitative responses. *Statistics in Medicine*, **28**, 3754–3758; discussion 3759–3760.

[26] Orme, M., Harry, J., Routledge, P. and Hobson, S. (1989) Healthy volunteer studies in Great Britain: the results of a survey into 12 months activity in this field. *British Journal of Clinical Pharmacology*, **27**, 125–133.

[27] Royle, J.M. and Snell, E.S. (1986) Medical research on normal volunteers. *British Journal of Clinical Pharmacology*, **21**, 548–549.

[28] Sibille, M., Deigat, N., Janin, A. *et al.* (1998) Adverse events in phase-1 studies: a report in 1015 healthy volunteers. *European Journal of Clinical Pharmacology*, **54**, 13–20.

[29] Julious, S. (2007) A personal perspective on the Royal Statistical Society report of the working party on statistical issues in first-in-man studies. *Pharmaceutical Statistics*, **6**, 75–78.

[30] Julious, S., Tan, S.B. and Machin, D. (2010) *An Introduction to Statistics in Early Phase Trials*, Wiley-Blackwell, Chichester.

[31] Milton, M.N. and Horvath, C.J. (2009) The EMEA guideline on first-in-human clinical trials and its impact on pharmaceutical development. *Toxicologic Pathology*, **37**, 363–371.

[32] Baillie, T.A. (2009) Approaches to the assessment of stable and chemically reactive drug metabolites in early clinical trials. *Chemical Research in Toxicology*, **22**, 263–266.

[33] Brennan, F.R., Morton, L.D., Spindeldreher, S.K.A. *et al.* (2010) Safety and immunotoxicity assessment of immunomodulatory monoclonal antibodies. *MAbs*, **2**, 233–255.

[34] Francillon, A., Pickering, G. and Belorgey, C. (2009) Exploratory clinical trials: implementation modes & guidelines, scope and regulatory framework. *Thérapie*, **64**, 149–159.

[35] Ivy, S.P., Siu, L.L., Garett-Mayer, E. and Rubenstein, L. (2010) Approaches to phase 1 clinical trial design focused on safety, efficiency, and selected patient populations: a report from the clinical trial design task force of the National Cancer Institute investigational drug steering committee. *Clinical Cancer Research*, **16**, 1726–1736.

[36] Muller, P.Y. and Brennan, F.R. (2009) Safety assessment and dose selection for first-in-human clinical trials with immunomodulatory monoclonal antibodies. *Clinical Pharmacology and Therapeutics*, **85**, 247–258.

[37] Pasqualetti, G., Gori, G., Blandizzi, C. and Del Tacca, M. (2010) Healthy volunteers and early phases of clinical experimentation. *European Journal of Clinical Pharmacology*, **66**, 647–653.

# 5

# Phase 1 trials

## A. Lawrence Gould
*Merck Research Laboratories, 770 Sumneytown Pike, West Point, PA 19486, USA*

## 5.1 Introduction

The main goal of Phase 1 trials, especially those of anticancer drugs, is to determine the dose or doses to carry forward into Phase 2. Conventional anticancer drugs rely on cytotoxicity for their effect, so that a balance must be achieved between administering enough drug to have the desired effect of killing cancer cells, yet not so much as to cause intolerable toxic adverse effects. Phase 1 trials of these drugs therefore seek to determine the maximum tolerated dose (MTD), that is, the maximum dose that does not lead to unacceptable dose-limiting severe toxicity, which must be defined carefully in the trial protocol. Once this dose has been found, the next step is to see if this dose provides acceptable efficacy, which also must be carefully defined. This step can occur in the same trial or separately in a Phase 2 trial. Regardless of the design that is used, careful attention to the definition of "toxicity" is important because observation errors, especially incorrectly recording as a toxicity an event that really is not a toxicity, can affect the probability of correctly identifying the MTD substantially [1].

Phase 1 oncology trials primarily address toxicity in practice; antitumor activity usually is a secondary objective. Antitumor response rates, at least in early stage development, generally have been low, possibly because Phase 1 oncology trials often include patients with different tumor types that have been refractory to standard treatments.

There are three general categories of design for Phase 1 cancer trial designs seeking to determine an appropriate dose to carry forward for future study based on expected toxicity. These are algorithmic (rule-based) approaches (especially the 3 + 3 design) that have been used in almost all such trials, model-based Bayesian designs, and model-free Bayesian designs. Methods other than standard rule-based approaches such as 3 + 3 have been used

*Statistical Methods for Evaluating Safety in Medical Product Development*, First Edition.
Edited by A. Lawrence Gould.
© 2015 John Wiley & Sons, Ltd. Published 2015 by John Wiley & Sons, Ltd.

infrequently if at all for various reasons, especially the difficulty in defining non-toxicity endpoints [2–5].

However, while the algorithmic designs are simple to communicate and implement, the Bayesian designs have a number of practical properties that make them better choices for Phase 1 trials than the commonly used algorithmic designs [6]: they provide estimates of a very specific (and relevant) measure of toxicity along with estimates of its precision; the precision of the estimates increases with the number of patients treated; the determination of the optimum dose uses all of the accumulated information; they are more flexible with regard to the shape of the dose–response relationship; they allow for dose skipping; and they are less affected by the number of doses in the schedule.

Increasing evidence supports the adoption of innovative dose–toxicity models, as these are safer and more efficient in meeting the challenges of modern investigational oncology than traditional models used in Phase I clinical trials. A literature review was carried out to provide an overview of current and innovative dose–toxicity models in oncology with an emphasis on recent clinical advances, including the benefits of a Bayesian framework [7]. Innovative dose–toxicity models attempt to minimize clinical risk and maximize research performance. Of these, the Bayesian continual reassessment method and the escalation with overdose control method are two successful contemporary designs that outperformed traditional models in clinical trials; they accounted for patient heterogeneity, combination therapy, and they appropriately assessed molecularly targeted agents.

Not all drugs, not even anticancer drugs, rely upon cytotoxicity for their efficacy. Molecularly targeted agents target specific pathways in tumor cells presumed to be essential for tumor growth and proliferation. The risk of toxicity with such drugs is assumed to increase with the dosage, but it is not necessarily true that their effects increase with dose. Le Tourneau *et al.* [3] address a number of issues arising in the Phase 1 evaluation of molecularly targeted drugs, which can be administered singly or in combination with other molecularly targeted drugs or with cytotoxic drugs. The key issue is the identification of pharmacodynamics biomarkers, that is, measures of pharmacologic response that can be used at early stages of drug development, that have been validated in Phase 3 clinical trials. As of the writing of the Le Tourneau *et al.* article, no such biomarkers had been validated, and the recommendation is that toxicity be the main focus of Phase 1 trials unless a validated efficacy biomarker is available.

This chapter describes a number of approaches to the design of Phase 1 trials aimed at determining appropriate doses of drugs to carry forward into later stages of development. The primary, but not exclusive, focus is on identifying maximal doses of drugs for treating various forms of cancer. Many designs are intended to identify doses corresponding to acceptable burdens of toxicity. These are sensible for identifying drugs for treating cancer because the effectiveness of these agents depends on their toxicity, to which rapidly growing cancer cells are expected to be more sensitive than healthy cells with lower metabolic rates. More recent designs, appropriate for molecularly targeted drugs, consider both efficacy and toxicity because the effectiveness of these agents is not necessarily monotonically related to dose, even though their toxicity may be. An interesting recent trend (with its own substantial literature), outside the scope of this chapter, is the combination of the Phase 1 and Phase 2 stages of drug development into a "seamless" Phase 1/2 design. The references provided in this chapter are by no means complete, but they do include a number of recently described approaches, and should be a useful starting point for readers interested in pursuing particular topics further. The references cited generally have extensive bibliographies of their own, so that the reader can obtain complete details about methods of interest and about refinements of these methods that were published subsequent to the original articles. In addition, a number of reviews of design strategies have recently been published, and these provide substantial links to earlier works on the design of Phase 1 trials; some also touch on combined Phase 1/2 trials [3, 6, 8–17].

## 5.2  Dose determined by toxicity

### 5.2.1  Algorithmic (rule-based) approaches

#### 5.2.1.1  3 + 3 designs

These are the designs that have been used most often in actual practice although, as discussed below, there certainly is room for improvement. A sequence of increasing dose levels generally will be fixed in advance, typically in a modified Fibonacci sequence in which the dose increments decrease with increasing dose; for example, given an initial dose, the next dose is double the first dose, the third dose increases the second by 67%, the fourth dose increases the third by 50%, and so on [8, 13]. Figure 5.1 outlines the implementation of a basic 3 + 3 design. The initial cohort of patients is treated with dose 1, presumed to be safe on the basis of information from, for example, animal toxicology studies. If two or more patients in the initial cohort of three experience unacceptable toxicity, then the trial is stopped with the conclusion that all of the proposed doses are unacceptably toxic. If the maximum dosage in the sequence has been reached and no more than one unacceptable toxicity has occurred, then the MTD is taken as the highest dose in the sequence. There are a number of variations of this design [13], including accelerated titration designs (ATDs) [18].

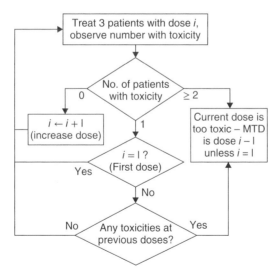

**Figure 5.1**   Outline of basic 3 + 3 design. MTD, the maximum tolerated dose, is the dose to carry forward in further studies. Dose 1 is the lowest dose in the prespecified sequence of doses. The design calls for treating successive cohorts of patients until either the maximum dose has been administered or two or more toxicities have been observed.

### 5.2.1.2    Up and down designs

Up-and-down designs are rule-based designs whose statistical properties can be determined explicitly. Gezmu and Flournoy [19] describe the properties of up-and-down designs for dose finding when successive doses are administered to groups of patients rather than to single patients (as commonly used). A typical trial proceeds as follows. Suppose that the cohort assigned to receive a dose at any stage contains $s$ subjects. Let $c_L$ and $c_U$ denote integers between 0 and $s$, $0 \leq c_L < c_U \leq s$; recommended values for $c_L$ and $c_U$ are provided in [19]. Suppose that a total of $K$ doses $d_1 < \ldots < d_K$ might be administered, and that the latest administered dose is $d_k (k = 2, \ldots, K - 1)$. If there are $c_U$ or more toxicities in this group, then the next group is treated with dose $d_{k-1}$. If there are $c_L$ or fewer toxicities, then the next group is treated at dose $d_{k+1}$. Otherwise, the next group is treated at dose $d_k$. Some boundary rules are necessary: if $d_k = d_1$, and there are no more than $c_L$ toxicities, then the next group is treated at dose $d_2$, otherwise the next group is treated at dose $d_1$. If $d_k = d_K$ and there are $c_U$ or more toxicities, the next group is treated at dose $d_{K-1}$, otherwise the next group is treated at dose $d_k$. This process amounts to a non-homogeneous (in the treatment space) random walk whose transition probabilities can be expressed explicitly. The result is a distribution across the dose levels that can be useful for selecting a target dose for further development. A recent simulation study [20] comparing a number of up-and-down designs (including the $3 + 3$ design) suggested that a variation of the up-and-down design that based dose-escalation decisions on the total numbers of patients treated at each dose [21] provided the best overall performance in terms of finding the MTD and assigning few patients to toxic doses.

### 5.2.1.3    Toxicity probability interval

The toxicity probability interval (TPI) [22] and modified toxicity probability interval (mTPI) [23] methods are rule-based methods that use accumulated information to guide dose selection (like model-based methods described below), but without requiring computation to determine the dose to administer to the next cohort of patients. The mTPI method differs from the TPI method in not requiring calibration; what follows therefore applies primarily to the mTPI method. All decisions about increasing or decreasing dosages, or terminating the trial if no dose is safe, can be identified at the outset and made available via a spreadsheet program [24] or even a printed table, which simplifies the dose determination process and, in principle, should be attractive to clinicians. The mTPI method requires only the specification of an "equivalence" interval (EI) for the toxicity rate that defines the MTD. That is, suppose that $p_{max}$ denotes the maximum acceptable toxicity rate for a drug; any dose for which the estimated toxicity rate lies in the EI $(p_{max} - \varepsilon_1, p_{max} + \varepsilon_2)$ is a candidate for being identified as the MTD to be carried forward into trials aimed at characterizing the dose–response properties of the drug. The values of $\varepsilon_1$ and $\varepsilon_2$ are specified by the clinical investigator, and may depend on the nature of the condition being treated. For example, if $p_{max} = 0.3$, then $(\varepsilon_1, \varepsilon_2) = (0.05, 0.05)$ implies that the EI is (0.25, 0.35) and $(\varepsilon_1, \varepsilon_2) = (0.1, 0.1)$ implies that the EI is (0.2, 0.4); which of these is the more appropriate would depend on the clinical context. The toxicity probability of a dose for which $x$ toxicities have been observed among $n$ treated patients has a Beta$(x + 1, n - x + 1)$ posterior distribution, assuming a uniform prior. The metric on which the algorithm is based is the maximum of what are called the unit probability masses (UPMs), defined as the posterior probabilities corresponding to the intervals $(0, p_{max} - \varepsilon_1)$, $(p_{max} - \varepsilon_1, p_{max} + \varepsilon_2)$, $(p_{max} + \varepsilon_2, 1)$ divided by their respective lengths. Given $p_{max}$, $\varepsilon_1$, and $\varepsilon_2$, values of the UPM for any collection of $x$ and $n$ values can be calculated and tabulated, or provided in a spreadsheet, before any data collection occurs. The algorithm proceeds as follows, with some necessary boundary adjustments. Suppose that there are $J$ potential doses, $(d_1 \leq \ldots \leq d_J)$ with corresponding toxicity probabilities $p_1 \leq \ldots \leq p_J$, that the latest cohort has received dose $d_i$, and that at this point $x_i$ toxicities have been observed among the $n_i$ patients who have received dose $d_i$ during the trial. Based on this information, and with no further computation, the interval with the largest UPM is identified. If the UPM for the first interval, $(0, p_{\max} - \varepsilon_1)$, is largest, then the next cohort will receive dose $d_{i+1}$. If the UPM for the second interval, $(p_{\max} - \varepsilon_1, p_{\max} + \varepsilon_2)$, is largest, then the next cohort will receive dose $d_i$. If the UPM for the third interval, $(p_{\max} + \varepsilon_2, 1)$, is largest, then the next cohort will receive dose $d_{i-1}$. Some boundary conditions are necessary. If $d_i$ happens to be the lowest dose $(d_1)$ and the posterior probability of the third interval exceeds some critical value $\xi(= 0.95, \text{say})$, then the trial is terminated due to excessive toxicity; otherwise, the trial continues to completion. If the UPM for the first interval is highest, then the dose should be escalated as noted unless the posterior probability of the third interval corresponding to the increased dose exceeds $\xi$; if this happens, then that dose and all higher doses will be eliminated from the set of considered doses and the next cohort will receive dose $d_i$ instead of dose $d_{i+1}$. The MTD at the end of the trial is the isotonic-transformed posterior mean of the dose-specific toxicity probabilities, $p_1, \ldots, p_J$. This is obtained when using Markov chain Monte Carlo methods by drawing realizations from the posterior distribution of the $p_i$ and then, for any set of realizations $(p_1, \ldots, p_J)$, obtaining corresponding isotonic (order-restricted) estimates $p_1^*, \ldots, p_J^*$; the result is the joint posterior distribution of the order-restricted estimates, from which various statistics can be calculated. The proposed method is equivalent to a Bayes rule in a decision-theoretic context with an appropriate choice of penalty functions.

The probability of selecting the right dose, the proportion of patients receiving toxic doses, and the average number of patients required to identify the MTD as determined using mTPI, TPI [22], the $3 + 3$ approach, and the continual reassessment method (CRM) were compared via simulation for a number of scenarios. The mTPI approach generally had the highest or nearly highest probability of selecting the correct dose, always higher than the $3 + 3$ method and often higher than the CRM approach, and about the same as the TPI approach. The proportions of patients receiving a dose above the MTD were about the same for all of the methods. The $3 + 3$ method required fewer patients to identify an MTD than the other methods, but identified the correct dose less frequently. Sensitivity analyses suggested that the analytic results were not sensitive to the choice of prior, so that a uniform prior distribution would generally be appropriate. The simulations presented in [23] showed that the sample sizes required to reach a dosage decision by the $3 + 3$ method always were smaller than those required by the mTPI. Ji and Wang [25] carried out simulations to compare the performance of mTPI and the $3 + 3$ method when the trials used similar sample sizes. They found that in most (40 of 42) cases considered, the $3 + 3$ method treated more patients at doses exceeding the MTD than did the mTPI. Also, the mTPI approach generally selected the correct MTD more often than did the $3 + 3$ approach, except when none of the candidate doses included the MTD or when the MTD was at the low or high end of the range of doses considered.

#### 5.2.1.4   Toxicity equivalence range

The toxicity (or target) equivalence range (TEQR) design [26] is a rule-based method similar to the mTPI [23]. The design is based on the empirical dose-limiting toxicity rates for the various dosages, defined for any dose as the proportions of the patients treated with that dose experiencing 0, 1, 2, 3, ... toxicities among the total numbers of patients treated with that dose. Thus, if the current cohort of patients was on dose $d$ and, among $n$ patients treated with dose $d$ in this and previous cohorts, $y$ demonstrated a toxicity, then the current value of the empirical dose-limiting toxicity rate is $r_d = y/n$. As with the mTPI, it is necessary to define $p_{max}$, the target toxicity rate, and small constants $\varepsilon_1$ and $\varepsilon_2$ such that a dosage that yields an $r_d$ value in the interval $(p_{max} - \varepsilon_1, p_{max} + \varepsilon_2)$ is regarded as a candidate for the MTD. In addition, the TEQR design requires specifying the smallest unacceptably high toxicity rate $p_X$, defined as the rate that clinicians would not want to exceed. The maximum sample size $N$ also needs to be specified. The three numbers, $p_{max} - \varepsilon_1, p_{max} + \varepsilon_2$, and $p_X$ define the procedure. If the latest cohort received dose $d$ then the dose to administer to the next cohort would be determined as follows. If $r_d < p_{max} - \varepsilon_1$ then the next cohort would receive the next highest dose unless the current value of $r_d$ for that dose exceeded $p_X$, in which case that dose would be removed from the trial and the new cohort would receive the same dose as the current cohort; if $d$ was the highest dose, then the trial should be terminated. If $p_{max} - \varepsilon_1 \le r_d \le p_{max} + \varepsilon_2$, then the next cohort also would receive dose $d$. If $r_d > p_{max} + \varepsilon_2$, then the next cohort would receive the next lowest dose; if, in fact, $r_d > p_X$ then the current dose would be removed from the trial and no further cohorts would receive it. At the end of the trial, the MTD would be the highest dose with a dose-limiting toxicity rate closest to $p_{max}$ following isotonic regression (as with mTPI). Modest simulations comparing the TEQR design with CRM, mTPI, and $3 + 3$ showed that the mTPI and TEQR designs had similar values of the various performance metrics, and both had superior values relative to $3 + 3$ designs. The TEQR and mTPI designs had somewhat smaller rates of correctly detecting the MTD than did the CRM design, but the CRM design required larger sample sizes to reach a decision.

## 5.3    Model-based approaches

Most model-based approaches are variations of the basic CRM [10, 16]. The CRM approach is (usually, but not necessarily exclusively) a Bayesian approach that updates a posterior distribution on the basis of the accumulated information about toxicity from successive cohorts of patients.

### 5.3.1    Basic CRM design

Suppose that the probability of unacceptable toxicity is related to the dose by a simple function, $Pr(\text{toxicity; dose}, \theta) = p(\text{dose}; \theta)$, for example, the logistic model

$$p(d; \theta) = (1 + \exp(-(a + b \times \text{ dose})))^{-1}$$

or the hyperbolic model

$$p(d; \theta) = ((\tanh(d) + 1)/2)^b.$$

The essential requirement is that $p(d; \theta)$ is invertible so that given a value $p^*$, a corresponding dosage value $d^*$ can be found such that $p(d^*; \theta) = p^*$ regardless of the value of $\theta$. Fixing the value of $a$ at $a = 3$ or 4 makes both of these one-parameter models, which O'Quigley and Pepe [16] suggest should be sufficient in practice. A prior distribution for $\theta$ also is required, and careful attention should be given to its definition (see [10] and references cited therein). As with the rule-based methods, a sequence of doses needs to be specified at the outset of the trial. Let $g(\theta; \xi_0)$ denote the prior distribution for $\theta$. Initially, suppose that $m$ patients are assigned to receive dose 1 (usually the lowest dose). If $y_1$ denotes the number of patients among this cohort who experience unacceptable toxicity, then the corresponding likelihood is proportional to

$$p(d_1; \theta)^{y_1} (1 - p(d_1; \theta))^{m-y_1}.$$

The product of the likelihood and the prior density for $\theta$ divided by the marginal probability of $y_1$ gives the posterior density $g(\theta; \xi_1)$ of $\theta$, where $\xi_1 = \{y_1, \xi_0\}$. This calculation can be carried out with readily available software. The value of the dosage is treated as a known constant. Let $\theta_1$ denote the mean of the posterior density $g(\theta; \xi_1)$. The objective is to find the dosage $d_{max}$ for which $p(d_{max}; \theta) \approx p_{max}$, the target probability of an unacceptable toxicity. The dosage that will be carried forward is the largest of the set of candidate doses that does not exceed $p_{max}$. Given the outcome from the initial cohort, suppose that the relationship between dosage and toxicity is specified by $p(\text{dose}; \theta_1)$, and let $d_2$ denote the dosage in the originally specified sequence such that $p(d_2; \theta_1)$ is closest to $p_{max}$. The next cohort of $m$ patients is then treated at dosage $d_2$, and the posterior density of $g(\theta; \xi_2), \xi_2 = (y_2, \xi_1)$, is determined as before, with posterior mean $\theta_2$. This is used to update the dose–toxicity relationship, which now becomes $p(\text{dose}; \theta_2)$. The next cohort of patients is treated as dosage $d_3$, which is the dosage in the originally specified sequence such that $p(d_3; \theta_2)$ is closest to $p_{max}$. There are several variations of rules determining when the process should stop. In general, the process continues until the maximum dose has been reached or until a sufficient number of patients have been treated at a particular dose. If the toxicity rate is too high even at the lowest dose, then the trial is terminated and another (lower) dosage sequence is specified. Actual implementation of the CRM requires attention to a number of details such as the choice of prior distribution, the dose–toxicity model, exactly how the sequence of dose–toxicity models corresponding to successive posterior distributions of the parameters of the models should be used to determine what dosage the next cohort of patients receives, and the sizes of successive cohorts [10].

## 5.3.2    Adaptive refinement of dosage list

Ji *et al.* [27] describe a simple model-based Bayesian version of CRM that can be useful for determining the MTD to carry forward in a Phase 1 oncology trial that has a limited sample size, for example because the treatment is very expensive or the disease studied is very rare, which is common in trials of adoptive immunogenicity. The probability of toxicity is related to dosage by a simple logistic model, $p(d) = (1 + \exp(-(c + ad)))^{-1}$, where $c$ is a known constant and $a$ is a parameter assumed to have a unit exponential prior density, $f_0(a) = \exp(-a)$. If $Y_i (= 0$ or $1)$ denotes the toxicity status of the $i$th subject in the trial, then the likelihood is the product $\prod_i p(d_i)^{Y_i} (1 - p(d_i))^{1-Y_i}$, where $d_i$ denotes the dose received by subject $i$. The dose-finding algorithm proceeds by assigning the first cohort (fewer than three subjects) to dose level 1 (the lowest dose). If the posterior probability given the data that $p(d_1) > p_T$, the maximum acceptable toxicity rate, exceeds 0.9, then the trial is stopped and no dose is chosen. If the posterior probability that $p(d_j) > p_T (j > 1)$ exceeds 0.9, then doses $d_j, d_{j+1}, \ldots$ are removed from consideration. Otherwise, the next cohort is treated at dose $d_k$, which (among the remaining doses) has the largest posterior probability associated with the statement $\{\text{abs}(p(d_k) - p_T) = \min_i(\text{abs}(p(d_i) - p_T))\}$. The process continues until the maximum number of subjects has been treated. Simulation studies under "realistic" clinical scenarios comparing the proposed method with the 3 + 3 algorithmic rule and CRM with and without a stopping rule (stop if dose 1 is toxic) indicated that the proposed method performed well in all situations, seldom continuing if all doses are toxic, quickly reaching the top dose if most doses are not toxic, and reaching the MTD most often if the MTD is within the dosage range.

### 5.3.3   Hybrid designs

Yuan and Yin [28] describe a "hybrid" dose-finding design based on toxicity that combines a rule-based method such as the standard 3 + 3 design with a model-based design such as CRM. The idea is to avoid possibly comprising the performance of the CRM approach because of misspecification of the dose–toxicity model relationship while basing dose selection on all accumulated data to improve design efficiency. The general strategy is to treat successive cohorts of patients at doses determined by either the finding from the previous cohort (standard method) or the accumulated findings from all cohorts (model-based method). Let $p_{max}$ denote the maximum acceptable toxicity rate, and let $p_j$ denote the true, unknown toxicity rate for the $j$th of $J$ predefined doses. Three hypotheses are considered: $H_1 : p_j < p_{max} - \delta$, $H_2 : p_{max} - \delta < p_j < p_{max} + \delta$, $H_3 : p_j > p_{max} + \delta$; $H_1$ corresponds to the $j$th dose being below the MTD, $H_3$ corresponds to the $j$th dose being above the MTD, and $H_2$ corresponds to the $j$th dose being "close to" the MTD. The aim is to find the index $j^*$ corresponding to the dose that is most likely to be "close to" the MTD, while avoiding exposing too many patients to doses that are likely to be toxic or too low. The posterior probabilities of these three hypotheses can be calculated using only the data from the current cohort or the data from all of the cohorts. A Bayes factor argument is used to determine that evidence is "compelling" for any of the hypotheses if the corresponding posterior probability exceeds 0.61. The process proceeds as follows. Let $y_{curr}$ denote the number of toxicities observed among the patients in the current cohort, and let $j_{curr}$ denote the index of the treatment administered to these patients. Also, let $\mathbf{J}_{curr}$ denote the indices of the doses that have been administered to the cohorts treated so far, and $\mathbf{Y}_{curr}$ denote the vector of toxicity counts for these doses. If the maximum sample size has been reached, then isotonic (order-restricted) estimates of the values of $p_j$ for the doses that have been used can be calculated, and the MTD is defined as the dose $j^*$ for which $p_{j*}$ is closest to $p_{max}$. If the maximum sample size has not been reached, then calculate the posterior probabilities of $H_1$, $H_2$, and $H_3$ given $y_{curr}$, say $q_1$, $q_2$, and $q_3$. If $q_1 > 0.61$, and $j_{curr} < J$ ($j_J$ indexes the highest dose), then treat the next cohort at the dose with index $j_{curr} + 1$; if $j_{curr} = J$, then stop the trial because the evidence is compelling that all doses are too low. If $q_3 > 0.61$ and $j_{curr} > 1$ ($j_1$ indexes the lowest dose), then treat the next cohort at the dose with index $j_{curr} - 1$; if $j_{curr} = 1$, then (although this is not made explicit in the paper) stop the trial because the evidence is compelling that all doses are toxic. If $q_2 > 0.61$, then treat the next cohort with the current dose. If $q_1$, $q_2$, and $q_3$ all are less than 0.61, then the CRM part of the process is invoked. Calculate the posterior probabilities of $H_1$, $H_2$, and $H_3$ using all of the accumulated data (i.e., $\mathbf{J}_{curr}$ and $\mathbf{Y}_{curr}$), say $r_1$, $r_2$, and $r_3$. If any of $r_1$, $r_2$, or $r_3$ exceeds 0.61, then determine the next dose as just described. Otherwise, use the CRM algorithm to calculate the dose "closest" to the MTD and assign that dose to the next cohort. Simulation studies carried out for a variety of scenarios suggested that the "hybrid" method led to the "correct" MTD more often, and had more patients treated at that dose, than the 3 + 3 method. Also, the "hybrid" approach had fewer episodes of toxicity and fewer patients treated with doses exceeding the MTD than did the CRM approach, and the "correct" dose was selected more often and more patients were treated at that dose in most of the scenarios. Additional simulations suggested that increasing the maximum allowable sample size had little effect on the results. Relaxing the restriction on skipping dose levels improved the recommendation rate for the optimal dose level, but more than doubled the rate at which patients received toxic dose combinations.

### 5.3.4  Comparisons with rule-based designs

Iasonos *et al.* [29] compare via simulation standard $3 + 3$ designs (standard methods) with four variations of CRM designs not allowing skipping doses on escalation. The standard method generally found the true MTD 10–30% fewer times than the CRM approaches, except in one case where the doses were closely spaced. The CRM methods generally treated more patients at the MTD dose than the standard approach. However, the CRM methods could require greater sample sizes to achieve desired precision of the MTD estimate than may be practical for Phase 1 trials.

Le Tourneau *et al.* [14] evaluated the properties of dose-escalation methods used in 84 Phase 1 oncology trials of single-component molecularly targeted agents. Almost half (49%) of the trials used the $3 + 3$ design, most of the rest (42%) used ATD and only 9% of the designs used modified continual reassessment method (mCRM) or pharmacologically guided dose escalation. More dose levels were explored with the mCRM and ATD designs than with the $3 + 3$ design. The mean MTD to starting dose ratio appeared to be at least twice as high for trials using mCRM or ATD designs as for trials using a standard $3 + 3$ design although the average number of patients exposed to doses below the MTD was similar for the three designs. The authors recommended more extensive use of innovative dose-escalation designs in Phase 1 oncology trials of molecularly targeted agents.

Oron and Hoff [30] compare the small-sample behavior of Bayesian and non-Bayesian Phase 1 dose-finding designs for determining MTD that used likelihood estimation based on accumulated information ("long-memory" designs) with that of short-memory "up-and-down" designs using information from published studies and via simulation. Although both strategies had similar success in finding the MTD, the number of cohorts of patients needed to be treated to find the MTD was substantially more variable with long-memory than with short-memory designs. In other words, although the long-memory designs may require fewer patients to identify a dose to carry forward, and although on average the number of cohorts that wind up being treated at the MTD is the same as with short-memory designs, many more cohorts wind up being treated at doses that are too low or too high. Detailed evaluation revealed that this behavior depended on the order of entry of participants into a trial and the fact that the long-memory designs use a "winner-take-all" rule that give disproportionate influence to the findings from early cohorts, especially if the dose sequence converges early, because the process always tries to assign the best estimate of the MTD to the next patient to enter. In addition, the prior predictive distribution over dose levels substantially affects the long-memory strategy performance even after the accumulation of substantial data. A theoretical investigation [31] established that designs seeking to identify the MTD in a sequential way (which includes long- memory designs) in fact cannot lead to consistent estimates of the MTD, but designs that do not require treatment at the current estimate of the MTD can yield consistent estimators. Azriel *et al.* [31] defined a dose-finding procedure that was asymptotically optimal, based on isotonic regression. Oron and Hoff examined this method, too, and found that it did not alleviate the excess variability problem. Their general conclusion was that it would be better to estimate the toxicity–dose relationship accurately and determine the MTD from the relationship rather than try to pinpoint the best candidate from a small number of arbitrary dose levels.

Subsequent discussion by Carlin *et al.* [32] and by Cheung [33] provided useful perspective. Carlin *et al.* pointed out that Bayesian Phase 1 methods, like all Bayesian methods, rely on the accuracy of the models that are used. They provide accurate insights when the models are accurate, and provide no guarantee of optimality or even relevance when they are not even approximately accurate, as was the case for some of the examples described by Oron and Hoff. This means using better priors for the starting dose to select, incorporating sensible restrictions on the dose paths, and using more than one patient at a time. Carlin *et al.* also point out that it may not be sensible to use the likelihood principle as a design strategy even though it should be sensible as an estimation principle, for example when using the posterior mean as a final MTD estimate. Cheung observed that the practical and ethical considerations of Phase 1 trials may not be reflected adequately by just counting the number of patients at the MTD, and that the number cohorts treated at a dose yielding an acceptable toxicity probability, for example between 25% and 35%, may be more appropriate. Choosing an appropriate CRM design can be difficult in the absence of guidance from theory because of the many design parameters that have to be specified. Cheung feels that the main consideration should be "whether a method can accommodate the complexity *in practice* that arises … including protocol amendments, delayed outcomes, efficacy-toxicity trade-off."

## 5.4 Model-based designs with more than one treatment (or non-monotonic toxicity)

Wages *et al.* [34] consider situations in which the dose–toxicity curve may not be monotonic, an increasingly common situation in Phase 1 trials that involve combinations of agents where the complete ordering of the probabilities of dose-limiting toxicity among the pairs of treatments cannot be known a priori. Their method involves laying out all possible orderings of toxicity probabilities that are consistent with the known orderings among treatment combinations and allowing the CRM to provide efficient estimates of the MTD within these orders. Suppose there are $J$ drug combinations, $d_1, \dots, d_J$ partially ordered with respect to toxicity in such a way that there are $M$ possible simple orders consistent with the partial ordering (this could be a large number if there are many dosage combinations). For example, if $d_1 \leq d_2$ and $d_3 \leq d_4$, then $(d_1, d_2, d_3, d_4)$, $(d_1, d_3, d_2, d_4)$, and $(d_1, d_3, d_4, d_2)$ are some simple orderings that are consistent with the known partial ordering. Each simple ordering can be thought of as a model. Let $p_{mj}$ denote the probability of dose-limiting toxicity at dose $d_{mj}$ in ordering $m$ (the dose among $d_1, \dots, d_J$ corresponding to $d_{mj}$ can depend on the ordering), and suppose that $p_{mj} \cong \psi_m(d_{mj}, a_m)$, for example $\psi_m(d_{mj}, a) = \alpha_{mj}^{a_m}$, where $0 < \alpha_{m1} < \dots < \alpha_{mJ} < 1$ represents the "skeleton" of the model, that is, the presumed toxicities corresponding to doses $d_{m1}, \dots, d_{mJ}$. Different orderings can have different skeletons. For ordering $m$, let $(y_{m1}, \dots, y_{mJ})$ denote at any stage of the trial the numbers of toxicities observed at doses $d_{m1}, \dots, d_{mJ}$. An estimate $\hat{a}_m$ of the parameter $a_m$ can be obtained, and the likelihood for that ordering, consisting of a product of Bernoulli probability functions, can be obtained. A weight corresponding to the $m$th ordering is the ratio of the current likelihood corresponding to the $m$th ordering divided by the sum of the likelihoods corresponding to all of the orderings. Generalized weights incorporating some prior beliefs about the plausibility of the various orderings can be incorporated by multiplying the likelihood by its prior plausibility and then constructing the (generalized) weights as just described. The current working model is taken to be the model with the largest weight. Standard CRM methods (the authors prefer the likelihood approach) can be applied to determine the combination of doses to be administered to the next cohort. A variation of an up-and-down method is used to start the process so that the accumulated data has some patients demonstrating toxicity and some not, which is required in order to get the estimates described above. The method was shown to perform well when compared to other suggested methods for partial orders. Wages and Conaway [35] provide some practical guidance for implementing the partially ordered CRM approach.

Wages and Conaway [35] discuss practical design considerations pertinent to the application of a CRM method based on the partial ordering for determining an appropriate combination of multiple dosages of multiple (actually, pairs of) agents in Phase 1 oncology trials when the dose–toxicity relationship may not be monotone for all combinations. This paper is a refinement of a previously described partial ordering method [34, 36]. The strategy entails arranging the dosages (and corresponding toxicity rates) of the agents in a matrix and then considering up to six (out of possibly a large number of) sequences of dosage pairs corresponding to various ways of choosing the matrix entries. The partially ordered combinations are arrayed in plausible complete orderings, CRM methods (likelihood [34, 36] or Bayesian [36]) are applied, and the dose for the next cohort is chosen using the ordering giving the largest likelihood. The method reduces to the CRM when the toxicity order is completely known with respect to dose. Simulation studies suggest that the method performs comparably to, sometimes better than, the CRM method when it can be applied.

Hirakawa *et al.* [37] describe an empirical Bayes method for selecting the MTD of a combination of drugs based on the occurrence of toxicity when the toxicity for either agent increases monotonically with dose when the dose of the other agent is held fixed. The logit of the probability of toxicity ($p(d_1, d_2)$) for a combination of doses ($d_1, d_2$) of the two agents can be expressed using a simple linear regression model, $\text{logit}(p(d_1, d_2; \boldsymbol{\beta})) = \beta_0 + \beta_1 d_1 + \beta_2 d_2 + \beta_3 d_1 d_2$, where $\boldsymbol{\beta} = (\beta_0, \beta_1, \beta_2, \beta_3)$. Given a vector of estimates $\widehat{\boldsymbol{\beta}}$ of the elements of $\boldsymbol{\beta}$, the quantity $p(d_1', d_2'; \widehat{\boldsymbol{\beta}})$ can be used to predict the toxicity of a new dose combination, $(d_1', d_2')$. The lack of information about joint effects makes specifying an informative prior and, therefore, using a Bayesian approach, difficult. The authors choose to use an empirical Bayes approach to estimating the parameters, with incorporation of shrinkage into the model [38, 39] to improve the accuracy of prediction. The logit of the toxicity probability is expressed as $\text{logit}(p(d_1, d_2; \boldsymbol{\beta}, \boldsymbol{\delta})) = \beta_0 + (1 - \delta_1)\beta_1 d_1 + (1 - \delta_2)\beta_2 d_2 + (1 - \delta_3)\beta_3 d_1 d_2$, where $\boldsymbol{\beta}$ is as before and $\boldsymbol{\delta} = (\delta_1, \delta_2, \delta_3)$. The determination of the MTD after the initial startup step proceeds conventionally. Suppose that $p_{\max}$ is the target MTD, and let $(\varepsilon_1, \varepsilon_2)$ denote small positive numbers. Let $(d_{1i}, d_{2i})$ denote the dosage combination administered to the $i$th (current) cohort, and let $p(d_{1i}, d_{2i}; \widehat{\boldsymbol{\beta}}, \widehat{\boldsymbol{\delta}})$ denote the predicted toxicity of that dosage combination based on all of the accumulated data. If $p_{\max} - \varepsilon_1 \leq p(d_{1i}, d_{2i}; \widehat{\boldsymbol{\beta}}, \widehat{\boldsymbol{\delta}}) \leq p_{\max} + \varepsilon_2$, then treat the next cohort of patients at the same dosage combination. If $(d_{1i}, d_{2i}) = (d_{11}, d_{21})$, the combination of the lowest doses on both agents, and $p(d_{1i}, d_{2i}; \widehat{\boldsymbol{\beta}}, \widehat{\boldsymbol{\delta}}) > p_{\max} + \varepsilon_2$, then stop the trial and conclude that none of the proposed doses is sufficiently safe. Otherwise, allocate the next cohort of patients to the dosage combination $(d_{1m}, d_{2m})$ such that $p(d_{1m}, d_{2m}; \widehat{\boldsymbol{\beta}}, \widehat{\boldsymbol{\delta}})$ is closest to $p_{\max}$ subject to the constraint that the dosage for the next cohort can be increased (if it is increased at all) only to either $(d_{1i+1}, d_{2i})$ or $(d_{1i}, d_{2i+1})$. The trial terminates when the maximum sample size is reached; the MTD is taken to be the dosage combination that would have been assigned to the next cohort. The initial startup step uses a conventional rule-based procedure such as $3 + 3$ or up-and-down with a particular ordering of the dosage combinations to assure that there never is more than a one-step increase in dosage of either agent or a one-step increase in both. Simulation studies were carried out comparing this approach with the approach described by Wages *et al.* [34–36] and those of Yin and Yuan [40, 41]. The proposed method increased the rates of recommendation of the true MTD combination and decreased the rates of recommendations of toxic dose combinations. The results suggest that the proposed method can be useful for dose finding involving combinations of drugs when there is little or no prior information about the dose–response relationship of combinations.

## 5.5    Designs considering toxicity and efficacy

Hoering *et al.* [12] propose a Phase 1/2 trial design to determine a dose level to carry forward in terms of toxicity and efficacy for cytostatic or targeted agents. A "maximum tolerated dose" is identified using a conventional Phase 1 design (e.g., 3 + 3, ATD, or CRM), and then a Phase 2 design is conducted using three doses: the MTD and the doses next below and above it. The rationale is that standard Phase 1 designs often terminate at a suboptimal dose, and it is worth exploring doses above and below the final Phase 1 dose to provide assurance that doses with better efficacy and acceptable toxicity are not missed. Simulation studies suggest that this strategy improves the probability of successfully identifying a "good" or "best" dose level, often without requiring larger sample sizes.

### 5.5.1    Binary efficacy and toxicity considered jointly

Wang and Day [42] describe a dose-finding approach that combines toxicity and efficacy and selects dose sequences using a simple Bayesian utility function approach. Toxicity and response (efficacy) are assumed to be binary, so that there are four possible outcomes for any patient and four corresponding utilities; the paper explores some alternative choices for utility values. Each patient is assumed to have threshold doses for toxicity and response, and the dose pairs for each patient are assumed to follow a bivariate lognormal distribution. The observation of toxicity following a given dose means that the patient's toxicity threshold was less than the dose, and so on. The probability of any of the four toxicity/efficacy outcomes corresponding to a given dose can be calculated as the probability content corresponding to threshold values above or below the dose. Given the likelihood based on accumulated toxicity/efficacy outcomes, the set of utilities, and a choice of prior, the expected utility of any dose that might be administered to the next patient can be calculated. The "optimal" dose, which will be administered to the next patient, is the dose that provides the largest expected utility. A number of practical issues are addressed via simulation in the paper, including the choice of utility values and priors for the parameters. Compared to the standard 3 + 3 MTD approach, the proposed approach put fewer patients on doses leading to undesirable outcomes. However, it would be interesting to see how the method would compare to strategies that used model-based dosing strategies.

   Dragalin and Fedorov [43] describe an adaptive procedure for dose finding in clinical trials based on binary efficacy and toxicity responses in which the binary endpoint is modeled using Gumbel bivariate logistic regression or a Cox bivariate binary model. The Fisher information matrix is used in either case to define optimum designs (choices of doses). The key idea is the use of penalized locally D-optimal designs (PLDODs) to choose doses. At the start, an up-and-down design (e.g., [44]) is used to get initial information about the relationship between doses and efficacy and toxicity. The maximum likelihood estimates of the parameters of the Cox or Gumbel models are then obtained and the dose for the next patient(s) is determined by means of a penalized adaptive D-optimal design subject to a condition that allocations at more than one step above the maximum tested are not allowed. The process is repeated until the entire suite of patients has been treated. The resulting design has good properties for finding an "optimal" dose and characterizing doses nearby, while avoiding assigning patients to highly toxic doses. The method as described is carried out for individually included patients, but there seems to be no reason why it could not be carried out for cohorts of patients.

Dragalin *et al.* [45] extend the optimal design principle to the problem of finding appropriate doses of combinations of two drugs using binary efficacy and toxicity responses. A bivariate probit model is used in this case to provide a natural measure of correlation. Analytic expressions for the Fisher information matrix are obtained and form the basis of locally optimal minimax, Bayesian, or adaptive designs. The method assumes that the available dose combinations and response variables have been defined, and that there is a known mathematical representation (model) relating the dose–response relationship (that is, the functional form is known but the parameter values need to be estimated from accumulated data). The acceptable dose combinations (design region) are determined to provide at least a minimal probability of efficacy and a maximal probability of toxicity, and an "optimal safe dose" is defined as the dose combination in the dose region that maximizes the probability of achieving a positive efficacy response and not experiencing toxicity. As in [43], an initial cohort of patients provides estimates of the model parameters, and this information is used to determine via the D-optimal design the dosage combination to give to the next patient(s).

Zhong *et al.* [46] extend bivariate binary toxicity/efficacy models described by Braun [47] and by Thall and Cook [48] that use toxicity and efficacy information to determine adaptively the sequences of doses to apply to successive cohorts of patients in Phase 1 cancer trials. The extensions consist of using binary toxicity, efficacy, and surrogate marker information to determine doses. The objective is to be able to use toxicity and surrogate marker information that is available quickly along with incomplete efficacy information to improve the dose-finding algorithm. The joint probabilities of the toxicity, surrogate marker, and efficacy outcomes are expressed as a product of a marginal toxicity probability, and conditional probabilities of an efficacy outcome given the toxicity outcome and a surrogate outcome given the efficacy outcome. The marginal probabilities are assumed to be expressible as logit transformations of simple linear functions of dose. Given target values for the probabilities of efficacy and toxicity that are determined by a clinician, the expected (posterior) probabilities of toxicity and efficacy are determined for each dose after observing a cohort of patients, and a function of the distance between the expected probabilities and the target values is determined, with the application of penalties for overdosing (toxicity) or underdosing (efficacy), and weights to allow for the toxicity and efficacy deviations from target to have different influences on the distance metric. The distance metric then is used to determine adaptively the dose to apply to the next cohort of patients. The dose-selection rule allows for early termination of the trial for toxicity or efficacy. Simulation studies demonstrated that the method can successfully improve dosage targeting efficiency and guard against excess toxicity over a range of true model settings and degrees of surrogacy.

Yin *et al.* [49] describe a two-stage dose-finding procedure for cytostatic agents, whose toxicity may increase with dose, but whose efficacy may not increase monotonically with dose. An algorithmic design (3 + 3 or ATD) is used to find the MTD, and then an "optimal" dose is determined when efficacy is measured in terms of time to event with fractional allocation of information for censored patients by stepping down to identify the dose below the

MTD that gives the "best" efficacy outcome. Simulation studies indicated that the method has "satisfactory" performance.

### 5.5.2    Use of surrogate efficacy outcomes

Efficacy outcomes may take a long time to observe and may require confirmation, which may not be practical in the context of Phase 1 trials that usually have relatively short observation periods. In this situation, quickly observed unconfirmed surrogate efficacy outcomes can be used in place of objective responses that take a long time to be observed to determine doses in Phase 1 trials that balance toxicity and efficacy satisfactorily [50]. Let $Y_{ei}$ denote the value of the "true" efficacy response for the $i$th subject, and let $S_{ei}$ denote the value of the surrogate response. The recommendation is to replace $Y_{ei}$ in the likelihood function with a modified quantity $\widetilde{Y}_{ei}$ that is equal to $c_0$ if $S_{ei} = 0$ and $Y_{ei}$ is unknown, or $c_1$ if $S_{ei} = 1$ and $Y_{ei}$ is unknown, or $Y_{ei}$ if $Y_{ei}$ is known. The recommended values for the constants are $c_0 = 0.25$ and $c_1 = 0.75$. Other values were studied, but simulation studies indicated that these choices seemed to provide dose selections most like what would have been obtained if all of the $Y_{ei}$ were known; in fact, the probabilities associated with the recommended doses were nearly the same.

### 5.5.3    Reduction of efficacy and toxicity outcomes to ordered categories

Zhang *et al.* [51] describe a modified CRM incorporating efficacy and toxicity responses in terms of three categories: (i) no efficacy, no toxicity; (ii) efficacy, acceptable or no toxicity; and (iii) toxicity, so that the responses follow a trinomial distribution. The design is a variation of an approach described by Thall and Russell [52]. The probabilities of these categories are related to dosage ($d$) by simple linear logistic (continuation ratio, CR) models. If $\psi_0 = \Pr(\text{no eff, no tox})$, $\psi_2 = \Pr(\text{tox})$, and $\psi_1 = \Pr(\text{eff, no tox})$, then $\text{logit}(\psi_2) = \alpha_2 + \beta_2 d$ and $\log(\psi_1/\psi_0) = \alpha_1 + \beta_1 d = \alpha_2 + \mu$. This formulation implies that $\psi_0$ is a monotone decreasing function of dose and that $\psi_2$ is a monotone increasing function of dose, that is, that the probability that nothing happens decreases with dose, and the probability that something happens increases with dose. The parameters are collected as $\theta = (\theta_1, \theta_2)$, where $\theta_1 = (\mu, \beta_1)$ and $\theta_2 = (\alpha_2, \beta_2)$, for convenience in the two-step estimation used in the paper. Prior distributions are needed for the parameters, and the paper uses independent uniform priors. The dosing strategy proceeds in a stagewise manner as follows, assuming that cohorts of $c$ patients are treated at each stage. The first cohort is treated at the lowest dose and the means of the joint posterior distribution of the parameters are obtained. These quantities are used to calculate the posterior expectations of $\psi_0$, $\psi_1$, and $\psi_2$. If the expected value of $\psi_2$ exceeds some maximum acceptable toxicity level ($\pi_0$) for the lowest dose, then the trial stops because the monotonicity of $\psi_2$ implies that no dose will lead to acceptably low toxicity; if the expected value of $\psi_2$ for the current dose (but not for the lowest dose) exceeds $\pi_0$, then the next cohort receives the next lowest dose level. Otherwise, if $\psi_2 \leq \pi_0$ for the current dose and $C$ denotes the set of doses with expected values of $\psi_2 \leq \pi_0$, then find the dose $d^*$ such that the expected value of $\delta = \psi_1 - \lambda\psi_2$ is the largest among the doses in $C$ and assign the next cohort of patients to $d^*$. The quantity $\lambda$ allows for tempering the probabilities of efficacy with probabilities of safety; the paper considers $\lambda = 0$ (no tempering) and $\lambda = 1$ (net improvement of efficacy over safety). Termination of the trial occurs when (i) at least $n_1$ patients are treated and at least $m$ have been treated at the currently recommended dosage level, (ii) at most $n_2$ subjects have been treated, or (iii) the expected value of $\psi_2$ exceeds $\pi_0$ at the lowest dosage. (Note: an interesting question in this context would be whether some other strategy for picking the next dose would be sensible, for example randomly picking from the collection, especially if the values of $\delta$ do not vary greatly among the doses.) Simulation studies were carried out for a variety of scenarios, that is, patterns of probabilities of efficacy or toxicity as functions of dosage. The simulations compared the proposed methods with a variation of the proposed method using values of $\psi_0$, $\psi_1$, and $\psi_2$ calculated using the proportional odds (PO) model employed by Thall and Russell [52]. The approach using the CR model described in this paper generally performed similarly to the approach using the PO model with respect to the proportion of times a dose was correctly identified as the "best" dose and the percentage of subjects treated at that dose level, although there were a few scenarios where the performance was better by at least 10 percentage points.

Mandrekar *et al.* [53] reviewed model-based approaches for dose finding, with a focus on designs placing binary efficacy and toxicity findings into one of three categories – no dose-limiting toxicity or efficacy, efficacy without dose-limiting toxicity, and dose-limiting toxicity – so that the likelihood for the observations is a trinomial distribution. The probabilities of this distribution are related to the dosage(s) by simple linear regressions in the context of either a PO model [52] or a CR model [51]. A trial is carried out using a basic continual reassessment plan in which the dose assigned to a cohort of patients depends on the information about toxicity and efficacy accumulated from the experience of previous cohorts; the calculations usually are based on a Bayesian approach that provides posterior distributions of the probabilities in the trivariate model. Two approaches use similar, but not identical, metrics for making the dose selection. The first is based on the posterior probability that the risk of dose-limiting toxicity for a patient is acceptably low, and the posterior probability that the likelihood of demonstrating efficacy is sufficiently high [52]. The second is based on whether the posterior expectation of the risk of dose-limiting toxicity is acceptably low, and on a penalized difference between the posterior expectations of the probability of demonstrating efficacy and the probability of dose-limiting toxicity [51, 54]. The authors conclude that although the simulation studies demonstrate at least theoretically that these model-based designs have considerable promise for identifying optimal doses, the evidence to date suggests that their penetration into routine clinical practice has been very limited [4, 5]. A number of pragmatic issues impede their routine use in practice, namely, lack of familiarity of clinicians and statisticians with the designs, fear of "black-box" decision-making of model-based rather than rule-based designs, potential loss of control of the data and the decision as to where to treat the next cohort of patients, fear of regulatory acceptance, and, possibly most importantly, resistance to change and reluctance to be the first to try something new.

### 5.5.4    Binary toxicity and continuous efficacy

Hirakawa [55] describes a Bayesian strategy for determining recommended doses from Phase 1 trials based on continuous efficacy measurements and binary toxicity observations. The probability of toxicity at dose $d$ is assumed to be a simple logistic function of dose, $\text{logit}(p_{(d)}) = a_0 + b_0 d$. The distribution of the efficacy measurement is assumed to be normal with a mean that depends on whether a patient given dose $d$ experienced toxicity or not. The mean is the sum of a four-parameter logistic model (conventional $E_{\max}$ model) and a multiple of the square of the difference between $p_{(d)}$ and a 0–1 variable indicating the absence or presence of toxicity. An extension of the model to accommodate a two-component combination therapy also is provided. A Bayesian approach is used with updating of the posterior distributions of the parameters as data accumulate. An indicator variable, $T(d)$, takes the value 1 if both the posterior mean of the efficacy measurement and the posterior probability of toxicity at dose $d$ have acceptable values, or 0 if not. For the set of doses for which $T(d) = 1$, the posterior distribution of the weighted Mahalanobis distance between the observed mean efficacy and probability of toxicity and their optimal value is determined, and the next dose to be administered is the one with the least posterior expected distance. A variety of simulation studies demonstrated that the "true" recommended dose was recommended more often by the proposed procedure than by the procedure described by Bekele and Shen [56] when the true recommended dose was relatively at the tail end among the tested doses, and was similar when the true recommended dose was relatively at the top end.

### 5.5.5 Time to occurrence of binary toxicity and efficacy endpoints

Traditional Phase 1 and Phase 2 dose-finding trials that incorporate both efficacy and toxicity usually assume that efficacy and toxicity are expressed as binary outcomes, without regard to when they occur after dosing, which may be important expressions of either effect. While this makes designs simple and easily implemented, there are at least three disadvantages. Firstly, when an event occurs may be important clinically: lowering toxicity risk is important, but so can be delaying the onset of toxicity. Secondly, waiting until sufficient information has been obtained from a cohort to provide guidance as to the treatment to assign to the next cohort may necessitate suspending a trial if accrual is rapid and the time required to observe efficacy or toxicity is long, which wastes resources and could unduly prolong a trial. Thirdly, moving to successive cohorts before obtaining complete information could lead to underestimation of both the toxicity and efficacy rates of a dosage and thereby cause excessive exposure to toxic doses or inappropriate early termination of a dosage or trial. Yuan and Yin [57] propose to address this problem by using models for the time to occurrence of toxicity and the time to occurrence of efficacy, both of which are binary responses. Toxicity time is modeled by a proportional hazard model [58] with the baseline hazard modeled using a Weibull distribution. Time to efficacy is modeled using a mixture cure rate model that allows for a proportion of the patients to be refractory to cure (i.e., never experience efficacy) [59]. The metric for selection of doses is the ratio of the areas under the survival curves for the occurrence of efficacy and toxicity, denoted by AUSC, between the initiation of treatment and some fixed time $T$ (e.g., the time by when a clinician would expect to see some evidence of effect). The survival curve for toxicity is denoted by $S_T(t|Z)$, so that the probability of the occurrence of toxicity by time $t$ is $1 - S_T(t|Z)$, where $Z$ denotes the covariate corresponding to the dose received. The survival curve for efficacy by time $t$, accounting for possible inability to demonstrate efficacy, is denoted by $S_E^*(t|Z)$. The likelihood for the trial is multinomial with probabilities that depend on the joint distribution of the efficacy and toxicity times, which uses a bivariate model due to Clayton [60]. For a typical trial, suppose that $J$ doses are to be considered and that every $M$ months a new cohort is to be entered into the trial ($M \leq T$). The first cohort receives the lowest dose, $d_1$. Following an essentially rule-based startup process, dosage assignments to subsequent cohorts proceed as follows. The $k$th cohort will be ready to initiate treatment after $k - 1$ cohorts have been treated, which will be at time $kM$ after the start of the trial. Let $d_h$ denote the highest dose tried at that point, $p_{max}$ the maximum acceptable probability of toxicity, and $q_{min}$ the minimum acceptable probability of demonstration of efficacy; $p_{max}$ and $q_{min}$ are determined on clinical grounds. Given the findings from the $k - 1$ cohorts entered so far, the dose level to be assigned to the $k$th cohort is determined by the following rule. If the posterior probability corresponding to the event "predicted probability of a toxic event by time $T$ is less than $p_{\max}$" is sufficiently high, say 0.85, then the $k$th cohort will receive dose $d_{h+1}$ (or dose $d_J$ if $h = J$). If the posterior probability is not sufficiently high, then a set $D$ of the doses so far considered for which the probability of the statement regarding toxicity still is high (greater than $p^*$, say, but less than 0.85) and the posterior probability of the statement "predicted probability of observing efficacy by time $T$ is greater than $q_{\min}$" is sufficiently high (greater than $q^*$, say). The trial is terminated if this set is empty. Otherwise, the $k$th cohort will be treated at the dose in $D$ for which the AUSC ratio is largest. On reaching the maximum sample size, the recommended dose will be the one from the current set $D$ that has the largest AUSC ratio. Simulations were carried out for a variety of scenarios and various assumptions about the hazard functions for toxicity and efficacy. In scenarios corresponding to the common situations of increasing toxicity and efficacy with dose, the proposed design always selected the target (correct) dose at least 67% of the time and had most of the patients at the target dose. These values were similar for the binary-only design, but the proposed design eliminated accrual suppression and had materially shorter total trial durations. The method also performed well in situations where toxicity suddenly increased with a modest increase in dosage, and where the correct dosage was at the beginning or the end of the collection of doses, and also where none of the dosages was effective or all were toxic. A minor tradeoff for the substantial savings in development times was a tendency for the proposed method to escalate the dose more aggressively and to treat more patients at toxic doses. However, if accrual is too rapid and too many observations are censored at the observation time, accrual could be suspended temporarily to observe more events.

### 5.5.6  Determining dosage and treatment schedule

Li *et al.* [61] describe a Bayesian approach for determining an optimum combination of dose and administration schedule using dose-schedule-finding trials that differ from conventional dose-finding trials in that they are aimed at finding a combination of dose and treatment schedule that has a large probability of efficacy yet a relatively small probability of toxicity. The key difference is that while the toxicity probabilities follow a simple non-decreasing order in dose-finding trials, the probabilities in dose-schedule-finding trials may adhere to a matrix order. The model assumes $D$ doses, each of which can be administered according to one of two schedules; the pair $(j, k)$ corresponds to dose $j$ administered according to schedule $k(j = 1, \ldots, D; k = 1, 2)$, and $(1,1)$ corresponds to the lowest dose under schedule 1. Suppose that $n_{jk}$ subjects have currently been treated at regimen $(j, k)$; let $X_{ijk}$ denote the binary toxicity outcome, and let $Y_{ijk}$ denote the binary efficacy outcome, for subject $i(i = 1, \ldots, n_{jk})$ receiving regimen $(j, k)$. Suppose that the marginal outcome probabilities are $\Pr(X_{ijk} = 1) = p_{jk}$ and $\Pr(Y_{ijk} = 1) = q_{jk}$, with corresponding logits $\mu_{jk} = \text{logit}(p_{jk})$ and $\gamma_{jk} = \text{logit}(q_{jk})$, that $\pi_{xy}^{(jk)} = \Pr(X_{ijk} = x, Y_{ijk} = y)(x, y = 0, 1)$ denote the joint outcome probabilities, and that the association between the toxicity and efficacy outcomes for regimen $(j, k)$ is expressed by the cross-product ratio $\theta_{jk} = \pi_{00}^{(jk)} \pi_{11}^{(jk)} / \pi_{01}^{(jk)} \pi_{10}^{(jk)}$. The individual joint outcome probabilities $\pi_{xy}^{(jk)}$ can be expressed in terms of the marginal probabilities and the cross-product ratio, so that the likelihood of trial outcomes corresponding to regimen $(j, k)$ can be expressed as a product of multivariate Bernoulli probability functions. The logits $\mu_{jk}$ and $\gamma_{jk}$ and the logarithm of $\theta_{jk}$ are assumed to have vague normal prior distributions.

Let $h_k$ denote the highest tried dose under schedule $k$ (0 if no dose has been tried), and start with $(1, 1)$ so $h_1 \geq 1$ and $h_2 \geq 0$. At any stage of the trial, denote by $\boldsymbol{\mu}^{(h_1,h_2)}$, $\boldsymbol{\gamma}^{(h_1,h_2)}$, and $\boldsymbol{\theta}^{(h_1,h_2)}$

the vectors of $\mu_{jk}$, $\gamma_{jk}$, and $\theta_{jk}$ values corresponding to dose–schedule combinations that have currently been tried. The objective is to make order-restricted inferences on $\boldsymbol{\mu}$. The marginal toxicity probabilities ($p_{jk}$) and their corresponding logits ($\mu_{jk}$) are assumed to be partially ordered, $\mu_{jk} \leq \mu_{j+1,k}$ and $\mu_{jk} \leq \mu_{j,k+1}$. Let $C = \{(j,k) : j = 1, \ldots, h_k, k = 1, 2\}$ denote the set of all dose–schedule combinations that have been tried, and define an ordering relation $\alpha$ on $C$ by $(j,k)\alpha(j',k')$ if $j \leq j'$ and $k \leq k'$. Directly sampling values $\widetilde{\boldsymbol{\mu}}$ of $\boldsymbol{\mu}$ from its posterior distribution can yield values that do not satisfy the partial ordering requirement; values $\widetilde{\boldsymbol{\mu}}^*$ that do satisfy the requirement can be obtained via isotonic regression, where the elements of $\widetilde{\boldsymbol{\mu}}^*$ minimize the weighted sum of squares $\sum_{(j,k)\in C} w_{jk}(\widetilde{\mu}_{jk} - \widetilde{\mu}_{jk}^*)^2$ subject to the constraint $\widetilde{\mu}_{jk}^* \leq \widetilde{\mu}_{j'k'}^*$ whenever $(j,k)\alpha(j',k')$; the weights $w_{jk}$ are taken to be the posterior precisions of the $\mu_{jk}$ values. The paper outlines the computational details. The order-restricted posterior samples of the $p_{jk}$ probabilities are obtained from the corresponding elements of $\widetilde{\mu}_{jk}^*$; the posterior samples of the $q_{jk}$ and $\theta_{jk}$ values are not order-restricted and can be obtained directly by sampling from their posterior distributions. The first step of the dose–schedule algorithm is the definition on clinical grounds of an upper bound $p_{max}$ on the toxicity probabilities and a lower bound $q_{min}$ on the efficacy probabilities. The algorithm seeks to identify at the end of the trial the dose–schedule combination that maximizes the posterior probability of the event $\{p_{jk} \leq p_{max}, q_{jk} \geq q_{min}\}$ given the data. Dose–schedule combinations can have negligible, acceptable, or unacceptable toxicity accordingly as the posterior probability that $p_{jk} \leq p_{max}$ exceeds $P_n$, is between $P_a$ and $P_n(P_a < P_n)$, or is less than $P_a$. In addition, a dose–schedule combination has *acceptable efficacy* if the posterior probability that $q_{jk} \geq q_{min}$ exceeds a small cutoff value $Q$. A dose–schedule combination is *acceptable* if its efficacy is acceptable and its toxicity is negligible or acceptable. At any stage of the trial, let $A$ denote the set of dose–schedule combinations that have been found so far. The posterior means of $p_{jk}$ (calculated from isotonic regression) and of $q_{jk}$ and $\theta_{jk}$ are available, from which estimates of the joint probabilities $\pi_{xy}^{(jk)}$ can be obtained; large values of $\pi_{01}^{(jk)}$, the probability of acceptable efficacy and negligible toxicity, are desirable. The first cohort of patients is treated at $(1, 1)$. If $(1, 1)$ has unacceptable toxicity, then the trial is terminated and no more patients are treated. If $(1, 1)$ has negligible toxicity, then the next cohort of patients is treated at $(1, 2)$. Recall that $h_k$ denotes the highest dose tested at schedule $k$. When $h_1 < D$ and $h_2 < D(D = $ index of maximum dose), then (i) if both $(h_1, 1)$ and $(h_2, 2)$ have negligible toxicity, the next cohort of patients is treated at $(h_1 + 1, 1)$ or $(h_2 + 1, 2)$ depending on which of the posterior probabilities that the toxicity for that regimen is less than $p_{max}$ is larger; (ii) if only one of $(h_1, 1)$ and $(h_2, 2)$ has negligible toxicity, then the next cohort of patients is treated at $(h_k + 1, k)$ where $k$ corresponds to the regimen with negligible toxicity; and (iii) if neither $(h_1, 1)$ nor $(h_2, 2)$ has negligible toxicity, then the next cohort of patients is treated at the dose–schedule combination in $A$ with the largest estimated value of $\pi_{01}^{(jk)}$. When $h_1 = D$ and $h_2 < D$, then the next cohort of patients is treated at $(h_2 + 1, 2)$ if $(h_2, 2)$ has negligible toxicity; otherwise (or if $h_2 = D$), the next cohort of patients is treated at the dose–schedule combination in $A$ with the largest estimated value of $\pi_{01}^{(jk)}$. The trial is terminated in either case if $A$ is empty. The algorithm will not allow treating a patient with a dose under schedule 2 that has not been found acceptable under schedule 1. Simulations comparing the proposed procedure with alternative designs over a number of scenarios found similar probabilities of selecting the correct dose and overall toxicity rates. However, the proposed procedure had more patients treated at the correct (target) dose–schedule combinations and slightly higher overall efficacy rates.

## 5.6   Combinations of active agents

Mandrekar *et al.* [54] extend the trivariate strategy of [51] to the case where the treatment consists of two agents whose doses could be adjusted separately. The same three categories of response (no efficacy, no toxicity; efficacy, acceptable or no toxicity; toxicity) are considered. The probabilities of these categories are related to the dosages of the combination therapy of two agents $d = \{d_1, d_2\}$ by simple linear logistic (CR) models. If $\psi_0 = \Pr\Pr(\text{no eff, no tox})$, $\psi_2 = \Pr(\text{tox})$, and $\psi_1 = \Pr(\text{eff, no tox})$, then $\text{logit}(\psi_2) = \alpha_2 + \beta_2 d_1 + \beta_4 d_2$ and $\log(\psi_1/\psi_0) = \alpha_1 + \beta_1 d_1 + \beta_3 d_2$. These equations can be solved for $\psi_0$, $\psi_1$, and $\psi_2$ as functions of $d_1$ and $d_2$ and the elements of the parameter vector $\boldsymbol{\theta} = (\alpha_1, \alpha_2, \beta_1, \beta_2, \beta_3, \beta_4)$, so that the probability of one of the three outcomes can be determined for any dose combination. Two decision functions are defined, $\delta_1(d; \boldsymbol{\theta}) = 1$ if $\psi_2(d; \boldsymbol{\theta}) < p_{\max}$, where $p_{\max}$ denotes a maximum acceptable risk of toxicity, and 0 otherwise; and $\psi_{1\max}(\boldsymbol{\theta}) = $ the maximum value of $\psi_1(d; \boldsymbol{\theta})$ among the set of acceptable doses $d$. A trial could be conducted as follows. Suppose that $d^{(1)}$ denotes the lowest combination dose level deemed safe enough be tested in combination; the doses $(d_{1a}, d_{2b})$ in $d^{(1)}$ do not both have to be at their lowest values for the two agents. Start by assigning cohorts of size $k$ to the three lowest levels of the combination, $(d_{1a}, d_{1b}), (d_{1,a+1}, d_{1b}), (d_{1a}, d_{1,b+1})$. Given the accumulated toxicity and efficacy responses at any stage of the process, update the posterior means of the elements of $\boldsymbol{\theta}$, and calculate $\delta(d; \boldsymbol{\theta})$ for each dosage combination and, for the dosage combinations for which $\delta_1(d; \boldsymbol{\theta}) = 1$, calculate $\psi_{1\max}(\boldsymbol{\theta})$ with respect to this set of dosage combinations.

## 5.7   Software

Table 5.1 lists some readily available free software for carrying out the calculations required by various Phase 1 designs. Software for calculations for some methods can be obtained upon request from the authors of publications describing the methods.

## 5.8   Discussion

The main goal of Phase 1 trials, especially those of anticancer drugs, is to determine the dose or doses to carry forward into Phase 2. This chapter has outlined a number of approaches that have been, and could be, used to determine the MTD to be carried forward, and has provided links to software for carrying out the necessary calculations. Determination of the MTD is critical in the development of oncologic drugs and drug combinations, but is of relevance for other therapeutic areas as well, even though drugs in those areas do not manifest their effects through their toxicities.

Even though there is abundant evidence from a variety of studies that appropriate dosages can be determined more efficiently and effectively by designs other than conventional rule-based designs such as the $3 + 3$ designs, these potentially more effective designs have made little penetration in the past [2–5]. A number of considerations may account for the poor penetration of better designs, including lack of familiarity of clinicians and statisticians with the designs, fear of "black-box" decision-making of model-based rather than rule-based designs, potential loss of control of the data and the decision as to where to treat the next

**Table 5.1**    Software for Phase 1 design calculations.

A. Software packages available for R [62]

| | |
|---|---|
| bcrm (Bayesian CRM designs) [63] | Implements a wide variety of one- and two-parameter Bayesian CRM designs. The program can run interactively to enter outcomes after each cohort has been recruited, or via simulation to assess operating characteristics |
| dfcrm (Dose Finding by CRM) [64] | Functions to run the CRM and time-to-event CRM in Phase 1 trials and calibration tools for trial planning purposes |
| CRM [16] | CRM simulator for clinical trials |
| TEQR (Target EQuivalence Range) [26] | Frequentist implementation of the modified toxicity probability interval (mTPI) design and a competitor to the standard $3 + 3$ design $(3 + 3)$ |

B. Programs available from MD Anderson (the websites corresponding to the individual URLs provide documentation and links to publications describing the methods. Substitute biostatistics.mdanderson.org/SoftwareDownload/SingleSoftware.aspx for Q in the URLs)

| Function | URL |
|---|---|
| Optimal interval design | https://Q?Software_Id=91 |
| Bayesian model averaging CRM | https://Q?Software_Id=81 |
| Toxicity probability intervals | https://Q?Software_Id=72 |
| Parallel Phase 1/2 clinical trial design | https://Q?Software_Id=85 |
| Dose schedule finder | https://Q?Software_Id=75 |
| Monitoring late onset toxicities | https://Q?Software_Id=69 |
| CRM simulator | https://Q?Software_Id=13 |
| Two-agent toxicity-based dose finder | https://Q?Software_Id=14 |
| Bivariate CRM | https://Q?Software_Id=15 |

cohort of patients, fear of regulatory acceptance, and, possibly most importantly, resistance to change and reluctance to be the first to try something new [53].

Regardless of how it is determined, the MTD determined in Phase 1 trials may be excessive. A retrospective study that considered the relationship of various doses to toxicities of various grades occurring after the first cycle of administration in Phase 1 dose-finding trials found that moderate and severe toxicities occurred regularly after the first cycle in the trials, so that the dose to carry forward to Phase 2 may not be the MTD found after the first cycle of administration [65].

# References

[1] Zohar, S. and O'Quigley, J. (2009) Sensitivity of dose-finding studies to observation errors. *Contemporary Clinical Trials*, **30**, 523–530.

[2] Jaki, T. (2013) Uptake of novel statistical methods for early-phase clinical studies in the UK public sector. *Clinical Trials*, **10**, 344–346.

[3] Le Tourneau, C., Dieras, V., Tresca, P. *et al.* (2010) Current challenges for the early clinical development of anticancer drugs in the era of molecularly targeted agents. *Targeted Oncology*, **5**, 65–72.

[4] Rogatko, A., Schoeneck, D., Jonas, W. *et al.* (2007) Translation of innovative designs into phase I trials. *Journal of Clinical Oncology*, **25**, 4982–4986.

[5] Zohar, S. and Chevret, S. (2007) Recent developments in adaptive designs for phase I/II dose-finding studies. *Journal of Biopharmaceutical Statistics*, **17**, 1071–1083.

[6] Jaki, T., Clive, S. and Weir, C.J. (2013) Principles of dose finding studies in cancer: a comparison of trial designs. *Cancer Chemotherapy and Pharmacology*, **71**, 1107–1114.

[7] Adamina, M. and Joerger, M. (2011) Dose-toxicity models in oncology. *Expert Opinion on Drug Metabolism & Toxicology*, **7**, 201–211.

[8] Ananthakrishnan, R. and Menon, S. (2013) Design of oncology clinical trials: a review. *Clinical Reviews in Oncology/Hematology*, **88**, 144–153.

[9] Brunetto, A.T., Kristeleit, R.S. and de Bono, J.S. (2010) Early oncology clinical trial design in the era of molecular-targeted agents. *Future Oncology*, **6**, 1339–1352.

[10] Garrett-Moyer, E. (2006) The continual reassessment method for dose-finding studies: a tutorial. *Clinical Trials*, **3**, 57–71.

[11] Guan, S.H. (2012) Statistical designs for early phases of cancer clinical trials. *Journal of Biopharmaceutical Statistics*, **22**, 1109–1126.

[12] Hoering, A., Mitchell, A., LeBlanc, M. and Crowley, J. (2013) Early phase trial design for assessing several dose levels for toxicity and efficacy for targeted agents. *Clinical Trials*, **10**, 422–429.

[13] Le Tourneau, C., Lee, J.J. and Siu, L.L. (2009) Dose escalation methods in phase I cancer clinical trials. *Journal of the National Cancer Institute*, **101**, 708–720.

[14] Le Tourneau, C., Gan, H.K., Razak, A.R.A. and Paoletti, X. (2012) Efficiency of new dose escalation designs in dose-finding phase I trials of molecularly targeted agents. *PLoS One*, **7**, e51039.

[15] Morabito, A., Di Maio, M., De Maio, E. *et al.* (2006) Methodology of clinical trials with new molecular-targeted agents: where do we stand? *Annals of Oncology*, **17**, VII128–VII131.

[16] O'Quigley, J., Pepe, M.S. and Fisher, L. (1990) Continual reassessment method: a practical design for phase-1 clinical trials in cancer. *Biometrics*, **46**, 33–48.

[17] Surnan, V.J., Dueck, A. and Sargent, D.J. (2008) Clinical trials of novel and targeted therapies: endpoints, trial design, and analysis. *Cancer Investigation*, **26**, 439–444.

[18] Simon, R.M., Freidlin, B., Rubinstein, L.V. *et al.* (1997) Accelerated titration designs for phase I clinical trials in oncology. *Journal of the National Cancer Institute*, **89**, 1138–1147.

[19] Gezmu, M. and Flournoy, N. (2006) Group up-and-down designs for dose finding. *Journal of Statistical Planning and Inference*, **136**, 1749–1764.

[20] Liu, S.Y., Cai, C.Y. and Ning, J. (2013) Up-and-down designs for phase I clinical trials. *Contemporary Clinical Trials*, **36**, 218–227.

[21] Ivanova, A., Flournoy, N. and Chung, Y.S. (2007) Cumulative cohort design for dose-finding. *Journal of Statistical Planning and Inference*, **137**, 2316–2327.

[22] Ji, Y., Li, Y. and Bekele, B.N. (2007) Dose-finding in phase I clinical trials based on toxicity probability intervals. *Clinical Trials*, **4**, 235–244.

[23] Ji, Y.A., Liu, P., Li, Y.S. and Bekele, B.N. (2010) A modified toxicity probability interval method for dose-finding trials. *Clinical Trials*, **7**, 653–663.

[24] Ji, Y. and Herrick, R. (2012) Toxicity Probability Intervals, https://biostatistics.mdanderson.org/SoftwareDownloadSingleSoftware.aspx?Software_Id=72, 2012.

[25] Ji, Y. and Wang, S.J. (2013) Modified toxicity probability interval design: a safer and more reliable method than the 3+3 design for practical phase I trials. *Journal of Clinical Oncology*, **31**, 1785–1791.

[26] Blanchard, M.S. and Longmate, J.A. (2011) Toxicity equivalence range design (TEQR): a practical phase I design. *Contemporary Clinical Trials*, **32**, 114–121.

[27] Ji, Y., Feng, L., Liu, P. *et al.* (2012) Bayesian continual reassessment method for dose-finding trials infusing T cells with limited sample size. *Journal of Biopharmaceutical Statistics*, **22**, 1206–1219.

[28] Yuan, Y. and Yin, G. (2010) Bayesian hybrid dose-finding design in phase I oncology clinical trials. *Statistics in Medicine*, **30**, 2098–2108.

[29] Iasonos, A., Wilton, A.S., Riedel, E.R. *et al.* (2008) A comprehensive comparison of the continual reassessment method to the standard 3+3 dose escalation scheme in phase I dose-finding studies. *Clinical Trials*, **5**, 465–477.

[30] Oron, A.P. and Hoff, P.D. (2013) Small-sample behavior of novel phase I cancer trial designs. *Clinical Trials*, **10**, 63–80.

[31] Azriel, D., Mandel, M. and Rinott, Y. (2011) The treatment versus experimentation dilemma in dose finding studies. *Journal of Statistical Planning and Inference*, **141**, 2759–2768.

[32] Carlin, B.P., Zhong, W. and Koopmeiners, J.S. (2013) Discussion of 'Small-sample behavior of novel phase I cancer trial designs' by Assaf P Oron and Peter D Huff. *Clinical Trials*, **10**, 81–85.

[33] Cheung, Y.K. (2013) Commentary on 'Small-sample behavior of novel phase I cancer trial designs'. *Clinical Trials*, **10**, 86–87.

[34] Wages, N.A., Conaway, M.R. and O'Quigley, J. (2011) Dose-finding design for multi-drug combinations. *Clinical Trials*, **8**, 380–389.

[35] Wages, N.A. and Conaway, M.R. (2013) Specifications of a continual reassessment method design for phase I trials of combined drugs. *Pharmaceutical Statistics*, **12**, 217–224.

[36] Wages, N.A., Conaway, M.R. and O'Quigley, J. (2011) Continual reassessment method for partial ordering. *Biometrics*, **67**, 1555–1563.

[37] Hirakawa, A., Hamada, C. and Matsui, S. (2013) A dose-finding approach based on shrunken predictive probability for combinations of two agents in phase I trials. *Statistics in Medicine*, **32**, 4515–4525.

[38] Copas, J.B. (1983) Regression, prediction and shrinkage. *Journal of the Royal Statistical Society, Series B*, **48**, 311–354.

[39] Copas, J.B. (1997) Using regression models for prediction: shrinkage and regression to the mean. *Statistical Methods in Medical Research*, **6**, 167–183.

[40] Yin, G. and Yuan, Y. (2009) A latent contingency table approach to dose finding for combinations of two agents. *Biometrics*, **65**, 866–875.

[41] Yin, G. and Yuan, Y. (2009) Bayesian dose finding for drug combinations by copula regression. *Applied Statistics*, **58**, 211–224.

[42] Wang, D.L. and Day, R. (2010) Adaptive Bayesian design for Phase I dose-finding trials using a joint model of response and toxicity. *Journal of Biopharmaceutical Statistics*, **20**, 125–144.

[43] Dragalin, V. and Fedorov, V. (2006) Adaptive designs for dose-finding based on efficacy-toxicity response. *Journal of Statistical Planning and Inference*, **136**, 1800–1823.

[44] Ivanova, A. (2003) A new dose-finding design for bivariate outcomes. *Biometrics*, **59**, 1001–1007.

[45] Dragalin, V., Fedorov, V. and Wu, Y. (2008) Adaptive designs for selecting drug combinations based on efficacy-toxicity response. *Journal of Statistical Planning and Inference*, **138**, 352–373.

[46] Zhong, W., Koopmeiners, J.S. and Carlin, B.P. (2012) A trivariate continual reassessment method for phase I/II trials of toxicity, efficacy, and surrogate efficacy. *Statistics in Medicine*, **31**, 3885–3895.

[47] Braun, T.A. (2002) The bivariate continual reassessment method: extending the CRM to phase I trials of two competing outcomes. *Controlled Clinical Trials*, **23**, 240–256.

[48] Thall, P.F. and Cook, J.D. (2004) Dose-finding based on efficacy-toxicity trade-offs. *Biometrics*, **60**, 684–693.

[49] Yin, G.S., Zheng, S.R. and Xu, J.J. (2013) Two-stage dose finding for cytostatic agents in phase I oncology trials. *Statistics in Medicine*, **32**, 644–660.

[50] Asakawa, T. and Hamada, C. (2013) A pragmatic dose-finding approach using short-term surrogate efficacy outcomes to evaluate binary efficacy and toxicity outcomes in phase I cancer clinical trials. *Pharmaceutical Statistics*, **12**, 315–327.

[51] Zhang, W., Sargent, D.J. and Mandrekar, S. (2006) An adaptive dose-finding design incorporating both toxicity and efficacy. *Statistics in Medicine*, **25**, 2365–2383.

[52] Thall, P.F. and Russell, K.E. (1998) A strategy for dose-finding and safety monitoring based on efficacy and adverse outcomes in phase I/II clinical trials. *Biometrics*, **54**, 251–264.

[53] Mandrekar, S.J., Qin, R. and Sargent, D.J. (2010) Model-based phase I designs incorporating toxicity and efficacy for single and dual agent drug combinations: Methods and challenges. *Statistics in Medicine*, **29**, 1077–1083.

[54] Mandrekar, S.J., Cui, Y. and Sargent, D.J. (2007) An adaptive phase I design for identifying a biologically optimal dose for dual agent drug combinations. *Statistics in Medicine*, **26**, 2317–2330.

[55] Hirakawa, A. (2012) An adaptive dose-finding approach for correlated bivariate binary and continuous outcomes in phase I oncology trials. *Statistics in Medicine*, **31**, 516–532.

[56] Bekele, B.N. and Shen, Y. (2005) A Bayesian approach to jointly modeling toxicity and biomarker expression in a phase I/II dose-finding trial. *Biometrics*, **61**, 344–354.

[57] Yuan, Y. and Yin, G. (2009) Bayesian dose finding by jointly modelling toxicity and efficacy as time-to-event outcomes. *Applied Statistics*, **58**, 719–736.

[58] Cox, D.R. (1972) Regression models and life tables (with discussion). *Journal of the Royal Statistical Society, Series B*, **34**, 187–220.

[59] Berkson, J. and Gage, R.P. (1952) Survival curve for cancer patients following treatment. *Journal of the American Statistical Association*, **47**, 501–515.

[60] Clayton, D.G. (1978) A model for association in bivariate life tables and its application in epidemiological studies of familial tendency in chronic disease incidence. *Biometrika*, **65**, 141–151.

[61] Li, Y.S., Bekele, B.N., Ji, Y. and Cook, J.D. (2008) Dose-schedule finding in phase I/II clinical trials using a Bayesian isotonic transformation. *Statistics in Medicine*, **27**, 4895–4913.

[62] R Development Core Team (2006) *R: A Language and Environment for Statistical Computing*, R Foundation for Statistical Computing, Vienna, http://www.R-project.org (accessed 24 June 2014).

[63] Sweeting M., Mander A., Sabin T. bcrm: Bayesian continual reassessment method designs for Phase I dose-finding trials. *Journal of Statistical Software* 2013; **54**, 1–26

[64] Cheung, Y.K. (2011) *Dose Finding by the Continual Reassessment Method*, Taylor & Francis, Boca Raton, FL.

[65] Postel-Vinay, S., Gomez-Roca, C., Molife, L.R. *et al.* (2011) Phase I trials of molecularly targeted agents: should we pay more attention to late toxicities? *Journal of Clinical Oncology*, **29**, 1728–1735.

# 6

# Summarizing adverse event risk

## A. Lawrence Gould
*Merck Research Laboratories, 770 Sumneytown Pike, West Point, PA 19486, USA*

## 6.1    Introduction

The analysis of adverse event frequency from clinical development projects includes summarization of important features of the occurrence of adverse events such as how often they occur, when they emerge, how often they recur, and how severely they are manifested. Comparisons of risks among treatment groups clearly are an essential part of this evaluation, particularly as expressed by confidence or credible intervals for measures of difference between or relative risk of adverse event occurrences among treatment groups.

Risk difference can be assessed by constructing confidence intervals separately for each event, ignoring the number of events for which the calculation is carried out. This is sensible if the set of events to which the calculation is applied is relatively small (the "Tier 1" events mentioned in Chapter 11). However, if there are many events (such as the "Tier 2" events), then it is possible to have "false alarms," with possible false interpretations of toxicity. In such cases, it is arguably more sensible to regard the evaluation of adverse event incidence as a screening exercise aimed at identifying particular adverse events whose possible causal relationship to the product being tested can be assessed using more detailed clinical and epidemiologic evaluation. Screening seeks to minimize both the false discovery rate (FDR), that is, the probability that an analysis incorrectly identifies a potential toxicity relationship between the product and the event, and the missed discovery rate, which is the probability that an analysis misses identifying a true toxicity relationship. These probabilities are familiar in the context of diagnostic testing: the FDR is 1 minus the positive predictive value, and the missed discovery rate is 1 minus the negative predictive value.

*Statistical Methods for Evaluating Safety in Medical Product Development*, First Edition.
Edited by A. Lawrence Gould.
© 2015 John Wiley & Sons, Ltd. Published 2015 by John Wiley & Sons, Ltd.

The purpose of this chapter is to describe briefly some means for summarizing and getting an understanding of the adverse event profile of the treatments in clinical development programs, most usually clinical trials. Adverse event occurrence can be evaluated by means other than the few considered in this chapter, and the analyses can become quite elaborate. Typical examples include survival-type analysis for adverse event emergence and recurrence, and various regression modeling strategies for identifying potential predictors of adverse event occurrence other than assigned treatment. Anything other than a very superficial examination of these approaches is outside the scope of this chapter, so they will not pursued in detail.

## 6.2   Summarization of key features of adverse event occurrence

Simple count tables of adverse event frequency comprise the first step in evaluating potential toxicity risk as manifested by the occurrence of adverse events. Figures 2.2 and 2.3 in the chapter on safety graphics provide tabular and graphical overall summaries of adverse event incidence. The programs that produce these figures also can be run on subsets of the data or for windows of time to provide insight into timing of adverse event occurrence. Likewise, Figures 2.4–2.6 provide additional information on timing and severity of specific adverse events. While these figures make the various dimensions of adverse event occurrence relatively easy to grasp, they focus only on single aspects of the occurrence. A more comprehensive understanding can be gained by an appropriate tabular presentation that combines the various aspects of adverse event occurrence. Table 6.1 illustrates one such tabular arrangement; it is produced by a SAS® macro that operates on an overall data file. The data are real, but old, and should be considered only illustrative. The macro is available on the website for this book. The table can be produced for combinations of adverse events, as illustrated in Table 6.1, or for events within a body or organ system, or for individual preferred terms. The macro has an option to produce the tables only for those adverse events with at least a minimum number of reports. A single invocation of the macro usually will be sufficient to generate a collection of adverse event tables for a study or set of studies.

The event occurrence pattern is broken down by time intervals that are selected when the macro is run. The pattern can be sorted by treatment group within each time interval, to highlight potential differences between treatment groups that may emerge over time. The pattern also can be sorted by time within each treatment group, to focus on the evolution of adverse event occurrence in each treatment group over time.

A distinction is made between first reports, that address emergence of adverse events over time and exposure, and any events, that address recurrence of adverse events over time and exposure. Exposure can be expressed in any convenient units; the table uses patient-weeks as the unit of exposure, but other units can be accommodated such as patient-months, patient-years, and so on. The first part of the table, that summarizes any exposure (ANY), provides in its first few columns what conventional count tables usually provide. The table is intended only as a summary, albeit a fairly comprehensive one. The information it provides can be useful for guiding specific inferential analyses such as analyses of time to occurrence or recurrence of events, and also can be useful for the interpretation of the results such analyses. For example, although the incidence of adverse events appears to be only modestly elevated in the control group relative to the test group (and persists within each time period), substantially more patients withdrew from the study in the control group than in the test

**Table 6.1**  Any adverse experiences: incidence, exposure, report count, and maximum intensity by treatment and time on treatment.

| Time on treatment | Treatment | First reports | | | | | Any reports | | | | | | Serious AE | | Maximum intensity | | | |
|---|---|---|---|---|---|---|---|---|---|---|---|---|---|---|---|---|---|---|
| | | Number of pats at risk | Number (%) of pats with first report | Exposure (pat-wks) | First reports/ exposure units | Average time to first event | Number of pats at risk | Number (%) of pats with any report | Total reports | Exposure (pat-wks) | Number of reports/ exposure units | Pats W/D due to AE | Number of Pats | Number of Reports | Mil | Mod | Sev | Number of data |
| Sorted by treatment within time period | | | | | | | | | | | | | | | | | | |
| ANY | TEST | 114 | 107 (94) | 73.6 | 1.5 | 0.5 | 114 | 107 (94) | 1637 | 722.4 | 2.3 | 31 | 58 | 188 | 5 | 10 | 19 | 7 |
| | CONTROL | 125 | 124 (99) | 75.9 | 1.6 | 0.6 | 125 | 124 (99) | 2592 | 849.6 | 3.1 | 44 | 76 | 286 | 7 | 4 | 13 | 10 |
| Days 1–7 | TEST | 114 | 95 (83) | 56.4 | 1.7 | 0.4 | 114 | 95 (83) | 492 | 109.3 | 4.5 | 14 | 28 | 50 | 12 | 22 | 10 | 5 |
| | CONTROL | 125 | 112 (90) | 48.7 | 2.3 | 0.3 | 125 | 112 (90) | 841 | 121.4 | 6.9 | 25 | 34 | 90 | 6 | 11 | 19 | 7 |
| Days 8–15 | TEST | 17 | 10 (59) | 8.6 | 1.2 | 0.2 | 104 | 83 (80) | 550 | 101.9 | 5.4 | 17 | 31 | 64 | 10 | 8 | 10 | 5 |
| | CONTROL | 13 | 8 (62) | 6.1 | 1.3 | 0.1 | 117 | 101 (86) | 913 | 125.9 | 7.3 | 20 | 30 | 84 | 6 | 7 | 8 | 8 |
| Days 16–30 | TEST | 5 | 2 (40) | 4.9 | 0.4 | 0.8 | 84 | 58 (69) | 353 | 160.9 | 2.2 | 1 | 21 | 48 | 7 | 8 | 8 | 3 |
| | CONTROL | 5 | 3 (60) | 8.4 | 0.4 | 1.4 | 104 | 77 (74) | 502 | 201.3 | 2.5 | 1 | 25 | 59 | 7 | 7 | 12 | 5 |
| Days 31–60 | TEST | 1 | 0 | 3.7 | | | 70 | 36 (51) | 174 | 261.7 | 0.7 | 0 | 11 | 25 | 6 | 4 | 8 | 1 |
| | CONTROL | 2 | 0 | 7.4 | | | 83 | 51 (61) | 264 | 301.4 | 0.9 | 0 | 22 | 48 | 8 | 7 | 9 | 2 |
| Days 61–120 | TEST | 0 | | 0 | | | 47 | 21 (45) | 68 | 88.7 | 0.8 | 0 | 1 | 1 | 1 | 2 | 7 | 1 |
| | CONTROL | 1 | 1 | 5.1 | 0.2 | 5.1 | 49 | 21 (43) | 72 | 95.1 | 0.8 | 0 | 3 | 5 | 3 | 0 | 0 | 1 |
| | CONTROL | 0 | | 0 | | | 0 | 0 | 0 | 4.4 | | | | | | | | |

(continued overleaf)

**Table 6.1** (continued)

| Time on treatment | Treatment | First reports | | | | | Any reports | | | | | | Serious AE | | Maximum intensity | | | |
|---|---|---|---|---|---|---|---|---|---|---|---|---|---|---|---|---|---|---|
| | | Number of pats at risk | Number (%) of pats with first report | Exposure (pat-wks) | First reports/exposure units | Average time to first event | Number of pats at risk | Number (%) of pats with any report | Total reports | Exposure (pat-wks) | Number of reports/exposure units | Pats W/D due to AE | Number of Pats | Number of Reports | Mil | Mod | Sev | Number of data |
| Sorted by time period within treatment | | | | | | | | | | | | | | | | | | |
| ANY | TEST | 114 | 107 (94) | 73.6 | 1.5 | 0.5 | 114 | 107 (94) | 1637 | 722.4 | 2.3 | 31 | 58 | 188 | 5 | 10 | 19 | 7 |
| Days 1–7 | TEST | 114 | 95 (83) | 56.4 | 1.7 | 0.4 | 114 | 95 (83) | 492 | 109.3 | 4.5 | 14 | 28 | 50 | 12 | 22 | 10 | 5 |
| Days 8–15 | TEST | 17 | 10 (59) | 8.6 | 1.2 | 0.2 | 104 | 83 (80) | 550 | 101.9 | 5.4 | 17 | 31 | 64 | 10 | 8 | 10 | 5 |
| Days 16–30 | TEST | 5 | 2 (40) | 4.9 | 0.4 | 0.8 | 84 | 58 (69) | 353 | 160.9 | 2.2 | 1 | 21 | 48 | 7 | 8 | 12 | 3 |
| Days 31–60 | TEST | 1 | 0 | 3.7 | | | 70 | 36 (51) | 174 | 261.7 | 0.7 | 0 | 11 | 25 | 6 | 4 | 9 | 1 |
| Days 61–120 | TEST | 0 | | 0 | | | 47 | 21 (45) | 68 | 88.7 | 0.8 | 0 | 1 | 1 | 1 | 2 | 1 | 1 |
| ANY | CONTROL | 125 | 124 (99) | 75.9 | 1.6 | 0.6 | 125 | 124 (99) | 2592 | 849.6 | 3.1 | 44 | 76 | 286 | 7 | 4 | 13 | 10 |
| Days 1–7 | CONTROL | 125 | 112 (90) | 48.7 | 2.3 | 0.3 | 125 | 112 (90) | 841 | 121.4 | 6.9 | 25 | 34 | 90 | 6 | 11 | 19 | 7 |
| Days 8–15 | CONTROL | 13 | 8 (62) | 6.1 | 1.3 | 0.1 | 117 | 101 (86) | 913 | 125.9 | 7.3 | 20 | 30 | 84 | 6 | 7 | 8 | 8 |
| Days 16–30 | CONTROL | 5 | 3 (60) | 8.4 | 0.4 | 1.4 | 104 | 77 (74) | 502 | 201.3 | 2.5 | 1 | 25 | 59 | 7 | 7 | 8 | 5 |
| Days 31–60 | CONTROL | 2 | 0 | 7.4 | | | 83 | 51 (61) | 264 | 301.4 | 0.9 | 0 | 22 | 48 | 8 | 7 | 7 | 2 |
| Days 61–120 | CONTROL | 1 | 1 | 5.1 | 0.2 | 5.1 | 49 | 21 (43) | 72 | 95.1 | 0.8 | 0 | 3 | 5 | 3 | 0 | 0 | 1 |
| Day 121+ | CONTROL | 0 | | 0 | | | 1 | 0 | 0 | 4.4 | | 0 | | | | | | |

group. Also, many more patients in the control group than in the test group reported a "serious" adverse event, and more "serious" adverse events were reported in the control group than in the test group. However, the maximum intensity of the events that did occur in the test group tended to be greater than the events occurring in the control group.

## 6.3  Confidence/credible intervals for risk differences and ratios

### 6.3.1  Metrics

There is a substantial literature on the subject of confidence or credible intervals for functions of event rates corresponding to event counts that follow a binomial distribution that can be applied when the events are evaluated separately. Recent reviews [1–9] compared the performance of several Bayesian and conventional alternatives and provided specific recommendations for calculations to carry out in practice. The particular measure of relative risk that is appropriate, that is, the difference between event rates, or ratio or odds ratio of event rates, may depend on the circumstances. Consequently the calculations for all of these measures are addressed. If the sample sizes are large and the event rates are relatively low, then a Poisson model may be appropriate, and calculations also are described for this model in Section 6.3.4.

### 6.3.2  Coverage and interpretation

The coverage provided by any confidence interval construction procedure is the probability that the confidence interval constructed given the data actually contains the true value of the quantity that is estimated. This probability can be calculated explicitly, without recourse to approximation or simulation. In general, the coverage probability is calculated as

$$\Pr(\text{LB} < m(p,q) < \text{UB}) = \sum_x \sum_y f(x,p)f(y;q)I(\text{LB}(x,y) < m(p,q) < \text{UB}(x,y)), \quad (6.1)$$

where LB and UB on the left-hand side denote the random confidence interval endpoints, $m(p,q)$ denotes a metric such as $p/q$, $p - q$, or $p(1-q)/q(1-p)$, $f(x; p)$ is the probability mass function corresponding to $x$ events when the true rate parameter is $p$, $f(y; q)$ is the probability mass function corresponding to $y$ events when the true rate parameter is $q$, and $I(\text{arg}) = 1$ if arg is a true statement and 0 otherwise. $\text{LB}(x, y)$ is the lower confidence bound computed when there are $x$ and $y$ events in the two groups, and $\text{UB}(x, y)$ is the corresponding upper bound. If $F_m(m(p,q))$ denotes the cumulative distribution fuction (cdf) of the metric evaluated at the (true) values $p$ and $q$ given $x$, $y$, and the prior information, then the computation of equation (6.1) can be made more efficient and stable by replacing the expression

$$I(\text{LB}(x,y) < m(p,q) < \text{UB}(x,y))$$

which requires inverting $F_m(m(p,q))$ for each value of $x$ and $y$, with the equivalent expression

$$I(F_m(\text{LB}(x,y)) < F_m(m(p,q)) < F_m(\text{UB}(x,y))),$$

which does not require the inversion. The alternative calculation is particularly efficient when central credible intervals are required, that is, when the intervals are required to have equal tail areas, when $F_m(\text{LB}(x, y)) = 1 - F_m(\text{UB}(x, y)) = \alpha/2$ for $100(1 - \alpha)\%$ intervals, because then $F_m(m(p, q))$ is the only calculation needed. Confidence/credible interval construction procedures can be assessed by other criteria, such as the interval width and the probability that they will lead to an interval with, say, coverage less than 93% when the goal is 95% confidence.

Interpreting the observation of a conventional $p$-value of less than 5% as evidence of a "significant" association between the administration of a test treatment and the occurrence of an adverse event is a common, but highly questionable, practice. The practice is scientifically invalid because it amounts to carrying out tests of hypotheses that have not been identified a priori, so that the observed data determine which tests are carried out. Moreover, there usually is no recognition of the fact that "significant" findings are almost inevitable if many tests are carried out because of the effect of multiplicity even if two treatments have exactly the same toxicity potential (or, for that matter, are the same treatment).

Because of this, significance tests have limited validity for the initial evaluation of potential safety issues, and better insight about potential risks can be obtained by providing estimates of effect along with measures of precision. This does not remove the invalidity issue because it is tempting to interpret a confidence or credible interval that excludes 0 (difference) or 1 (ratio or odds ratio) as the same as a significant $p$-value. However, it does make that interpretation a little less obvious and has the merit of quantifying the risk. Much of the problem can be avoided by looking at the evaluation of adverse event incidence from the standpoint of screening, and this will be addressed later in this chapter. For now, we consider methods for separately evaluating risk differences.

### 6.3.3    Binomial model

Suppose first that the numbers of events in each treatment group are generated from binomial distributions, so that the likelihood of the outcomes for a pair of treatment groups is the product of binomial probability functions for the numbers of events in each treatment group, say $X \sim f_{\text{bin}}(x; n_X, p_X)$ and $Y \sim f_{\text{bin}}(y; n_Y, p_Y)$, where

$$f_{\text{bin}}(x; n, p) = \binom{n}{x} p^x (1 - p)^{n-x}.$$

Comparisons of $p_X$ with $p_Y$ can be carried out using a variety of metrics, of which the most common are the difference $p_X - p_Y$, the risk ratio $p_X/p_Y$, and the odds ratio $p_X(1 - p_Y)/p_Y(1 - p_X)$. There are others [10]. The distributions of event counts in any real trial are mixtures of binomial distributions reflecting the different event risks associated with different subsets of the study population (e.g., elderly versus non-elderly), but the simple binomial approximation should be adequate for practical purposes, at least for an initial evaluation. The comparisons can be carried out using conventional (frequentist) methods, of which there are many (see, for example, [1, 3, 11–13]) or by Bayesian methods whose frequentist statistical properties can depend on the choice of prior [1]. Interestingly enough, the Bayesian methods are related to conventional frequentist methods by virtue of the fact that, at least in these applications, they are equivalent to fiducial methods for constructing tests and intervals [14].

### 6.3.3.1  Differences between risks

**Conventional (frequentist) intervals**   Inverted score tests appear to provide the most accurate conventional (frequentist) confidence intervals, based on numerical assessments of the various alternatives [1, 3]. Agresti and Min [1] recommended a score test described by Mee [15] that obtains the endpoints of a $100\gamma\%$ confidence interval for the difference $p_X - p_Y$ as the solutions of a score equation, or essentially equivalent tests described by Miettinen and Nurminen [16] and by Farrington and Manning [5], but with a slightly different variance (involving the factor $n/(n-1)$, where $n = n_X + n_Y$) which may improve coverage [7],

$$\frac{\hat{\pi}_X - \hat{\pi}_Y - \Delta}{\sqrt{(n/(n-1))(\tilde{\pi}_X(1-\tilde{\pi}_X)/n_X + \tilde{\pi}_Y(1-\tilde{\pi}_Y)/n_Y)}} = z_{(1+\gamma)/2};$$

for example, if $\gamma = 0.95$, then $z_{(1+0.95)/2} = 1.96$. The estimates $\hat{\pi}_X$ and $\hat{\pi}_Y$ are the usual estimates, $\hat{\pi}_X = x/n_X$ and $\hat{\pi}_Y = y/n_Y$, and the estimates $\tilde{\pi}_X$ and $\tilde{\pi}_Y$ are obtained by maximizing the likelihood ($f_{\text{bin}}(x; n_X, \pi_X) \times f_{\text{bin}}(y; n_Y, \pi_Y)$) subject to the constraint $\hat{\pi}_X - \hat{\pi}_Y = \Delta$. The calculations can be carried out using the diffscoreci function in the R system PropCIs package or the ciBinomial function in the R system gsDesign package [17], or the SAS® 9.3 FREQ procedure. Newcombe described a hybrid score based on Wilson score confidence intervals for $p_X$ and $p_Y$ that appears to have reasonable coverage properties [6],

$$d_L, d_U = \hat{\pi}_X - \hat{\pi}_Y - \sqrt{(\hat{\pi}_X - L_X)^2 + (\hat{\pi}_Y - U_Y)^2} \ , \ \hat{\pi}_X - \hat{\pi}_Y + \sqrt{(\hat{\pi}_X - U_X)^2 + (\hat{\pi}_Y - L_Y)^2},$$

where $L_i, U_i, i = X, Y$, are Wilson score confidence intervals for $\pi_X$ and $\pi_Y$ [18],

$$L_i, U_i = \hat{\pi}_i \left( \frac{n_i}{n_i + z_{\alpha/2}^2} \right) + 0.5 \left( \frac{z_{\alpha/2}^2}{n_i + z_{\alpha/2}^2} \right)$$

$$\pm z_{\alpha/2}^2 \sqrt{\left[ \hat{\pi}_i \left(1 - \hat{\pi}_i\right) \left( \frac{n_i}{n_i + z_{\alpha/2}^2} \right) + 0.25 \left( \frac{z_{\alpha/2}^2}{n_i + z_{\alpha/2}^2} \right) \right] / \left( n_i + z_{\alpha/2}^2 \right)}.$$

Brown and Li [2] proposed additional estimates that appeared to have desirable coverage properties and, in addition, were fairly simple to compute. One is a "Jeffreys CI" confidence interval inspired by the performance of a Bayes estimator of the response rate using a Jeffreys prior,

$$L, U \ = \breve{\pi}_X - \breve{\pi}_Y \pm z_{\alpha/2} \sqrt{(\breve{\pi}_X(1-\breve{\pi}_X)/n_X + \breve{\pi}_Y(1-\breve{\pi}_Y)/n_Y)},$$

where $\breve{\pi}_X = (x + 1/2)/(n_X + 1)$ and $\breve{\pi}_Y = (y + 1/2)/(n_Y + 1)$. The other is a truncated recentered interval with limits

$$\frac{\hat{\Delta}}{1 + \kappa^2/(n_X + n_Y)} \pm \frac{\kappa \sqrt{(1 + \kappa^2/(n_X + n_Y))(1/n_X + 1/n_Y)\tilde{p}(1 - \tilde{p}) - \hat{\Delta}^2/(n_X + n_Y)}}{1 + \kappa^2/(n_X + n_Y)},$$

where $\kappa$ is the upper $\alpha/2$ quantile of a standard $t$ distribution with $n_X + n_Y - 2$ degrees of freedom and

$$\tilde{p} = \begin{cases} \dfrac{\Delta n_Y}{n_X + n_Y} & \text{if } \hat{p} < \dfrac{n_Y}{n_X + n_Y} \\ \hat{p} = \dfrac{n_Y\dfrac{x}{n_X} + n_X\dfrac{y}{n_Y}}{n_X + n_Y} & \text{if } \dfrac{\Delta n_Y}{n_X + n_Y} \le \hat{p} \le 1 - \dfrac{n_X}{n_X + n_Y} \\ 1 - \dfrac{\Delta n_X}{n_X + n_Y} & \text{if } \hat{p} \ge 1 - \dfrac{\Delta n_X}{n_X + n_Y}. \end{cases}$$

The calculations for the score test intervals can be carried out using the SAS® 9.3 FREQ procedure or the software included in Appendix 6.A. The Agresti–Caffo approach [19] also appears to have desirable coverage properties [3]. The calculations for the Agresti–Caffo approach also can be carried out using the R system pairwiseCI package. Agresti and Min [1] advise against the use of highest posterior density intervals, primarily because they are not invariant to choice of metric.

**Bayesian intervals**  As before, the likelihood is the product of binomial probability functions. Bayesian analyses require prior distributions, and for the present analyses we assume that each parameter $p$ has a Beta$(a, b)$ distribution,

$$f_{\text{beta}}(u; a, b) = B^{-1}(a, b)u^{a-1}(1 - u)^{b-1},$$

where $B(a, b) = \Gamma(a)\Gamma(b)/(\Gamma(a + b))$ denotes the usual beta function and $\Gamma(a)$ denotes the usual gamma function, so that the posterior distribution of the rate parameter for each group also is a beta distribution, but with parameters $(a + x, b + n_X - x)$ for the $X$ observations and $(a + y, b + n_Y - y)$ for the $Y$ observations. Note that although it is conventional and convenient to use the same prior for both groups, this is not necessary for constructing credible intervals. Agresti and Min [1] found that binomial credible intervals based on the posterior distributions of any of the metrics, not just the differences between the event rates, provided coverage level closer to the nominal level and with a lesser incidence of low coverage intervals with a Jeffreys prior (Beta$(1/2, 1/2)$) than with a uniform prior (Beta$(1,1)$).

The joint posterior density for the rate parameters therefore is the product of two beta densities,

$$f_{\text{post}}(p_X, p_Y; a, b, n_X, x, n_Y, y) = f_{\text{beta}}(p_X; a + x, b + n_X - x) \times f_{\text{beta}}(p_Y; a + y, b + n_Y - y). \tag{6.2}$$

The endpoints $\Delta_L$, $\Delta_U$ of equal-tail $100\gamma\%$ credible intervals for the difference $\Delta = p_X - p_Y$ are

$$P_{\text{post}}(\Delta < \Delta_L; a, b, n_X, x, n_Y, y) = P_{\text{post}}(\Delta > \Delta_U; a, b, n_X, x, n_Y, y) = \dfrac{1 - \gamma}{2}.$$

That is, the posterior probability that $\Delta < \Delta_L$ is the same as the posterior probability that $\Delta > \Delta_U$, and each is equal to $(1 - \gamma)/2$. The region of $\Delta$ values for which $\Delta > \delta > 0$ is the

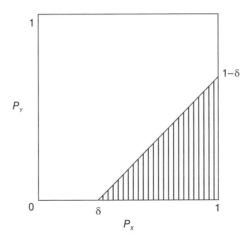

**Figure 6.1**    Region of the $(p_X, p_Y)$ plane for which $\Delta = p_X - p_Y > \delta > 0$.

shaded area in Figure 6.1. For $\delta > 0$, let

$$H_{\mathrm{diff}}(\delta, a, b, n_X, x, n_Y, y) = \int_{u=\delta}^{1} f_{\mathrm{beta}}(u; a+x, b+n_X-x)F_{\mathrm{beta}}(u-\delta; a+y, b+n_Y-y)du,$$

where $F_{\mathrm{beta}}(u; a, b) = I_u(a, b)$ denotes the usual beta cdf ($I_u(a, b)$ = incomplete beta function). The posterior cdf of $\Delta$ takes the form

$$F_{\mathrm{post}}(\delta; a, b, n_X, x, n_Y, y) = \begin{cases} 1 - H_{\mathrm{diff}}\left(\delta, a, b, n_X, x, n_Y, y\right) & \text{if } \delta > 0 \\ H_{\mathrm{diff}}(-\delta; a, b, n_Y, y, n_X, x) & \text{if } \delta < 0. \end{cases} \quad (6.3)$$

The calculation of equation (6.3) can be carried out in R using BetaMetricCDF.fn in Appendix 6.A, which also can calculate the posterior cdf of the ratio $p_X/p_Y$ and the odds ratio $p_X(1 - p_Y)/p_Y(1 - p_X)$.

### 6.3.3.2    Relative risks

**Conventional (frequentist) intervals**    Confidence intervals for the ratio $\pi_X/\pi_Y$ based on score tests [5, 16, 20] appeared to have the best coverage properties among a number of procedures [3]. The endpoints of the confidence interval for $\phi = \pi_X/\pi_Y$ are the roots of the expression

$$\frac{\hat{p}_X - \phi\hat{p}_Y}{\sqrt{\tilde{p}_X\left(1 - \tilde{p}\tilde{\pi}_X\right)/n_X + \tilde{p}_Y\left(1 - \tilde{p}_Y\right)/n_Y}} = z_{(1+\gamma)/2},$$

where $\tilde{p}_X$ and $\tilde{p}_Y$ are the maximum likelihood estimates of $p_X$ and $p_Y$ subject to the condition that their ratio equals $\phi$. Nam [21] provided a non-iterative method for calculating the endpoints of the interval for $\phi$ based on the roots of a cubic polynomial. The riskscoreci function in the R package PropCIs and the ciBinomial function in the R package gsDesign implement the score function described by Miettinen and Nurminen [16], which also is implemented in the SAS® 9.3 FREQ procedure. Calculations using the Gart and Nam approach [22] can be carried out using the software in Appendix 6.A.

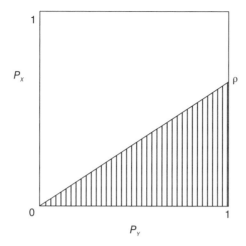

**Figure 6.2**  Region of the $(p_X, p_Y)$ plane for which $R = p_X/p_Y < \rho < 1$.

**Bayesian intervals**  The joint posterior distribution of the rate parameters $p_X$ and $p_Y$ is given by equation (6.2). The difference is that interest lies in the posterior distribution of the ratio $R = p_X/p_Y$. The posterior distribution of $R$ can be obtained by integration similar to the approach used to obtain the posterior cdf of the difference $\Delta$. Figure 6.2 illustrates the integration region. If

$$H_{\mathrm{rat}}(\rho,\ a,\ b,\ n_X,\ x,\ n_Y,\ y) = \int_{u=0}^{1} f_{\mathrm{beta}}(u; a+y, b+n_Y-y)F_{\mathrm{beta}}(\rho u; a+x, b+n_X-x)du,$$

then the posterior cdf of the ratio R takes the form

$$F_{\mathrm{post}}(\rho;\ a,\ b,\ n_X,\ x,\ n_Y,\ y) = \begin{cases} H_{\mathrm{rat}}\left(\rho,\ a,\ b,\ n_X,\ x,\ n_Y,\ y\right) & \text{if } \rho < 1 \\ 1 - H_{\mathrm{rat}}(1/\rho;\ a,\ b,\ n_Y,\ y,\ n_X,\ x) & \text{if } \rho > 1. \end{cases}$$

The R functions BetaMetricCDF.fn and BetaMetricCDFInv.fn in Appendix 6.A calculate, respectively, the posterior cdf and inverse cdf for the event rate ratio.

The posterior cdf of $R$ also can be obtained explicitly rather than by numerical integration. When $b$ is an integer, the cdf of the ratio of two beta variates, $X/Y$, $X \sim \mathrm{Beta}(a,b)$, $Y \sim \mathrm{Beta}(c,d)$, can be written as [23, 24]

$$F_{\mathrm{ratio}}(u; a, b, c, d) = \begin{cases} \dfrac{\Gamma(a+b)\,\Gamma(c+d)}{\Gamma(a+b+c+d-1)\Gamma(c)\Gamma(d)} \\[2em] \displaystyle\sum_{j=1}^{b}\dfrac{\Gamma(a+c+j-1)\Gamma(b+d-j)}{\Gamma(a+j)\Gamma(b+1-j)}I_u(a,j) & \text{if } u \leq 1 \\[2em] 1 - F_{\mathrm{ratio}}(1/u;\ c,\ d,\ a,\ b) & \text{if } u > 1. \end{cases}$$

(6.4)

Expression (6.4) is easily and efficiently calculated by recursion. If

$$w_j = \frac{\Gamma(a+b)\Gamma(c+d)}{\Gamma(a+b+c+d-1)\Gamma(c)\Gamma(d)} \times \frac{\Gamma(a+c+j-1)\Gamma(b+d-j)}{\Gamma(a+j)\Gamma(b+1-j)}$$

then

$$w_1 = B^{-1}(a,b)B^{-1}(c,d)B(a+c,b+d-1)/a$$

and

$$w_{j+1} = \frac{(a+c+j-1)(b-j)}{(b+d-j-1)(a+j)}w_j = h_jw_j$$

so that $w_2 = h_1w_1, w_3 = h_1h_2w_1$, and so on. The entire sequence of $w_j$ values therefore can be calculated using simple rational operations, and the potentially expensive computation of gamma function values needs to be done only once.

### 6.3.3.3 Odds ratios

**Conventional (frequentist) intervals**  The mid-$p$ variation of the Baptista–Pike exact conditional interval for odds ratios [25] appears to be the best choice for conventional confidence intervals [3, 4]. The conditional probability of observing $x$ "successes" in a $2 \times 2$ table with row totals $n_X$ and $n_Y$, the total number of successes $m$ fixed, is the probability function of a non-central hypergeometric distribution,

$$f(x;\ \psi,\ n_X,\ n_Y,\ m) = \frac{\binom{n_X}{x}\binom{n_Y}{m-x}\psi^x}{\sum\limits_{i=n_{\max}}^{n_{\min}}\binom{n_X}{i}\binom{n_Y}{m-i}\psi^i},$$

where $n_{\max} = \max(0,\ m-n_Y)$ and $n_{\min} = \min(n_X,\ m)$. The $100(1-\alpha)\%$ confidence limits $(\psi_L, \psi_U)$ are the solutions of

$$\sum_{i=n_{\max}}^{n_{\min}} f(i;\psi_L,\ n_X,n_Y,m) \times I\{f(i;\psi_L,n_X,n_Y,m) \le f(x;\ \psi_L,n_X,n_Y,m)\}$$

$$- f(x;\ \psi_L,\ n_X,n_Y,m) = \alpha/2,$$

$$\sum_{i=n_{\max}}^{n_{\min}} f(i;\psi_U,\ n_X,n_Y,m) \times I\{f(i;\psi_U,\ n_X,n_Y,m) \le f(x;\ \psi_U,n_X,n_Y,m)\}$$

$$- f(x;\ \psi_U,\ n_X,n_Y,m) = \alpha/2. \tag{6.5}$$

Calculation of the limits in equation (6.5) can be accomplished easily using an algorithm described by Liao and Rosen [26]. The BPmidp.fn function in Appendix 6.A provides the R code for carrying out the calculation.

Fagerland and Newcombe recently described an asymptotic approach based on the inverse hyperbolic sine transform [4]. The odds ratio is estimated by

$$\widetilde{\psi} = \frac{(x+\xi_1)(n_Y-y+\xi_1)}{(n_X-x+\xi_1)(y+\xi_1)}$$

and the confidence interval endpoints are obtained from

$$\log(\widetilde{\psi}) \pm 2\ \sinh^{-1}\left(\frac{z_{\alpha/2}}{2}\sqrt{\frac{1}{x+\xi_2} + \frac{1}{n_X-x+\xi_2} + \frac{1}{y+\xi_2} + \frac{1}{n_Y-y+\xi_2}}\right),$$

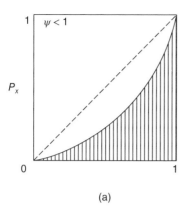
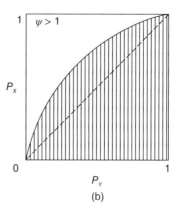

(a)                                    (b)

**Figure 6.3**   (a,b) Regions of the $(p_X, p_Y)$ plane for which $\Psi = p_X/p_Y < \psi$ when (a) $\psi > 1$ and (b) $\psi < 1$.

with $(\xi_1, \xi_2) = (0.45,\ 0.25)$ or $(0.6,\ 0.4)$. Expressions for relative risk confidence limits also are provided. The calculations can be carried out using the R code provided in Appendix 6.A. Confidence intervals for the odds ratio using a score-based approach can be calculated using the ciBinomial function in the gsDesign R package [17].

**Bayesian intervals**   As with the difference and risk ratio, the posterior distribution of the odds ratio

$$\Psi = \frac{p_X(1 - p_Y)}{p_Y(1 - p_X)}$$

can be obtained by integration. Figure 6.3 illustrates typical integration regions. The posterior cdf of the odds ratio is given by

$$F_{\text{post}}(\psi, a, b, n_X, x, n_Y, y)$$

$$= \int_{u=0}^{1} f_{\text{beta}}(u; c + y, d + n_Y - y) F_{\text{beta}}\left(\frac{\psi u}{1 - u + \psi u}; a + x, b + n_X - x\right) du.$$

### 6.3.3.4   Computational results

All of the intervals described above were calculated for the adverse events with non-zero event occurrences in the test and control groups tabulated in Mehrotra and Heyse [27]. The results for the conventional approaches are summarized in Table 6.2, and the results for the Bayesian approaches are summarized in Table 6.3. The R code for producing Table 6.2 is included in Appendix 6.A. The results for the Miettinen–Nurminen and Gart–Nam approaches were essentially identical, so the latter are omitted from Table 6.2. The intervals for the recommended conventional score tests based on risk differences are nearly the same, so in a practical setting it may not matter which one is used. The odds ratio intervals for the Baptista–Pike mid-$p$ approach were wider than the score-based intervals, which suggests more conservative coverage.

**Table 6.2** Summary of conventional confidence intervals for the difference, ratio, and odds ratio of event rates using adverse event counts from Mehrotra and Heyse [27].

| Original data | | | | | Differences | | | | | | | | | | | Ratios | | | Odds ratios | | | | | | |
|---|---|---|---|---|---|---|---|---|---|---|---|---|---|---|---|---|---|---|---|---|---|---|---|---|---|
| | nT | nC | | | | Score test | | Agresti–Caffo | | Brown–Li Jeffreys | | Brown–Li Recentered | | Newcombe Hybrid | | | Koopman Score test | | | Score test | | Baptista-Pike Mid-$p$ | | Fagerland-Newcombe Asymptotic | |
| AE | 148 | 132 | $x_T$ | $x_C$ | Difference | LD | UD | LD | UD | LD | UD | LD | UD | LD | UD | Ratio | LR | UR | OR | LO | UO | LO | UO | LO | UO |
| 1 | | | 57 | 40 | 0.082 | −0.03 | 0.191 | −0.03 | 0.192 | −0.03 | 0.192 | −0.03 | 0.192 | −0.029 | 0.19 | 1.271 | 0.918 | 1.772 | 1.441 | 0.876 | 2.368 | 0.813 | 2.534 | 0.552 | 3.734 |
| 2 | | | 34 | 26 | 0.033 | −0.065 | 0.129 | −0.065 | 0.128 | −0.06 | 0.129 | −0.063 | 0.128 | −0.064 | 0.127 | 1.166 | 0.745 | 1.835 | 1.216 | 0.686 | 2.155 | 0.641 | 2.329 | 0.407 | 3.607 |
| 4 | | | 3 | 1 | 0.013 | −0.023 | 0.051 | −0.021 | 0.045 | −0.02 | 0.043 | −0.015 | 0.04 | −0.024 | 0.051 | 2.676 | 0.389 | 18.57 | 2.71 | 0.38 | 19.17 | 0.284 | 71.87 | 0.112 | 41.27 |
| 5 | | | 27 | 20 | 0.031 | −0.059 | 0.119 | −0.058 | 0.118 | −0.06 | 0.118 | −0.057 | 0.118 | −0.058 | 0.118 | 1.204 | 0.716 | 2.037 | 1.25 | 0.667 | 2.342 | 0.606 | 2.595 | 0.379 | 4.078 |
| 6 | | | 7 | 2 | 0.032 | −0.012 | 0.081 | −0.013 | 0.075 | −0.01 | 0.074 | −0.008 | 0.072 | −0.013 | 0.081 | 3.122 | 0.754 | 13.09 | 3.227 | 0.743 | 13.92 | 0.641 | 22.94 | 0.253 | 31.09 |
| 9 | | | 24 | 10 | 0.086 | 0.01 | 0.164 | 0.008 | 0.161 | 0.01 | 0.161 | 0.011 | 0.16 | 0.009 | 0.162 | 2.141 | 1.085 | 4.274 | 2.361 | 1.097 | 5.074 | 1.006 | 5.707 | 0.556 | 9.532 |
| 10 | | | 3 | 1 | 0.013 | −0.023 | 0.051 | −0.021 | 0.045 | −0.02 | 0.043 | −0.015 | 0.04 | −0.024 | 0.051 | 2.676 | 0.389 | 18.57 | 2.71 | 0.38 | 19.17 | 0.284 | 71.87 | 0.112 | 41.27 |
| 11 | | | 2 | 7 | −0.04 | −0.094 | 0.002 | −0.086 | 0.007 | −0.08 | 0.005 | −0.081 | 0.003 | −0.093 | 0.004 | 0.255 | 0.061 | 1.057 | 0.245 | 0.057 | 1.062 | 0.034 | 1.233 | 0.025 | 3.123 |
| 12 | | | 19 | 19 | −0.02 | −0.099 | 0.066 | −0.098 | 0.066 | −0.1 | 0.065 | −0.096 | 0.065 | −0.099 | 0.065 | 0.892 | 0.498 | 1.599 | 0.876 | 0.445 | 1.724 | 0.409 | 1.875 | 0.245 | 3.13 |
| 13 | | | 3 | 2 | 0.005 | −0.036 | 0.045 | −0.032 | 0.04 | −0.03 | 0.038 | −0.026 | 0.036 | −0.036 | 0.044 | 1.338 | 0.271 | 6.626 | 1.345 | 0.263 | 6.854 | 0.197 | 11.45 | 0.092 | 17.31 |
| 16 | | | 2 | 2 | −0 | −0.042 | 0.035 | −0.036 | 0.031 | −0.03 | 0.029 | −0.029 | 0.026 | −0.041 | 0.034 | 0.892 | 0.159 | 5.004 | 0.89 | 0.154 | 5.137 | 0.092 | 8.657 | 0.056 | 14.09 |
| 17 | | | 75 | 43 | 0.181 | 0.065 | 0.291 | 0.065 | 0.292 | 0.066 | 0.293 | 0.065 | 0.292 | 0.065 | 0.29 | 1.556 | 1.169 | 2.096 | 2.126 | 1.308 | 3.458 | 1.228 | 3.654 | 0.83 | 5.391 |
| 18 | | | 4 | 1 | 0.019 | −0.017 | 0.061 | −0.017 | 0.054 | −0.01 | 0.052 | −0.011 | 0.049 | −0.018 | 0.06 | 3.568 | 0.545 | 23.6 | 3.639 | 0.535 | 24.54 | 0.449 | 90.68 | 0.154 | 50.48 |
| 19 | | | 4 | 1 | 0.019 | −0.017 | 0.061 | −0.017 | 0.054 | −0.01 | 0.052 | −0.011 | 0.049 | −0.018 | 0.06 | 3.568 | 0.545 | 23.6 | 3.639 | 0.535 | 24.54 | 0.449 | 90.68 | 0.154 | 50.48 |
| 20 | | | 1 | 2 | −0.01 | −0.048 | 0.024 | −0.04 | 0.022 | −0.04 | 0.019 | −0.033 | 0.016 | −0.047 | 0.024 | 0.446 | 0.059 | 3.371 | 0.442 | 0.057 | 3.436 | 0.015 | 5.886 | 0.025 | 11.15 |

| | | | | | | | | | | | | | | | | | | | | | | |
|---|---|---|---|---|---|---|---|---|---|---|---|---|---|---|---|---|---|---|---|---|---|---|
| 21 | 13 | 8 | 0.027 | −0.038 | 0.092 | −0.037 | 0.09 | −0.04 | 0.089 | −0.034 | 0.088 | −0.038 | 0.091 | 1.449 | 0.637 | 3.32 | 1.493 | 0.612 | 3.638 | 0.514 | 4.503 | 0.289 7.403 |
| 22 | 28 | 20 | 0.038 | −0.052 | 0.126 | −0.052 | 0.125 | −0.05 | 0.126 | −0.05 | 0.125 | −0.052 | 0.125 | 1.249 | 0.746 | 2.103 | 1.307 | 0.699 | 2.439 | 0.642 | 2.696 | 0.398 4.235 |
| 23 | 2 | 1 | 0.006 | −0.029 | 0.041 | −0.026 | 0.036 | −0.02 | 0.033 | −0.018 | 0.03 | −0.03 | 0.041 | 1.784 | 0.236 | 13.54 | 1.795 | 0.231 | 13.88 | 0.135 | 53.31 | 0.071 32.3 |
| 24 | 13 | 8 | 0.027 | −0.038 | 0.092 | −0.037 | 0.09 | −0.04 | 0.089 | −0.034 | 0.088 | −0.038 | 0.091 | 1.449 | 0.637 | 3.32 | 1.493 | 0.612 | 3.638 | 0.514 | 4.503 | 0.289 7.403 |
| 25 | 15 | 14 | −0.01 | −0.08 | 0.068 | −0.079 | 0.068 | −0.08 | 0.067 | −0.076 | 0.067 | −0.08 | 0.068 | 0.956 | 0.486 | 1.883 | 0.951 | 0.445 | 2.029 | 0.39 | 2.276 | 0.232 3.878 |
| 26 | 3 | 1 | 0.013 | −0.023 | 0.051 | −0.021 | 0.045 | −0.02 | 0.043 | −0.015 | 0.04 | −0.024 | 0.051 | 2.676 | 0.389 | 18.57 | 2.71 | 0.38 | 19.17 | 0.284 | 71.87 | 0.112 41.27 |
| 27 | 2 | 1 | 0.006 | −0.029 | 0.041 | −0.026 | 0.036 | −0.02 | 0.033 | −0.018 | 0.03 | −0.03 | 0.041 | 1.784 | 0.236 | 13.54 | 1.795 | 0.231 | 13.88 | 0.135 | 53.31 | 0.071 32.3 |
| 28 | 3 | 1 | 0.013 | −0.023 | 0.051 | −0.021 | 0.045 | −0.02 | 0.043 | −0.015 | 0.04 | −0.024 | 0.051 | 2.676 | 0.389 | 18.57 | 2.71 | 0.38 | 19.17 | 0.284 | 71.87 | 0.112 41.27 |
| 31 | 2 | 1 | 0.006 | −0.029 | 0.041 | −0.026 | 0.036 | −0.02 | 0.033 | −0.018 | 0.03 | −0.03 | 0.041 | 1.784 | 0.236 | 13.54 | 1.795 | 0.231 | 13.88 | 0.135 | 53.31 | 0.071 32.3 |
| 32 | 13 | 3 | 0.065 | 0.012 | 0.125 | 0.008 | 0.119 | 0.011 | 0.118 | 0.012 | 0.116 | 0.01 | 0.124 | 3.865 | 1.217 | 12.47 | 4.141 | 1.23 | 13.87 | 1.018 | 18.44 | 0.466 29.79 |
| 33 | 6 | 2 | 0.025 | −0.018 | 0.073 | −0.018 | 0.067 | −0.02 | 0.065 | −0.013 | 0.063 | −0.019 | 0.072 | 2.676 | 0.631 | 11.47 | 2.746 | 0.619 | 12.12 | 0.503 | 20.01 | 0.211 27.55 |
| 34 | 8 | 1 | 0.046 | 0.007 | 0.097 | 0.002 | 0.089 | 0.004 | 0.087 | 0.007 | 0.085 | 0.003 | 0.096 | 7.135 | 1.184 | 43.7 | 7.486 | 1.188 | 46.73 | 0.889 | 168.6 | 0.334 89.02 |
| 35 | 4 | 2 | 0.012 | −0.03 | 0.054 | −0.027 | 0.049 | −0.03 | 0.047 | −0.022 | 0.045 | −0.03 | 0.054 | 1.784 | 0.389 | 8.244 | 1.806 | 0.378 | 8.589 | 0.315 | 14.26 | 0.13 20.65 |
| 37 | 1 | 2 | −0.01 | −0.048 | 0.024 | −0.04 | 0.022 | −0.04 | 0.019 | −0.033 | 0.016 | −0.047 | 0.024 | 0.446 | 0.059 | 3.371 | 0.442 | 0.057 | 3.436 | 0.015 | 5.886 | 0.025 11.15 |
| 39 | 18 | 14 | 0.016 | −0.062 | 0.092 | −0.061 | 0.091 | −0.06 | 0.09 | −0.059 | 0.09 | −0.062 | 0.091 | 1.147 | 0.602 | 2.195 | 1.167 | 0.561 | 2.424 | 0.489 | 2.812 | 0.296 4.536 |
| 40 | 2 | 1 | 0.006 | −0.029 | 0.041 | −0.026 | 0.036 | −0.02 | 0.033 | −0.018 | 0.03 | −0.03 | 0.041 | 1.784 | 0.236 | 13.54 | 1.795 | 0.231 | 13.88 | 0.135 | 53.31 | 0.071 32.3 |

Highlighted rows identify cases where difference or ratio CIs exclude 0 or 1, respectively. Lx, and Ux are respective lower and upper bounds for metric x, where x = D for difference and R for ratio.

**Table 6.3**  Summary of 95% Bayesian credible intervals for the difference, ratio, and odds ratio of event rates using adverse event counts from Mehrotra and Heyse [27].

| | Original counts | | | | Difference | | | Ratio | | | Odds ratio | | |
|---|---|---|---|---|---|---|---|---|---|---|---|---|---|
| AE | $n_T$ | $x_T$ | $n_C$ | $x_C$ | Difference | LD | UD | Ratio | LR | UR | OR | LO | UO |
| 1 | 148 | 57 | 132 | 40 | 0.082 | −0.029 | 0.191 | 1.27 | 0.92 | 1.78 | 1.44 | 0.88 | 2.37 |
| 2 | 148 | 34 | 132 | 26 | 0.033 | −0.064 | 0.127 | 1.17 | 0.75 | 1.85 | 1.22 | 0.69 | 2.17 |
| 4 | 148 | 3 | 132 | 1 | 0.013 | −0.018 | 0.045 | 2.68 | 0.36 | 30.2 | 2.71 | 0.35 | 31.1 |
| 5 | 148 | 27 | 132 | 20 | 0.031 | −0.057 | 0.117 | 1.20 | 0.71 | 2.06 | 1.25 | 0.67 | 2.37 |
| 6 | 148 | 7 | 132 | 2 | 0.032 | −0.009 | 0.076 | 3.12 | 0.76 | 17.0 | 3.23 | 0.76 | 18.0 |
| 9 | 148 | 24 | 132 | 10 | 0.086 | 0.011 | 0.161 | 2.14 | 1.10 | 4.44 | 2.36 | 1.11 | 5.3 |
| 10 | 148 | 3 | 132 | 1 | 0.013 | −0.018 | 0.045 | 2.68 | 0.36 | 30.2 | 2.71 | 0.35 | 31.1 |
| 11 | 148 | 2 | 132 | 7 | 0.040 | −0.088 | 0.001 | 0.26 | 0.05 | 1.04 | 0.25 | 0.04 | 1.04 |
| 12 | 148 | 19 | 132 | 19 | 0.016 | −0.097 | 0.064 | 0.89 | 0.49 | 1.61 | 0.88 | 0.44 | 1.74 |
| 13 | 148 | 3 | 132 | 2 | 0.005 | −0.030 | 0.039 | 1.34 | 0.24 | 8.46 | 1.35 | 0.23 | 8.73 |
| 16 | 148 | 2 | 132 | 2 | 0.002 | −0.035 | 0.029 | 0.89 | 0.13 | 6.29 | 0.89 | 0.12 | 6.44 |
| 17 | 148 | 75 | 132 | 43 | 0.181 | 0.066 | 0.291 | 1.56 | 1.17 | 2.10 | 2.13 | 1.31 | 3.47 |
| 18 | 148 | 4 | 132 | 1 | 0.019 | −0.013 | 0.055 | 3.57 | 0.54 | 38.3 | 3.64 | 0.53 | 39.9 |
| 19 | 148 | 4 | 132 | 1 | 0.019 | −0.013 | 0.055 | 3.57 | 0.54 | 38.3 | 3.64 | 0.53 | 39.9 |
| 20 | 148 | 1 | 132 | 2 | 0.008 | −0.040 | 0.018 | 0.45 | 0.04 | 4.10 | 0.44 | 0.04 | 4.18 |
| 21 | 148 | 13 | 132 | 8 | 0.027 | −0.035 | 0.089 | 1.45 | 0.63 | 3.48 | 1.49 | 0.61 | 3.80 |
| 22 | 148 | 28 | 132 | 20 | 0.038 | −0.051 | 0.125 | 1.25 | 0.75 | 2.13 | 1.31 | 0.70 | 2.47 |
| 23 | 148 | 2 | 132 | 1 | 0.006 | −0.023 | 0.035 | 1.78 | 0.19 | 21.9 | 1.80 | 0.19 | 22.4 |
| 24 | 148 | 13 | 132 | 8 | 0.027 | −0.035 | 0.089 | 1.45 | 0.63 | 3.48 | 1.49 | 0.61 | 3.80 |
| 25 | 148 | 15 | 132 | 14 | 0.005 | −0.078 | 0.067 | 0.96 | 0.48 | 1.91 | 0.95 | 0.44 | 2.06 |
| 26 | 148 | 3 | 132 | 1 | 0.013 | −0.018 | 0.045 | 2.68 | 0.36 | 30.2 | 2.71 | 0.35 | 31.1 |
| 27 | 148 | 2 | 132 | 1 | 0.006 | −0.023 | 0.035 | 1.78 | 0.19 | 21.9 | 1.80 | 0.19 | 22.4 |
| 28 | 148 | 3 | 132 | 1 | 0.013 | −0.018 | 0.045 | 2.68 | 0.36 | 30.2 | 2.71 | 0.35 | 31.1 |
| 31 | 148 | 2 | 132 | 1 | 0.006 | −0.023 | 0.035 | 1.78 | 0.19 | 21.9 | 1.80 | 0.19 | 22.4 |
| 32 | 148 | 13 | 132 | 3 | 0.065 | 0.013 | 0.120 | 3.87 | 1.26 | 14.8 | 4.14 | 1.28 | 16.5 |
| 33 | 148 | 6 | 132 | 2 | 0.025 | −0.014 | 0.067 | 2.68 | 0.63 | 14.8 | 2.75 | 0.62 | 15.7 |
| 34 | 148 | 8 | 132 | 1 | 0.046 | 0.008 | 0.091 | 7.14 | 1.28 | 71.0 | 7.49 | 1.30 | 76.1 |
| 35 | 148 | 4 | 132 | 2 | 0.012 | −0.025 | 0.049 | 1.78 | 0.36 | 10.6 | 1.81 | 0.36 | 11.0 |
| 37 | 148 | 1 | 132 | 2 | 0.008 | −0.040 | 0.018 | 0.45 | 0.04 | 4.10 | 0.44 | 0.04 | 4.18 |
| 39 | 148 | 18 | 132 | 14 | 0.016 | −0.060 | 0.090 | 1.15 | 0.60 | 2.24 | 1.17 | 0.56 | 2.47 |
| 40 | 148 | 2 | 132 | 1 | 0.006 | −0.023 | 0.035 | 1.78 | 0.19 | 21.9 | 1.80 | 0.19 | 22.4 |

Highlighted rows identify cases where difference or ratio CIs exclude 0 or 1, respectively. Lx, Ux are respective lower and upper confidence bounds for metric x, where x = D for difference, R for ratio, and O for odds ratio (OR).

The Bayesian intervals for the differences in Table 6.3 are similar to the intervals for the score test in Table 6.2, but tend to be slightly narrower than the score test intervals. On the other hand, the Bayesian intervals for the ratios and for the odds ratios tend to be wider than those for the score test. All of the Bayesian intervals for the odds ratios were narrower than the corresponding intervals based on the Baptista–Pike mid-$p$ test. At least for the data considered here, it seems reasonable to conclude that the Bayesian and conventional score test intervals would provide about the same inferences, and all would be less conservative than the Baptista–Pike mid-$p$ test, which is an exact conditional (on the marginal totals) test.

### 6.3.3.5  Coverage comparisons

A better picture of the statistical properties of the various approaches for constructing confidence or credible intervals can be provided by a number of statistics that consider the entire set of possible outcomes. We focus here on the coverage probabilities, especially toward the lower values of the event rates that one would expect for adverse event occurrence.

Tables 6.4 and 6.5 illustrate the coverage probabilities for combinations of $p_X$ and $p_Y$ values likely to occur in evaluations of adverse event occurrence. Three sample sizes are considered: 5, 25, and 50 per group. The first sample size is intended for "stress testing" since few if any trials will be this small; this is a much smaller sample than coverage evaluations ordinarily assume. The scale of rate values is not uniform across the axes. The rate values increase by 0.01 from 0.01 to 0.1, and then by 0.1 to 0.5. These values provide increased resolution of the coverage rates when the event rates are small and also give a general picture of how the coverage rates vary for greater event rates. Adverse event rates exceeding 0.5 are unusual in clinical development, so only rates less than 0.5 are considered in the coverage comparisons. Calculations were carried out for each of the interval construction methods used in Table 6.2. Coverages of conventional confidence intervals for the difference between event rates are provided only for the Newcombe hybrid score method [6], which tended to have the least undercoverage without undue conservatism, at least for the cases considered here.

Conventional and Bayesian intervals for differences between event rates appeared to have similar coverage properties, with the Bayesian intervals being somewhat less conservative than the conventional intervals, again for the cases considered here (Table 6.3). However, the Bayesian intervals for the ratio of event rates appear to be preferable because they tended to have more accurate coverage and to be less conservative.

If the true event rates are less than 0.3 in both groups, then the coverages of the intervals obtained using both the conventional and Bayesian approaches tend to be conservative, which is not surprising because of the discreteness of the possible set of outcomes. This is a useful finding because adverse event rates exceeding 30% in any treatment group in a clinical trial would be a cause for concern.

Using 50 observations per group smooths the coverage contour considerably. Intervals for event rate differences based on the conventional score test tend to be somewhat more conservative than those based on the Bayesian approach, which sometimes becomes a bit liberal (coverage less than the nominal 95%).

The case of 25 observations per group is interesting because the differences in coverage patterns between the conventional and Bayesian approaches depend on the metric (difference or ratio). The conventional approach seems to provide intervals for the event rate difference with somewhat better coverage patterns than the Bayesian approach, while the opposite is true for intervals for the ratio of event rates.

**Table 6.4**  Coverage probabilities of conventional and Bayes intervals for the difference between two rates.

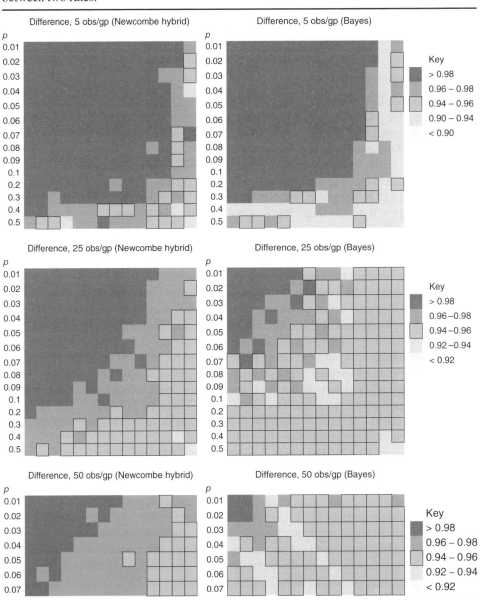

The column labels in each subtable are the same as the row labels.

**Table 6.5**  Coverage probabilities of conventional and Bayes intervals for the ratio of two rates.

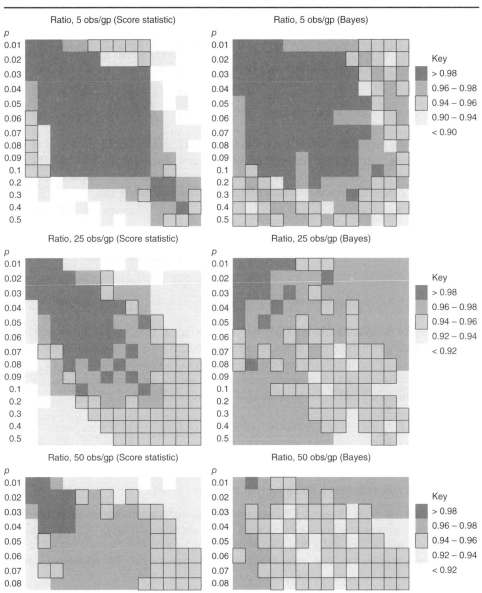

The column labels in each subtable are the same as the row labels.

The general conclusion is that the Bayesian (or fiducial [14]) intervals work well and can be considered as supplements or alternatives for the differences between, or ratios of, event rates or (results omitted) odds ratios.

### 6.3.4 Poisson model

When the sample sizes $(n_X, n_Y)$ are "large" and events are rare, the event counts can be regarded as having been generated from Poisson distributions rather than binomial distributions. Therefore, let $X$ and $Y$ denote event counts (with observed values $x$ and $y$, respectively) with exposures $t_X$ and $t_Y$, respectively, so that

$$X \sim \frac{(t_X \lambda_X)^x e^{-t_X \lambda_X}}{x!} \quad \text{and} \quad Y \sim \frac{(t_Y \lambda_Y)^y e^{-t_Y \lambda_Y}}{x!}.$$

Including the exposures means that the event rates $\lambda_X$ and $\lambda_Y$ can be expressed in standardized terms such as per 1000 person-years of exposure. In addition, if the values of $n_X$ and $n_Y$ are large, but not equal, the exposures provide a way to correct for the disparity in sample sizes. The maximum likelihood estimates of the event rate parameters are

$$\widehat{\lambda}_X = x/t_X \quad \text{and} \quad \widehat{\lambda}_Y = y/t_Y.$$

For Bayesian analyses, gamma conjugate priors for $\lambda_X$ and $\lambda_Y$ usually are employed,

$$f_{\text{gam}}(\lambda; \, a, \, b) = \frac{e^{-b\lambda} b^a \lambda^{a-1}}{\Gamma(a)}. \tag{6.6}$$

The density in equation (6.6) is fairly flat over a wide range of values for $\lambda$ when $b = 1$ and $a$ is "small" so that we take $b = 1$ in equation (6.6) for the prior densities for $\lambda_X$ and $\lambda_Y$. The product of the likelihood and the priors turns out to be the product $f_{\text{gam}}(\lambda_X; x + a, t_X + 1) f_{\text{gam}}(\lambda_Y; y + c, t_Y + 1) \times$ marginal probability function of $X$ and $Y$, so that the joint posterior density of $\lambda_X$ and $\lambda_Y$ is the product of gamma densities,

$$f_{\text{post}}(\lambda_X, \lambda_Y; a, c, x, y, t_X, t_Y) = f_{\text{gam}}(\lambda_X; x + a, t_X + 1) f_{\text{gam}}(\lambda_Y; y + c, t_Y + 1)$$

$$= f_{\text{gam}}(\lambda_X; \, a_X, b_X) \times f_{\text{gam}}(\lambda_Y; a_Y, b_Y).$$

#### 6.3.4.1 Differences between Poisson event rates

**Conventional intervals** Li *et al.* [28] described explicit asymptotic two-sided intervals for the difference between two Poisson event rates using variations of a hybrid method similar to Newcombe's method (see also [29]). Two of the variations turned out to have attractive coverage and length properties, and were recommended for general use. The confidence interval endpoints for all of the variations were of the form

$$L = \widehat{\lambda}_X - \widehat{\lambda}_Y - \sqrt{(\widehat{\lambda}_X - L_X)^2 + (\widehat{\lambda}_Y - U_Y)^2},$$

$$U = \widehat{\lambda}_X - \widehat{\lambda}_Y + \sqrt{(\widehat{\lambda}_X - U_X)^2 + (\widehat{\lambda}_Y - L_Y)^2}.$$

and differed only in how the quantities $L_X$, $U_X$, $L_Y$, and $U_Y$ were defined. The two variations that performed particularly well were the Freeman–Tukey interval [30]

$$L_X = \frac{\left(\sqrt{x} + \sqrt{x+1} - z_{\alpha/2}\right)^2 - 1}{4t_X}, \quad U_X = \frac{\left(\sqrt{x} + \sqrt{x+1} + z_{\alpha/2}\right)^2 - 1}{4t_X},$$

with $L_Y$ and $U_Y$ similarly defined; and the Jeffreys interval [31]

$$L_X = F_{\text{gam}}^{-1}(\alpha/2; x+1/2, t_X), \quad U_X = F_{\text{gam}}^{-1}(1 - \alpha/2; x+1/2, t_X),$$

where $F_{\text{gam}}(x; a, b)$ denotes the cdf of a gamma distribution,

$$f_{\text{gam}}(x; a, b) = \frac{e^{-bx}b^a x^{a-1}}{\Gamma(a)}.$$

**Bayesian intervals**  The region in the $(\lambda_X, \lambda_Y)$ plane for which the difference $\Delta = \lambda_X - \lambda_Y$ exceeds a fixed quantity $\delta$ looks like the region illustrated in Figure 6.1 for the $(p_X, p_Y)$ plane except that the upper limit of the $\lambda_X$-axis is infinite. As in Section 6.3.3.1.2, if

$$H_{\text{diff}}(\delta, a_X, b_X, a_Y, b_Y, x, y, t_X, t_Y) = \int_{u=\delta}^{\infty} f_{\text{gam}}(u; a_X, b_X) F_{\text{gam}}(u - \delta; a_Y, b_Y) du,$$

then the posterior cdf of $\Delta$ is obtained as

$$P_{\text{post}}(\Delta \leq \delta; a_X, b_X, a_Y, b_Y, x, y, t_X, t_Y) = \begin{cases} 1 - H_{\text{diff}}\left(\delta, a_X, b_X, a_Y, b_Y, x, y, t_X, t_Y\right) & \text{if } \delta \geq 0 \\ H_{\text{diff}}(-\delta; a_Y, b_Y, a_X, b_X, y, x, t_Y, t_X) & \text{if } \delta < 0. \end{cases}$$

#### 6.3.4.2   Ratios of Poisson event rates

**Conventional intervals**  Graham *et al.* [32] described approximate limits based on a score test that appear to provide reasonable coverage without being overly conservative. The limits are

$$R_L, R_U = \frac{t_Y}{t_X} \left\{ \frac{2xy + (x+y)z_\alpha^2 \pm \sqrt{(x+y)z_\alpha^2(4xy + (x+y)z_\alpha^2)}}{y^2} \right\}.$$

The lower limit ordinarily would be set to zero if $x = 0$, and the upper limit would be set to infinity if $y = 0$. If both $x$ and $y$ equal zero, then there is no information about the ratio of event rates and the corresponding interval for the ratio would be the entire positive real line.

**Bayesian intervals**  The ratio $R = \lambda_X / \lambda_Y$ has essentially a beta posterior distribution, that is, the quantity $W = Rb_X/(Rb_X + b_Y)$ has a Beta$(a_X, a_Y)$ density, so that percentage points of the posterior distribution of $R$ can be obtained easily. If $(L_\beta, U_\beta)$ denote the endpoints of an equal-tailed $100(1 - \alpha)\%$ credible interval for $W$, then the corresponding $100(1 - \alpha)\%$ credible interval for $R$ is

$$R_L, R_U = \frac{b_Y L_\beta}{b_x(1 - L_\beta)}, \frac{b_Y U}{b_x(1 - U_\beta)}.$$

### 6.3.5    Computational results

All of the intervals described above were calculated for the adverse events with non-zero event occurrences in the test and control groups tabulated in Mehrotra and Heyse [27]. The results for all of the approaches considered are summarized in Table 6.6. The R code for producing Table 6.6 is included in Appendix 6.A. The intervals for the differences (Table 6.6) and for the ratios (Table 6.7) produced by the various methods are nearly the same for these data.

## 6.4    Screening for adverse events

The intervals described above are constructed without regard to how many different adverse events actually were reported. However, adverse event frequencies need to be evaluated differently from how efficacy ordinarily is assessed. Efficacy often is evaluated in terms of multiple outcome measures that are specified in the trial protocol and are analyzed separately. The analyses must account explicitly for the number of assessments so that a conclusion of efficacy will not result if statistical significance at, say, a 5% level, is reached for only a few of several outcomes. Safety is different. What constitutes an acceptable or unacceptable potential safety burden generally is not defined in the protocol but, except for "Tier 1" adverse events, depends on the emergence of unspecified adverse events. Hypothesis testing in this context therefore means that the same data used in the test calculations identify the hypotheses being tested, which is scientifically invalid. Consequently, apparently significant differences in incidence of adverse events not identified a priori must be regarded at best as potential associations whose causal nature needs to be established by clinical and biological evaluation.

Multiplicity adjustments that are suitable for evaluating efficacy usually will not be appropriate for evaluating safety. A product might affect liver function, renal function, hematology, bone marrow, neurologic function, or cardiovascular function singly or in combination. A product's toxic effects could be very specific, and manifested by only a few adverse events occurring with different frequencies in the test and control group. Multiplicity adjustments suitable for efficacy evaluations could fail to detect instances of such toxic effects.

Nonetheless, multiplicity needs to be considered to reduce the likelihood of potential "false alarms." Two approaches, one frequentist, one Bayesian, have been proposed for addressing this issue. Mehrotra and Heyse [27] described the application of a "double FDR" approach that reduces the effect of multiplicity by subdividing the observed events into body systems and making adjustments to p-values reflecting the numbers of events in each body system, which are much smaller than the total number of events across all body systems. Berry and Berry [33] used a similar hierarchical scheme, but with a Bayesian approach employing a two-level random-effects model that generates posterior distributions of risk difference measures.

We describe in what follows a different approach [34, 35] that regards the collection of adverse event incidences as realizations from a mixture of distributions and seeks to identify the element of the mixture corresponding to each adverse event. This is a screening strategy rather than a testing strategy, with two objectives: identifying the drug–adverse event associations that should be evaluated further, and quantifying the strength of the evidence. Neither

**Table 6.6** Conventional and Bayesian confidence intervals for the difference and ratio of event counts assuming that event counts follow Poisson distributions using adverse event counts from Mehrotra and Heyse [27].

| | | | | | | Difference | | | | | | Ratio | | | | |
|---|---|---|---|---|---|---|---|---|---|---|---|---|---|---|---|---|
| | | | | | | Freeman–Tukey | | Jeffreys | | Bayes | | | Graham [32] | | Bayes | |
| AE | $x_T$ | $x_C$ | $\lambda_T$ | $\lambda_C$ | Difference | LD | UD | LD | UD | LD | UD | Ratio | LR | UR | LR | LR |
| 1 | 57 | 40 | 0.385 | 0.303 | 0.082 | −0.06 | 0.22 | −0.06 | 0.22 | −0.06 | 0.22 | 1.27 | 0.85 | 1.90 | 0.85 | 1.91 |
| 2 | 34 | 26 | 0.230 | 0.197 | 0.033 | −0.08 | 0.14 | −0.08 | 0.14 | −0.08 | 0.14 | 1.17 | 0.70 | 1.93 | 0.70 | 1.95 |
| 4 | 3 | 1 | 0.020 | 0.008 | 0.013 | −0.02 | 0.05 | −0.02 | 0.05 | −0.02 | 0.05 | 2.68 | 0.38 | 18.7 | 0.35 | 30.5 |
| 5 | 27 | 20 | 0.182 | 0.152 | 0.031 | −0.07 | 0.13 | −0.07 | 0.13 | −0.07 | 0.13 | 1.20 | 0.68 | 2.13 | 0.68 | 2.16 |
| 6 | 7 | 2 | 0.047 | 0.015 | 0.032 | −0.01 | 0.08 | −0.01 | 0.08 | −0.01 | 0.08 | 3.12 | 0.74 | 13.2 | 0.75 | 17.2 |
| 9 | 24 | 10 | 0.162 | 0.076 | 0.086 | 0.005 | 0.17 | 0.01 | 0.17 | 0.01 | 0.17 | 2.14 | 1.04 | 4.41 | 1.05 | 4.61 |
| 10 | 3 | 1 | 0.020 | 0.008 | 0.013 | −0.02 | 0.05 | −0.02 | 0.05 | −0.02 | 0.05 | 2.68 | 0.38 | 18.7 | 0.35 | 30.5 |
| 11 | 2 | 7 | 0.014 | 0.053 | −0.04 | −0.09 | 0.00 | −0.09 | 0.00 | −0.09 | 0.00 | 0.26 | 0.06 | 1.08 | 0.05 | 1.06 |
| 12 | 19 | 19 | 0.128 | 0.144 | −0.02 | −0.11 | 0.07 | −0.11 | 0.07 | −0.11 | 0.07 | 0.89 | 0.48 | 1.67 | 0.47 | 1.69 |
| 13 | 3 | 2 | 0.020 | 0.015 | 0.005 | −0.03 | 0.04 | −0.03 | 0.04 | −0.03 | 0.04 | 1.34 | 0.27 | 6.69 | 0.24 | 8.56 |
| 16 | 2 | 2 | 0.014 | 0.015 | −0 | −0.04 | 0.03 | −0.04 | 0.03 | −0.04 | 0.03 | 0.89 | 0.16 | 5.05 | 0.13 | 6.38 |
| 17 | 75 | 43 | 0.507 | 0.326 | 0.181 | 0.03 | 0.33 | 0.03 | 0.33 | 0.03 | 0.33 | 1.56 | 1.07 | 2.26 | 1.08 | 2.28 |
| 18 | 4 | 1 | 0.027 | 0.008 | 0.019 | −0.01 | 0.06 | −0.01 | 0.06 | −0.04 | 0.06 | 3.57 | 0.54 | 23.7 | 0.53 | 38.8 |
| 19 | 4 | 1 | 0.027 | 0.008 | 0.019 | −0.01 | 0.06 | −0.01 | 0.06 | −0.01 | 0.06 | 3.57 | 0.54 | 23.7 | 0.53 | 38.8 |
| 20 | 1 | 2 | 0.007 | 0.015 | −0.01 | −0.04 | 0.02 | −0.04 | 0.02 | −0.04 | 0.02 | 0.45 | 0.06 | 3.40 | 0.04 | 4.16 |

*(continued overleaf)*

**Table 6.6** (continued)

|  |  |  |  |  |  | Difference | | | | | | | Ratio | | | |
| | | | | | | Freeman–Tukey | | Jeffreys | | Bayes | | | Graham [32] | | Bayes | |
| AE | $x_T$ | $x_C$ | $\lambda_T$ | $\lambda_C$ | Difference | LD | UD | LD | UD | LD | UD | Ratio | LR | UR | LR | LR |
|---|---|---|---|---|---|---|---|---|---|---|---|---|---|---|---|---|
| 21 | 13 | 8 | 0.088 | 0.061 | 0.027 | −0.04 | 0.09 | −0.04 | 0.09 | −0.04 | 0.09 | 1.45 | 0.62 | 3.41 | 0.61 | 3.58 |
| 22 | 28 | 20 | 0.189 | 0.152 | 0.038 | −0.06 | 0.14 | −0.06 | 0.14 | −0.06 | 0.13 | 1.25 | 0.71 | 2.20 | 0.71 | 2.24 |
| 23 | 2 | 1 | 0.014 | 0.008 | 0.006 | −0.02 | 0.04 | −0.02 | 0.04 | −0.02 | 0.04 | 1.78 | 0.23 | 13.6 | 0.19 | 22.1 |
| 24 | 13 | 8 | 0.088 | 0.061 | 0.027 | −0.04 | 0.09 | −0.04 | 0.09 | −0.04 | 0.09 | 1.45 | 0.62 | 3.41 | 0.61 | 3.58 |
| 25 | 15 | 14 | 0.101 | 0.106 | −0.01 | −0.08 | 0.07 | −0.08 | 0.07 | −0.08 | 0.07 | 0.96 | 0.47 | 1.95 | 0.46 | 1.99 |
| 26 | 3 | 1 | 0.020 | 0.008 | 0.013 | −0.02 | 0.05 | −0.02 | 0.05 | −0.02 | 0.05 | 2.68 | 0.38 | 18.7 | 0.35 | 30.5 |
| 27 | 2 | 1 | 0.014 | 0.008 | 0.006 | −0.02 | 0.04 | −0.02 | 0.04 | −0.02 | 0.04 | 1.78 | 0.23 | 13.6 | 0.19 | 22.1 |
| 28 | 3 | 1 | 0.020 | 0.008 | 0.013 | −0.02 | 0.05 | −0.02 | 0.05 | −0.02 | 0.05 | 2.68 | 0.38 | 18.7 | 0.35 | 30.5 |
| 31 | 2 | 1 | 0.014 | 0.008 | 0.006 | −0.02 | 0.04 | −0.02 | 0.04 | −0.02 | 0.04 | 1.78 | 0.23 | 13.6 | 0.19 | 22.1 |
| 32 | 13 | 3 | 0.088 | 0.023 | 0.065 | 0.01 | 0.13 | 0.01 | 0.13 | 0.01 | 0.12 | 3.87 | 1.18 | 12.6 | 1.23 | 15.1 |
| 33 | 6 | 2 | 0.041 | 0.015 | 0.025 | −0.02 | 0.07 | −0.02 | 0.07 | −0.02 | 0.07 | 2.68 | 0.62 | 11.6 | 0.62 | 15.1 |
| 34 | 8 | 1 | 0.054 | 0.008 | 0.046 | 0.006 | 0.09 | 0.01 | 0.10 | 0.01 | 0.09 | 7.14 | 1.16 | 43.9 | 1.26 | 71.9 |
| 35 | 4 | 2 | 0.027 | 0.015 | 0.012 | −0.03 | 0.05 | −0.03 | 0.05 | −0.03 | 0.05 | 1.78 | 0.38 | 8.33 | 0.36 | 10.7 |
| 37 | 1 | 2 | 0.007 | 0.015 | −0.01 | −0.04 | 0.02 | −0.04 | 0.02 | −0.04 | 0.02 | 0.45 | 0.06 | 3.40 | 0.04 | 4.16 |
| 39 | 18 | 14 | 0.122 | 0.106 | 0.016 | −0.07 | 0.10 | −0.07 | 0.10 | −0.07 | 0.10 | 1.15 | 0.58 | 2.28 | 0.57 | 2.33 |
| 40 | 2 | 1 | 0.014 | 0.008 | 0.006 | −0.02 | 0.04 | −0.02 | 0.04 | −0.02 | 0.04 | 1.78 | 0.23 | 13.6 | 0.19 | 22.1 |

Highlighted rows identify cases where difference or ratio CIs exclude 0 or 1, respectively. $n_T = 148$, $n_C = 132$ for all adverse events.

**Table 6.7**   Coverage probabilities of conventional and Bayes intervals for the ratio of two rates.

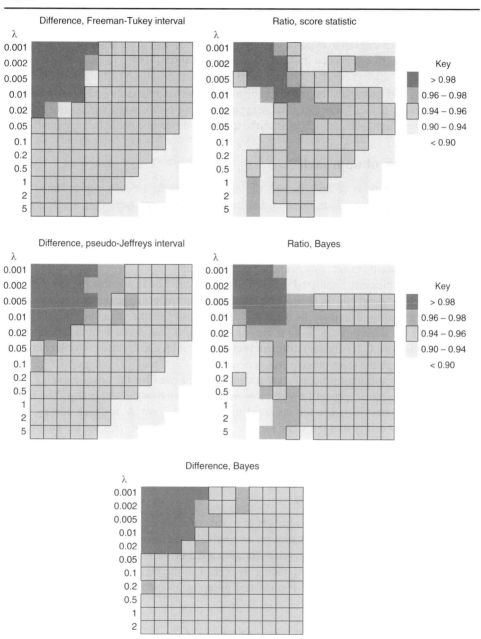

The column labels in each sub-table are the same as the row labels.

of these establishes causality or even plausible association by the occurrence of nominally "significant" findings. Both objectives are important, especially the latter:

> In most trials the safety and tolerability implications are best addressed by applying descriptive statistical methods to the data, supplemented by calculation of confidence intervals wherever this aids interpretation. [The] use of confidence intervals is preferred to hypothesis testing … imprecision often arising from low frequencies of occurrence is clearly demonstrated [36].

Detection and quantification are not equivalent. Large sample sizes could cause the posterior probability of a difference in adverse event incidence between test and control products to be to be very high, even though in absolute terms the difference could be very small.

### 6.4.1  Outline of approach

As in previous sections of this chapter, the adverse event frequencies are assumed to be realizations from binomial or Poisson distributions with event rates that are specific to the adverse event and may differ between the control and test groups. Each event rate is assumed to be a realization from a parent distribution, beta for binomial parameters, gamma for Poisson parameters. These parent distributions define the processes that generate the adverse-event-specific event rates in each treatment group.

Two possibilities are considered for each adverse event. The first is that the same process that generated the event rate for the adverse event in the control group generated the rate for the event in the test group. This does not mean that the event rates are the same, only that they were generated by the same process. Even if the control and test treatments were in fact identical, it still could happen that (slightly) different event rates could lead to different observed event counts even though the same process was generating the event rate for both groups. The other possibility is that different processes generated the event rates for the adverse events in the test and control groups, generally with more events expected in the test group. The aim of the screening process is to use the observed information to provide for each adverse event a (posterior) probability that the same process generated the event rates for the control and test groups. Small values of this probability would identify adverse events requiring further follow-up to evaluate a potential associative or causal relationship.

### 6.4.2  Distributional model

Let $X_i$ and $Y_i$ denote the (random) numbers of reports of event $i, i = 1, \ldots, N$, among $n_C$ and $n_T$ subjects in the control and test groups, respectively; the corresponding observed counts are $x_i$ and $y_i$. The observations can arise from binomial or Poisson distributions. Denote by $f(x_i; n_C, \theta_{iC}^{(X)})$ the likelihood corresponding to event $i$ in the control group, but express the likelihood corresponding to event $i$ in the test group as a random mixture of two possible likelihoods,

$$f_T(y_i; n_T, \theta_{iC}^{(y)}, \theta_{iT}, \gamma_i) = (1 - \gamma_i) f(y_i; n_T, \theta_{iC}^{(y)}) + \gamma_i f(y_i; n_T, \theta_{iT}),$$

the random mixing indicator $\gamma_i$ taking the value 0 if the likelihood for the test group is essentially the same as that for the control group, and 1 if the likelihoods are different. A distinction is made between the values of $\theta_{iC}$ corresponding to the two groups because the fact that they are generated separately from the same process means that their actual values could differ. Let

$$g_\gamma(\gamma;\pi) = \pi^{1-\gamma}(1-\pi)^\gamma$$

denote the prior probability function of $\gamma$ and let $g_\pi(\pi,\xi)$ denote the prior density of $\pi$ with known parameter $\xi$. Finally, suppose that the likelihood parameters $\theta_{iC}^{(y)}$ and $\theta_{iT}$ are random draws from respective prior densities $g_\theta(\theta_C;\Theta_C)$ and $g_\theta(\theta_T;\Theta_T)$, with known values of the possibly vector-valued quantities $\Theta_C$ and $\Theta_T$. If $g_\theta$ is a conjugate prior density, as is assumed here, then the product $f(y;n,\theta)g_\theta(\theta;\Theta)$ can be written as

$$f(y;n,\theta)g_\theta(\theta;\Theta) = h(y;n,\Theta)g_\theta(\theta;\Theta(y)),$$

where $h(y;n,\Theta)$ denotes the marginal probability function of Y and $g_\theta(\theta;\Theta(y))$ is the posterior density of $\theta$ with the same functional form as the prior density, but with a parameter that reflects both the initial assumptions ($\Theta$) and the observed data ($y$). The product of the joint likelihoods and the prior distributions is

$$f(\mathbf{x},\mathbf{y},\boldsymbol{\theta}_C^{(y)},\boldsymbol{\theta}_T,\boldsymbol{\gamma},\ \pi;\ n_C,\ n_T,\boldsymbol{\Theta}_C,\boldsymbol{\Theta}_T,\ \xi) = g_\pi(\pi;\xi)\prod_{i=1}^N f(x_i;\ n_C,\ \theta_{iC}^{(X)})$$

$$\times \prod_{i=1}^N \{(1-\gamma_i)\pi\ h(y_i;n_T,\ \boldsymbol{\Theta}_C)g_\theta(\theta_{iC}^{(y)};\boldsymbol{\Theta}_C(y_i)) + \gamma_i(1-\pi)\ h(y_i;n_T,\ \boldsymbol{\Theta}_T)g_\theta(\theta_{iT};\boldsymbol{\Theta}_T(y_i))\}$$

$$\text{(6.7)}$$

where $\mathbf{x} = (x_1,x_2,\ \dots\ )$ and $\mathbf{y} = (y_1,y_2,\ \dots\ )$. The random mixing parameter $\gamma_i$ provides automatic adjustment for the effect of having many adverse events [37]. Straightforward integration and division yields the quantities of interest: the conditional (on $\pi$) probability that $\gamma_i = 0$,

$$P(\gamma_i = 0;\mathbf{y},\pi,n_T,\boldsymbol{\Theta}_C,\boldsymbol{\Theta}_T) = \left\{1 + \frac{1-\pi}{\pi} \times \frac{h\left(y_i;n_T,\boldsymbol{\Theta}_T\right)}{h(y_i;n_T,\boldsymbol{\Theta}_C)}\right\}^{-1};$$

the posterior density of $\pi$,

$$f(\pi;\mathbf{y},n_T,\boldsymbol{\Theta}_C,\boldsymbol{\Theta}_T,\ \xi) \propto g_\pi(\pi;\xi) \times \prod_{i=1}^N \{\pi h(y_i;n_T,\boldsymbol{\Theta}_C) + (1-\pi)\ h(y_i;n_T,\boldsymbol{\Theta}_T)\};$$

and the unconditional probability that $\gamma_i = 0$,

$$\int_{\pi=0}^1 f(\pi;\mathbf{y},n_T,\boldsymbol{\Theta}_C,\boldsymbol{\Theta}_T,\ \xi)\left\{1 + \frac{1-\pi}{\pi} \times \frac{h\left(y_i;n_T,\ \boldsymbol{\Theta}_T\right)}{h(y_i;n_T,\ \boldsymbol{\Theta}_C)}\right\}^{-1} d\pi.$$

The analysis is Bayesian when the values of $\Theta_C$ and $\Theta_T$ do not depend on the event counts in the test group, even when they are functions of the control group counts. This is sensible and desirable because defining the prior distributions for the test group event rates in terms of both the prior parameters and the control group counts provides a better perspective in which to interpret the test group findings than does using just the prior parameters.

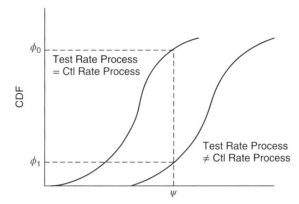

**Figure 6.4** Relationships between the posterior cdfs of the metric when the same and different processes generate the event rates in the test and control group, and the critical values used to construct them.

Suppose that the prior density of $\theta_{iC}^{(y)}$ is $g_\theta(\theta_{iC}^{(y)}; \Theta_C(x_i))$ and the prior density of $\theta_{iT}^{(y)}$ is $g_\theta\left(\theta_{iT}^{(y)}; \Theta_T(x_i)\right)$. The posterior distributions have the same form, except that $\Theta_C(x_i)$ is replaced with $\Theta_C(x_i, y_i)$, and $\Theta_T(x_i)$ is replaced with $\Theta_T(x_i, y_i)$. The posterior density of $\theta_{iC}^{(X)}$ is $g_\theta\left(\theta_{iC}^{(X)}; \Theta_C(x_i)\right)$. Let $R$ denote an appropriate metric (odds ratio when the counts arise from binomial distributions, ratio when the counts arise from Poisson distributions). Since the posterior distribution of the rate parameter for the test group is a mixture distribution, the same is true of the posterior distribution of $R$. Hence, if $F_R(r; \Theta_A, \Theta_B)$ denotes the posterior distribution of the ratio or odds ratio of event rates $\theta_A$ and $\theta_B$ whose posterior distributions have parameters $\Theta_A$ and $\Theta_B$, respectively, then the posterior distribution of the actual ratio or odds ratio also is a mixture of two distributions,

$$F_R(r; x_i, y_i, n_C, n_T, \Theta_C, \Theta_T, \xi) = \pi F_R(r; \Theta_C(x_i, y_i), \Theta_C(x_i))$$
$$+ (1 - \pi)F_R(r; \Theta_T(x_i, y_i), \Theta_C(x_i)).$$

### 6.4.3  Specification of priors

The details involved in determining $\Theta_C, \Theta_T$ can get complicated, but the principle is simple. Figure 6.4 illustrates the principle. The idea is to choose the parameters so that if $\psi$ denotes a maximally acceptable metric (ratio or odds ratio) value, for example $\psi = 2$, then the likelihood of a metric value greater than $\psi$ is "small" $(1 - \phi_0)$ if the same process generated the control and test group event rates, and the likelihood of an odds ratio value *less* than $\psi$ also is "small" $(\phi_1)$ if different processes generated the event rates.

A few details will be helpful for understanding how the software that carries out the calculations works. We start with $\Theta_C = (a_C, b_C)$. The initial requirement that

$$P(R \le \psi; \Theta_C, \Theta_C) \ge \phi_0$$

defines a curve in the $(a_C, b_C)$ plane. In order to select an appropriate point on this curve, and thus provide a specific value for $\Theta_C$, an additional condition is needed, preferably one that is consistent with the overall event rate evidence provided by the control group. To this end, let $\Theta_*$ denote the maximum likelihood or moment estimate of the parameters of the marginal distribution of the event counts in the control group,

$$\Theta^* = \arg\max_{\Theta} \prod_{i=1}^{N} h(x_i; n_C, \Theta).$$

Next, define $\theta_{C_\kappa}$ as the $100\kappa\%$ upper percentage point of the prior distribution of $\theta_C$ when the prior parameter vector is $\Theta_*$,

$$G_\theta(\theta_{C_\kappa}; \Theta_*) = \kappa.$$

This assures that the theoretical range of control group event rate values is consistent with the observed range of values. Finally, define $(a_C, b_C)$ as the point that comes closest to satisfying

$$G_\theta(\theta_{C_\kappa}; \Theta_C = (a_C, b_C)) = \kappa.$$

The software uses this relationship to calculate $\Theta_C$. The value of $\Theta_C$ is modified for each particular adverse event by incorporating the event counts in the control group, so that $\Theta_C$ is replaced by $\Theta_C(x_i)$ for the $i$th adverse event, that is,

$$\Theta_C(x_i) = \begin{cases} (a_C + x_i, b_C + n_C - x_i) & \text{for binomial models} \\ (a_C + x_i, b_C + n_C) & \text{for Poisson models.} \end{cases}$$

We assume that the value of $\Theta_T = (a_T, b_T)$ is a function of the value of $\Theta_C$ and the control group outcomes. For convenience, set $b_T = b_T(x_i) = b_C(x_i)$. Then $a_T = a_T(x_i)$ is the value that satisfies the condition

$$F_R(\psi; \Theta_T = (a_T(x_i), b_T(x_i)) \le \phi_1.$$

## 6.4.4   Example

Table 6.8 displays the results of carrying out the calculations for the adverse events whose confidence intervals in Tables 6.2 and 6.3 did not include 0 (difference) or 1 (ratio, odds ratio) using two values of the maximum acceptable odds ratio value $\psi$ ($\psi = 2$ or 4) when the same process generates the test and control rates, and critical probabilities $\phi_0 = 0.0, 0.95, 0.99$ and $\phi_1 = 0.01, 0.05$, and 0.1. The screening process identified only event 17 as worth subsequent follow-up. Table 6.9 displays selected values of the posterior cdf of the odds ratio corresponding to event 17. Although it is clear from Table 6.8 that different processes generated the rates for event 17, it also is clear from Table 6.9 that the increase in risk was fairly modest, almost certainly less than a doubling of the risk, regardless of the values of $\psi$, $\phi_0$, and $\phi_1$.

Analyses carried out using the methods described by Mehrotra and Heyse [27] and by Berry and Berry [33] also wound up selecting just event 17 for further follow-up. However, neither also provided the posterior distribution of the odds ratio to quantify the extent of the difference between the test and control groups.

**Table 6.8**  $Pr(\gamma_i = 0)$ for rows from Tables 6.2 and 6.3 as a function of $\phi_0$, $\phi_1$, and critical odds ratio values ($\psi$).

| | $\psi = 2$ | | | $\psi = 2$ | | | $\psi = 2$ | | |
|---|---|---|---|---|---|---|---|---|---|
| | $\phi_0 = 0.9$ | | | $\phi_0 = 0.95$ | | | $\phi_0 = 0.99$ | | |
| Event | $\phi_1 = 0.01$ | 0.05 | 0.1 | $\phi_1 = 0.01$ | 0.05 | 0.1 | $\phi_1 = 0.01$ | 0.05 | 0.1 |
| 9 | 0.78 | 0.65 | 0.62 | 0.93 | 0.82 | 0.76 | 0.99 | 0.97 | 0.95 |
| 17 | 0.01 | 0.04 | 0.09 | 0.00 | 0.01 | 0.01 | 0 | < 0.01 | < 0.01 |
| 32 | 1.00 | 0.97 | 0.94 | 1.00 | 1.00 | 0.99 | 1 | 1 | 1 |
| 34 | 1.00 | 1.00 | 0.99 | 1 | 1 | 1 | 1 | 1 | 1 |
| | $\psi = 4$ | | | $\psi = 4$ | | | $\psi = 4$ | | |
| | $\phi_0 = 0.9$ | | | $\phi_0 = 0.95$ | | | $\phi_0 = 0.99$ | | |
| Event | $\phi_1 = 0.01$ | 0.05 | 0.1 | $\phi_1 = 0.01$ | 0.05 | 0.1 | $\phi_1 = 0.01$ | 0.05 | 0.1 |
| 9 | 0.82 | 0.53 | 0.47 | 0.95 | 0.71 | 0.58 | 1.00 | 0.96 | 0.90 |
| 17 | 0.05 | 0.13 | 0.22 | 0.01 | 0.04 | 0.08 | < 0.01 | < 0.01 | 0.01 |
| 32 | 0.99 | 0.85 | 0.69 | 1.00 | 0.98 | 0.93 | 1 | 1 | 1 |
| 34 | 1.00 | 0.99 | 0.94 | 1 | 1 | 1 | 1 | 1 | 1 |

**Table 6.9**  Posterior cdf of the odds ratio $p_T(1 - p_C)/p_C(1 - p_T)$ for event 17 as a function of the values of $\phi_0$ and $\phi_1$ when the critical odds ratio value was set at $\psi = 2$ or 4.

| $\psi = 2$ | | Posterior CDF of the odds ratio evaluated at | | | | | | |
|---|---|---|---|---|---|---|---|---|
| $\phi_0$ | $\phi_1$ | 1 | 1.1 | 1.2 | 1.3 | 1.4 | 1.5 | 2 |
| 0.9 | 0.01 | 0.01 | 0.04 | 0.10 | 0.19 | 0.31 | 0.44 | 0.90 |
| 0.9 | 0.05 | 0.04 | 0.10 | 0.19 | 0.32 | 0.46 | 0.59 | 0.95 |
| 0.9 | 0.1 | 0.06 | 0.14 | 0.26 | 0.40 | 0.54 | 0.67 | 0.97 |
| 0.95 | 0.01 | 0.04 | 0.08 | 0.16 | 0.26 | 0.38 | 0.50 | 0.91 |
| 0.95 | 0.05 | 0.10 | 0.20 | 0.32 | 0.45 | 0.58 | 0.70 | 0.97 |
| 0.95 | 0.1 | 0.15 | 0.27 | 0.41 | 0.55 | 0.68 | 0.78 | 0.98 |
| 0.99 | 0.01 | 0.00 | 0.01 | 0.03 | 0.08 | 0.16 | 0.27 | 0.82 |
| 0.99 | 0.05 | 0.01 | 0.03 | 0.08 | 0.17 | 0.28 | 0.42 | 0.91 |
| 0.99 | 0.1 | 0.02 | 0.05 | 0.12 | 0.22 | 0.36 | 0.50 | 0.94 |
| $\psi = 4$ | | Posterior CDF of the odds ratio evaluated at | | | | | | |
| 0.9 | 0.01 | 0 | 0 | 0.00 | 0.01 | 0.03 | 0.08 | 0.63 |
| 0.9 | 0.05 | 0 | 0 | 0.01 | 0.04 | 0.09 | 0.17 | 0.79 |
| 0.9 | 0.1 | 0.00 | 0.01 | 0.02 | 0.06 | 0.13 | 0.25 | 0.85 |
| 0.95 | 0.01 | 0.00 | 0.00 | 0.01 | 0.02 | 0.05 | 0.10 | 0.58 |
| 0.95 | 0.05 | 0.00 | 0.01 | 0.03 | 0.07 | 0.14 | 0.24 | 0.77 |
| 0.95 | 0.1 | 0.01 | 0.02 | 0.06 | 0.12 | 0.22 | 0.33 | 0.84 |
| 0.99 | 0.01 | 0.01 | 0.02 | 0.06 | 0.12 | 0.22 | 0.33 | 0.84 |
| 0.99 | 0.05 | 0.01 | 0.03 | 0.07 | 0.13 | 0.22 | 0.33 | 0.83 |
| 0.99 | 0.1 | 0.04 | 0.09 | 0.17 | 0.28 | 0.41 | 0.53 | 0.93 |

## 6.5  Discussion

This chapter has described a number of ways to construct confidence or credible intervals for measures of difference between adverse event incidences in a test and a control group. Many such approaches have been proposed for this purpose, but several review articles comparing their performance have identified a small number that have desirable statistical properties such as accurate coverage and small interval width. These approaches include conventional frequentist and Bayesian methods, methods assuming binomial and Poisson likelihoods, and various difference measures, particularly the arithmetic difference between event rates, the ratio of the rates and, for binomially distributed data, odds ratios. A Bayesian screening method that adjusts for the potential multiplicity issue that arises when many events occur also is described.

The descriptions are drawn from source publications. Software for calculating the various measures is provided or at least referenced. In addition, coverage comparisons of the various approaches are presented, focusing on accuracy of coverage especially for event rates in the 0–0.1 range.

The coverages of all of the approaches improve with sample size. The coverages of the various conventional methods are similar, but not identical. The coverages of the Bayesian approaches compare favorably with conventional approach coverages.

## Appendix 6.A  R Functions

```
BayesBinLims.fn <- function(nxny,conflim=c(.025,.5,.975),
    abcd=rep(.5,4),adj=.5)
{
#  Calculates the posterior mean and confidence intervals for the
#  differences, ratios, and odds ratios of a set of observations from
#  binomial distributions.
#
#  INPUT
#     nxny = (nX,x,nY,y) = 4-column array (or 4-elt vector) of trial
#     outcomes:
#        nX = sample size, x = no. of events, likewise for nY, y
#  conflim = percentiles of the posterior distribution to calculate
#     abcd = parameters of prior distns of event rates (pX, pY) for X and Y
#            (default is Jeffreys prior, abcd = rep(.5,4)
#      adj = additional offset added to x, n-x, y, and n-y when x or y = 0 to
#            to stabilize the calculations).
#
#  OUTPUT
#     call = command sequence to invoke program
#     date = date when run was made
#   result = matrix of outcomes
#                                      A. L. Gould   March 2013

  if (length(dim(nxny))==0) nxny <- array(nxny,c(1,4))
  ncases <- dim(nxny)[1]
  i0 <- (1:ncases)[nxny[,2]*nxny[,4] == 0]
  nxny[i0,] <- nxny[i0,] + adj*c(2,1,2,1)
```

```
xy <- cbind(nxny[,2],nxny[,1]-nxny[,2],nxny[,4],nxny[,3]-nxny[,4])
result <- matrix(0,ncases,18)
result[,1:4] <- as.matrix(nxny)
result[,5:6] <- result[,c(2,4)]/result[,c(1,3)]
result[,7] <- result[,5] - result[,6]
result[,8] <- result[,5]/(result[,6] + .001*(result[,4]==0))
result[,9] <- result[,8]*(1-result[,6])/
              (1-result[,5] + .001*(result[,1]==result[,2]))
for (i in 1:ncases)
{
  abcdxy <- abcd + xy[i,]
  result[i,10:12] <- BetaMetricCDFInv.fn(1,conflim,abcdxy)$metric
  result[i,13:15] <- BetaMetricCDFInv.fn(2,conflim,abcdxy)$metric
  result[i,16:18] <- BetaMetricCDFInv.fn(3,conflim,abcdxy)$metric
}
result[,5:18] <- round(result[,5:18],3)
result <- as.data.frame(result)
dimnames(result)[[2]] <- c("nX","x","nY","y","pX","pY","Diff","Ratio",
                           "OddsRat", "Diff.L","Diff.Med","Diff.U","Rat.L",
                           "Rat.Med","Rat.U", "OR.L","OR.Med","OR.U")
return(list(call=sys.call(),date=date(),conflim=conflim,result=result))
}


FreqBinLims.fn <- function(nxny,conf=0.95,eps=1e-4)
{
#  Calculates a variety of frequentist-based confidence intervals for
#  difference, ratio, and odds ratio of binomial rate parameters
#
#  INPUT
#  nxny = a 4-element vector of outcomes (n1, x1, n2, x2) from
#  distributions with rate parameters p1 and p2, or an m x 4 matrix
#  whose rows are values of
#         (n1, x1, n2, x2).
#  conf = confidence level -- default is 95% (0.95)
#
#  OUTPUT
#  lims = a 23-element vector whose elements (or an m x 23 matrix
#          whose rows) are
#    n1, x1, n2, x2 = original data
#              Diff = actual difference x1/n1 - x2/n2
#        LDsc, UDsc = score-based confidence limits for difference
#        LDAC, UDAC = Agresti-Caffo score limits
#          LDN, UDN = Newcombe hybrid Wilson score confidence limits
#      LDBLJ, UDBLJ = Jeffreys pseudo confidence limits (Brown & Li,
#                      JSPI 2005)
#    LDBLrc, UDBLrc = recentered confidence limits (Brown & Li, JSPI 2005)
#             Ratio = actual ratio (x1/n1 / x2/n2)
#        LRsc,URsc = score-based confidence limits for ratio
#               OR = actual odds ratio (x1*(n2-x2)/x2*(n1-x1))
#        LOsc,UOsc = score-based confidence limits for odds ratio
#        LOFN,UOFN = Fagerland-Newcombe asymptotic confidence limits for
#                      odds ratio
```

```
#         LOBP,UOPB = confidence limits based on Baptista-Pike mid-p test
#
#  Requires the PropCIs and pairwiseCI packages.
#                                                   A. L. Gould  March 2013
  za <- qnorm((1+conf)/2)
  if (length(dim(nxny))==0) nxny <- array(nxny,c(1,length(nxny)))
  n1 <- nxny[,1];  n2 <- nxny[,3];  x1 <- nxny[,2];  x2 <- nxny[,4]
  ncases <- length(n1)
  p1 <- x1/n1
  p2 <- x2/n2
  diff <- p1 - p2                                  # Get estimates of
  i <- (x2 > 0)                                    # the various
  rat <- 0*x1                                      # metrics (diff,
                                                   # ratio, OR)
  orat <- rat
  rat[i] <- p1[i]/p2[i]
  rat[!i] <- Inf
  i <- (x2 > 0) & (x1 < n1)
  orat[i] <- x1[i]*(n2[i]-x2[i])/(x2[i]*(n1[i]-x1[i]))
  orat[!i] <- Inf
  z.sc.diff <- NULL                               # Get score-based CI
  z.sc.rat <- NULL
  z.sc.orat <- NULL
  clim <- NULL
  for (i in 1:ncases)                  # Get arrays of lower and
                                       # upper bounds
  {
    z.sc.diff <- rbind(z.sc.diff,diffscoreci(x1[i],n1[i],x2[i],n2[i],
                      conf.level=conf)$conf.int[1:2])
    z.sc.rat <- rbind(z.sc.rat,riskscoreci(x1[i],n1[i],x2[i],n2[i],
                      conf.level=conf)$conf.int[1:2])
    z.sc.orat <- rbind(z.sc.orat,orscoreci(x1[i],n1[i],x2[i],n2[i],
                      conf.level=conf)$conf.int[1:2])
    clim <- rbind(clim,BPmidp.fn(x1[i],n1[i],n2[i],x1[i]+x2[i],
                      alpha=1-conf,eps=eps))
  }
  lims <- AgrestiBrownLiDiff.fn(nxny,conf)             # Agresti-Caffo &
                                                      # Brown-Li CI
  lims <- cbind(lims,Newcombe.fn(nxny,conf))          # Newcombe hybrid
                                                      # score CI
  lims <- cbind(nxny,round(cbind(diff,z.sc.diff,lims,rat,z.sc.rat,orat,
                      z.sc.orat,clim[,2:3]),3))
  lims <- cbind(lims,round(FagNew.fn(nxny,conf),3))   # Fagerland-Newcombe
                                                      # asymp. CI
  dimnames(lims)[[2]][5:25] <- c("Diff","LDsc","UDsc","LDAC",
                      "UDAC","LDBLJ","UDBLJ",
                      "LDBLrc","UDBLrc","LDN","UDN","Ratio",
                      "LRsc","URsc",
                      "OR","LOsc","UOsc","LOBP","UOBP",
                      "LOFN","UOFN")
  return(list(call=sys.call(),Date = date(),lims=lims))
}
```

```
ConfCredB.fn <- function(n,p=c(.01*1:9,.1*1:5),abcd=c(.5,.5,.5,.5),
                         conflim=c(0.025,0.975),inclOR=FALSE,eps=1e-8,
                         eta=1e-8)
{
#  Calculates coverage probabilities for Bayesian credible intervals for
#  difference between or ratio of binomial probabilities as a
#  function of the true event rates
#  and the sample size.  Also optionally calculates coverage
#  probabilities for credible intervals for the odds ratio.
#
#  Given values pX and pY of the event rates and a per-group sample
#  size of n, the credible intervals are calculated for all
#  possible binomial sample outcomes X ~ binom(n,pX)
#  and Y ~ binom(n,pY) are calculated and the probabilities of those
#  outcomes for which the true value of the difference or ratio falls in the
#  credible interval are accumulated.  The sum of these probabilities is the
#  coverage probability corresponding to the sample size and the
#  values of pX & pY.
#
#  INPUT
#      n = per-group sample sizes
#      p = vector of event rates: coverage probabilities are calculated
#          for all combinations of pairs of values contained in p.
#   abcd = parameters of the prior distribution of the event rate(s).
#          Default is Jeffreys prior
# conflim = lower and upper confidence probabilities
#  inclOR = TRUE to calculate coverage probabilities for odds ratios,
#          FALSE if not (default)
# OUTPUT
#
#  CovProbD = Coverage probabilities of credible intervals for the difference
#             between each possible pair of values in p
#  CovProbR = Coverage probabilities of credible intervals for the
#             ratio of each possible pair of values in p
#  CovProbO = Coverage probabilities of credible intervals for the
#             odds ratio of each possible pair of values in p
#             (if inclOR = TRUE -- not included otherwise)
#                                       A. L. Gould  April 2013
  step1.fn <-function(p,n,eps)
  {
    np <- length(p)
    LU <- array(0,c(np,2))
    for (ip in 1:np)
    {
      if (pbinom(0,n,p[ip]) > eps) L <- 0 else L <- qbinom
          (eps,n,p[probabilities of those ip])
      if (pbinom(0,n,1-p[ip]) > eps) U <- n  else U <- qbinom(1-eps,n,p[ip])
      LU[ip,] <- c(L,U)
    }
    return(LU)
  }
```

```
t1 <- proc.time()[3]
np <- length(p)
LUx <- step1.fn(p,n,eps)
LUy <- LUx
CovProbD <- array(0,c(np,np))                  # Initialize accumulation
                                               # arrays
CovProbR <- CovProbD
TrueDiff <- outer(p,p,"-")                      # Set up arrays of true
                                               # differences,
TrueRatio <- outer(p,p,"/")                     # ratios, and odds ratios
if (inclOR)
{
  CovProbO <- CovProbD
  TrueOddsRatio <- outer(p,1-p,"*")/outer(1-p,p,"*")
}
for (iX in 1:np)
{
  X <- LUx[iX,1]:LUx[iX,2]                       # Get range of
                                               # X values with
  fX <- dbinom(X,n,p[iX])                        # "positive"
                                               # likelihoods and
  for (iY in 1:np)                               # get corresponding
                                               # likelihoods
  {
    Y <- LUy[iY,1]:LUy[iY,2]                      # Same for Y values
    fY <- dbinom(Y,n,p[iY])
    XY <- growarray.fn(list(X,Y))                # All (X,Y)
                                               # outcomes in ranges
    fXY <- apply(growarray.fn(list(fX,fY)),1,prod)   # Corresp. joint
                                               # likelihoods
    nXY <- length(fXY)
    iXY <- (1:nXY)[fXY > eta]                    # Retain outcomes and
                                               # likelihoods
    nnXY <- length(iXY)                          # with non-trivial
                                               # likelihood values
    XXYY <- XY[iXY,]
    ffXY <- fXY[iXY]
    abcdxy <- abcd + cbind(XXYY[,1],n-XXYY[,1],XXYY[,2],n-XXYY[,2])  # Post
                                               # params
    for (jXY in 1:nnXY)                          # Calculate
                                               # credible intervals
    {                                           # and coverage
                                               # probabilities
      diffcdf <- BetaMetricCDF.fn(1,TrueDiff[iX,iY],abcdxy[jXY,])$cdf
      if ((diffcdf >= conflim[1]) & (diffcdf <= conflim[2]))
        CovProbD[iX,iY] <- CovProbD[iX,iY] + ffXY[jXY]
      ratcdf <- BetaMetricCDF.fn(2,TrueRatio[iX,iY],abcdxy[jXY,])$cdf
      if ((ratcdf >= conflim[1]) & (ratcdf <= conflim[2]))
        CovProbR[iX,iY] <- CovProbR[iX,iY] + ffXY[jXY]
      if (inclOR)
```

```
          {
            oratcdf <- BetaMetricCDF.fn(3,TrueOddsRatio[iX,iY],
            abcdxy[jXY,])$cdf
            if ((oratcdf >= conflim[1]) & (oratcdf <= conflim[2]))
              CovProbO[iX,iY] <- CovProbO[iX,iY] + ffXY[jXY]
          }
        }
      }
    }
  CovProbD <- rbind(p,round(CovProbD,3))          # Add labels to coverage
  CovProbD <- cbind(c(0,p),CovProbD)              # arrays to identify pX,
                                                  #   pY values

  CovProbR <- rbind(p,round(CovProbR,3))
  CovProbR <- cbind(c(0,p),CovProbR)
  if (inclOR)
  {
    CovProbO <- rbind(p,round(CovProbO,3))
    CovProbO <- cbind(c(0,p),CovProbO)
  }
  t1 <- Elapsed.time.fn(t1)
  if (inclOR)
    return(list(call=sys.call(), date=date(), Elapsed.Time=t1,
            CovProbD = CovProbD, CovProbR = CovProbR, CovProbO = CovProbO,
            CovProbD = CovProbD, CovProbR = CovProbR))
  else
    return(list(call=sys.call(), date=date(), Elapsed.Time=t1,
            CovProbD = CovProbD, CovProbR = CovProbR))
}

ConfFreqB.fn <- function(n,p=c(.01*1:9,.1*1:5),abcd=c(.5,.5,.5,.5),
    conflim=c(0.025,0.975),conflev=0.95,eps=0.00001)
{
  t1 <- proc.time()[3]
  np <- length(p)
  Lsc.D <- matrix(0,n+1,n+1)              # Set up accumulation arrays
  Usc.D <- Lsc.D
  DHitssc <- matrix(0,np,np)
  LNH.D <- Lsc.D
  UNH.D <- Lsc.D
  DHitsNH <- DHitssc
  LAC.D <- Lsc.D
  UAC.D <- Lsc.D
  DHitsAC <- DHitssc
  LBLJ.D <- Lsc.D
  UBLJ.D <- Lsc.D
  DHitsBLJ <- DHitssc
  LBLrc.D <- Lsc.D
  UBLrc.D <- Lsc.D
  DHitsBLrc <- DHitssc
  Lsc.R <- Lsc.D
  Usc.R <- Lsc.D
  RHitssc <- DHitssc
  Lsc.O <- Lsc.D
  Usc.O <- Lsc.D
  OHitssc <- DHitssc
```

```
LFN.O <- Lsc.D
UFN.O <- Lsc.D
OHitsFN <- DHitssc
LBP.O <- Lsc.D
UBP.O <- Lsc.D
Wsc.D <- Lsc.D
WAC.D <- Lsc.D
WNH.D <- Lsc.D
WBLrc.D <- Lsc.D
WBLJ.D <- Lsc.D
Wsc.R <- Lsc.D
Wsc.O <- Lsc.D
WFN.O <- Lsc.D
WBP.O <- Lsc.D
DWidthsc <- DHitssc
DWidthAC <- DHitssc
DWidthNH <- DHitssc
DWidthBLJ <- DHitssc
DWidthBLrc <- DHitssc
RWidthsc <- DHitssc
OWidthsc <- DHitssc
OWidthFN <- DHitssc
OWidthBP <- DHitssc
OHitsBP <- DHitssc
for (x in 0:n)
  for (y in 0:n)
  {
    abcdxy <- abcd + c(x, n-x, y, n-y)       # Get arrays of lower and upper
    nx <- abcdxy[1]+abcdxy[2]                # confidence bounds on the
                                             # differences
    ny <- abcdxy[3]+abcdxy[4]
    zz <- diffscoreci(abcdxy[1],nx,abcdxy[3],ny,
        conf.level=conflev)$conf.int[1:2]
    Lsc.D[x+1,y+1] <- zz[1]
    Usc.D[x+1,y+1] <- zz[2]
    Wsc.D[x+1,y+1] <- zz[2] - zz[1]
    zz <- Newcombe.fn(array(c(n,x,n,y),c(1,4)),conflev)
    LNH.D[x+1,y+1] <- zz[1]
    UNH.D[x+1,y+1] <- zz[2]
    WNH.D[x+1,y+1] <- zz[2] - zz[1]
    zz <- AgrestiBrownLiDiff.fn(array(c(n,x,n,y),c(1,4)),conflev)
    LAC.D[x+1,y+1] <- zz[1]
    UAC.D[x+1,y+1] <- zz[2]
    WAC.D[x+1,y+1] <- zz[2] - zz[1]
    LBLJ.D[x+1,y+1] <- zz[3]
    UBLJ.D[x+1,y+1] <- zz[4]
    WBLJ.D[x+1,y+1] <- zz[4] - zz[3]
    LBLrc.D[x+1,y+1] <- zz[5]
    UBLrc.D[x+1,y+1] <- zz[6]
    WBLrc.D[x+1,y+1] <- zz[6] - zz[5]
    zz <- riskscoreci(abcdxy[1],nx,abcdxy[3],ny,
        conf.level=conflev)$conf.int[1:2]
    Lsc.R[x+1,y+1] <- zz[1]
    Usc.R[x+1,y+1] <- zz[2]
    Wsc.R[x+1,y+1] <- zz[2] - zz[1]
```

```
        zz <- orscoreci(abcdxy[1],nx,abcdxy[3],ny,
                        conf.level=conflev)$conf.int[1:2]
      Lsc.O[x+1,y+1] <- zz[1]
      Usc.O[x+1,y+1] <- zz[2]
      Wsc.O[x+1,y+1] <- zz[2] - zz[1]
      zz <- FagNew.fn(c(n,x,n,y),conflev)
      LFN.O[x+1,y+1] <- zz[1]
      UFN.O[x+1,y+1] <- zz[2]
      WFN.O[x+1,y+1] <- zz[2] - zz[1]
      zz <- BPmidp.fn(x,n,n,x+y,alpha=1-conflev,eps=eps)
      LBP.O[x+1,y+1] <- zz[2]
      UBP.O[x+1,y+1] <- zz[3]
      if (zz[3] < 1e8) WBP.O[x+1,y+1] <- zz[3] - zz[2]  else
                       WBP.O[x+1,y+1] <- 0
    }
  for (ip in 1:np)                       # Get the probabilities
                                         # of sample
    for (jp in 1:np)                     # outcomes for all
                                         # combinations of
      {                                  # true event rates, and
                                         # calculate
      TrueD <- p[ip] - p[jp]             # the probabilities of
                                         # sample outcomes
      TrueR <- p[ip]/p[jp]               # leading to confidence
                                         # intervals
      TrueOR <- p[ip]*(1-p[jp])/(p[jp]*(1-p[ip]))   # that cover the diffs,
                                                    # ratios,
      xden <- dbinom(0:n,n,p[ip])        # and odds ratios of the
                                         # true event
      yden <- dbinom(0:n,n,p[jp])        # rates for each pair of
                                         # event rates
      xyden <- outer(xden,yden,"*")

      ULsc.D <- 0+((TrueD >= Lsc.D) & (TrueD <= Usc.D))
      DHitssc[ip,jp] <- sum(ULsc.D*xyden)
      DWidthsc[ip,jp] <- sum(Wsc.D*xyden)
      ULNH.D <- 0+((TrueD >= LNH.D) & (TrueD <= UNH.D))
      DHitsNH[ip,jp] <- sum(ULNH.D*xyden)
      DWidthNH[ip,jp] <- sum(WNH.D*xyden)
      ULAC.D <- 0+((TrueD >= LAC.D) & (TrueD <= UAC.D))
      DHitsAC[ip,jp] <- sum(ULAC.D*xyden)
      DWidthAC[ip,jp] <- sum(WAC.D*xyden)
      ULBLJ.D <- 0+((TrueD >= LBLJ.D) & (TrueD <= UBLJ.D))
      DHitsBLJ[ip,jp] <- sum(ULBLJ.D*xyden)
      DWidthBLJ[ip,jp] <- sum(WBLJ.D*xyden)
      ULBLrc.D <- 0+((TrueD >= LBLrc.D) & (TrueD <= UBLrc.D))
      DHitsBLrc[ip,jp] <- sum(ULBLrc.D*xyden)
      DWidthBLrc[ip,jp] <- sum(WBLrc.D*xyden)
      ULsc.R <- 0+((TrueR >= Lsc.R) & (TrueR <= Usc.R))
      RHitssc[ip,jp] <- sum(ULsc.R*xyden)
      RWidthsc[ip,jp] <- sum(Wsc.R*xyden)
      ULsc.O <- 0+((TrueOR >= Lsc.O) & (TrueOR <= Usc.O))
      OHitssc[ip,jp] <- sum(ULsc.O*xyden)
      OWidthsc[ip,jp] <- sum(Wsc.O*xyden)
      ULFN.O <- 0+((TrueOR >= LFN.O) & (TrueOR <= UFN.O))
      OHitsFN[ip,jp] <- sum(ULFN.O*xyden)
```

```
      OWidthFN[ip,jp] <- sum(WFN.O*xyden)
      ULBP.O <- 0+((TrueOR >= LBP.O) & (TrueOR <= UBP.O))
      OHitsBP[ip,jp] <- sum(ULBP.O*xyden)
      pFin <- sum(xyden[WBP.O > 0])
      OWidthBP[ip,jp] <- sum(WBP.O*xyden)/pFin
    }
  xy <- growarray.fn(list(p,p))
  DHitssc <- rbind(c(NA,p),cbind(p,round(DHitssc,3)))
  DHitsNH <- rbind(c(NA,p),cbind(p,round(DHitsNH,3)))
  DHitsAC <- rbind(c(NA,p),cbind(p,round(DHitsAC,3)))
  DHitsBLJ <- rbind(c(NA,p),cbind(p,round(DHitsBLJ,3)))
  DHitsBLrc <- rbind(c(NA,p),cbind(p,round(DHitsBLrc,3)))
  RHitssc <- rbind(c(NA,p),cbind(p,round(RHitssc,3)))
  OHitssc <- rbind(c(NA,p),cbind(p,round(OHitssc,3)))
  OHitsFN <- rbind(c(NA,p),cbind(p,round(OHitsFN,3)))
  OHitsBP <- rbind(c(NA,p),cbind(p,round(OHitsBP,3)))
  DWidthsc <- rbind(c(NA,p),cbind(p,round(DWidthsc,3)))
  DWidthNH <- rbind(c(NA,p),cbind(p,round(DWidthNH,3)))
  DWidthAC <- rbind(c(NA,p),cbind(p,round(DWidthAC,3)))
  DWidthBLJ <- rbind(c(NA,p),cbind(p,round(DWidthBLJ,3)))
  DWidthBLrc <- rbind(c(NA,p),cbind(p,round(DWidthBLrc,3)))
  RWidthsc <- rbind(c(NA,p),cbind(p,round(RWidthsc,3)))
  OWidthsc <- rbind(c(NA,p),cbind(p,round(OWidthsc,3)))
  OWidthFN <- rbind(c(NA,p),cbind(p,round(OWidthFN,3)))
  OWidthBP <- rbind(c(NA,p),cbind(p,round(OWidthBP,3)))
  t1 <- Elapsed.time.fn(t1)
  return(list(call=sys.call(), date=date(), Elapsed.Time=t1,abcd=abcd,
              conflim=conflim,conflev=conflev, DHitssc=DHitssc,
              DHitsNH=DHitsNH, DHitsAC=DHitsAC, DHitsBLJ=DHitsBLJ,
              DHitsBLrc=DHitsBLrc, RHitssc=RHitssc, OHitsBP=OHitsBP,
              OHitssc=OHitssc, OHitsNF=OHitsFN, DWidthsc=DWidthsc,
              DWidthNH=DWidthNH, DWidthAC=DWidthAC, DWidthBLJ=DWidthBLJ,
              DWidthBLrc=DWidthBLrc, RWidthsc=RWidthsc, OWidthBP=OWidthBP,
              OWidthsc=OWidthsc, OWidthFN=OWidthFN))
}


PoisLims.fn <- function(nxny,conflim=c(.025,.975),ab=c(.5,1,.5,1))
{
#  Calculates the posterior mean and confidence intervals for the
#  differences and ratios of a set of observations from
#  Poisson distributions.
#
#  INPUT
#     nxny = (nX,x,nY,y) = 4-column array (or 4-elt vector)
#              of trial outcomes:
#            nX = sample size or exposure, x = no. of events,
#                likewise for nY, y
#  conflim = percentiles of the posterior distribution to calculate
#     abcd = parameters of prior distns of event rates (lambdaX,
#            lambdaY) for X & Y
#
#  OUTPUT
#     call = command sequence to invoke program
#     date = date when run was made
#   result = matrix of outcomes
#    n1, x1, n2, x2 = original data
```

```
#          lamX, lamY = estimates of Poisson parameters
#                Diff = actual difference x1/n1 - x2/n2
#               Ratio = actual ratio (x1/n1 / x2/n2)
#       LFT.D, UFT.D = confidence limits for difference using
#                      Freeman-Tukey interval
#          LJ.D, UJ.D = confidence limits for difference using Jeffries
#                       interval
#            L.R, U.R = confidence limits for ratio using Graham interval
#          LB.D, UB.D = credible interval for difference
#          LB.R, UB.R = credible interval for ratio
#                                                           A. L. Gould
#                                                           March 2013
  step.fn <- function(diff,Lx,Ux,Ly,Uy)
  {
    LB <- diff - sqrt((result[,5]-Lx)^2 + (result[,6]-Uy)^2)
    UB <- diff + sqrt((result[,5]-Ux)^2 + (result[,6]-Ly)^2)
    return(cbind(LB,UB))
  }

  if (length(dim(nxny))==0) nxny <- array(nxny,c(1,4))
  ncases <- dim(nxny)[1]
  abXY <- t(ab + t(nxny[,c(2,1,4,3)]))    # x + 1/2, nX + 1, y + 1/2, nY + 1
  za <- qnorm(conflim[1])
  za2 <- za^2
  result <- NULL
  result <- as.matrix(nxny)
  result <- cbind(result,result[,c(2,4)]/result[,c(1,3)])
  result <- cbind(result,result[,5] - result[,6])
  result <- cbind(result,result[,5]/(result[,6] + .001*(result[,4]==0)))
  LxFT <- 0.25*((sqrt(nxny[,2]) + sqrt(nxny[,2] + 1) + za)^2 - 1)/nxny[,1]
  LyFT <- 0.25*((sqrt(nxny[,4]) + sqrt(nxny[,4] + 1) + za)^2 - 1)/nxny[,3]
  UxFT <- 0.25*((sqrt(nxny[,2]) + sqrt(nxny[,2] + 1) - za)^2 - 1)/nxny[,1]
  UyFT <- 0.25*((sqrt(nxny[,4]) + sqrt(nxny[,4] + 1) - za)^2 - 1)/nxny[,3]
  LxJ <- qgamma(conflim[1],abXY[,1],nxny[,1])
  LyJ <- qgamma(conflim[1],abXY[,3],nxny[,3])
  UxJ <- qgamma(conflim[2],abXY[,1],nxny[,1])
  UyJ <- qgamma(conflim[2],abXY[,3],nxny[,3])
  result <- cbind(result,step.fn(result[,7],LxFT,UxFT,LyFT,UyFT))
  result <- cbind(result,step.fn(result[,7],LxJ,UxJ,LyJ,UyJ))

  L.R <- array(0,ncases)
  U.R <- array(Inf,ncases)
  ii <- (1:ncases)[nxny[,4] > 0]
  if (length(ii) > 0)
  {
    xpy <- nxny[ii,2] + nxny[ii,4]
    xty <- nxny[ii,2]*nxny[ii,4]
    w1 <- 2*xty + xpy*za2
    w2 <- sqrt(xpy*za2*(4*xty + xpy*za2))
    L.R[ii] <- 0.5*(nxny[ii,3]/nxny[ii,1])*(w1 - w2)/nxny[ii,4]^2
    U.R[ii] <- 0.5*(nxny[ii,3]/nxny[ii,1])*(w1 + w2)/nxny[ii,4]^2
  }
```

```
  result <- cbind(result,L.R,U.R)
  w <- NULL
  for (i in 1:ncases)
  {
    w <- rbind(w,c(GammaMetricCDFInv.fn(1,conflim,abXY[i,])$metric,
                   GammaMetricCDFInv.fn(2,conflim,abXY[i,])$metric))
  }
  result <- cbind(result,w)
  result[,5:18] <- round(result[,5:18],3)
  dimnames(result)[[2]] <- c("nX","x","nY","y","lamX","lamY","Diff",
                       "Ratio","LFT.D","UFT.D","LJ.D","UJ.D","L.R","U.R",
                       "LB.D","UB.D","LB.R","UB.R")
  return(list(call=sys.call(),date=date(),conflim=conflim,result=result))
}


ConfCredG.fn <- function(lambda,abcd=c(.5,1,.5,1),n=100,
                         conflim=c(0.025,0.975),eps=1e-8,eta=1e-4)
{
#  Calculates coverage probabilities for Bayesian credible intervals for
#  difference between or ratio of Poisson event rates as functions of the
#  true event rates.
#
#  Given values lambdaX and lambdaY of the event rates and a per-group
#  sample size or exposure denoted by n, credible intervals are
#  calculated for all possible Poisson sample outcomes X ~ poiss(n lambdaX)
#  and Y ~ binom(n lambdaY) and the
#  probabilities of those outcomes for which the true value of the
#  differences lambdaX - lambdaY or or ratios lambdaX/lambdaY falls in the
#  credible interval are
#  accumulated.  The sum of these probabilities is the coverage probability f
#  corresponding to the values olambdaX and lambdaY.
#
#  INPUT
#  lambda = vector of event rates per exposure unit: coverage probs are
#           calculated for all combinations of pairs of values
#           contained in lambda.
#     abcd = parameters of the prior distribution of the event rate(s).
#           Default is Jeffreys prior
#        n = per-group sample sizes or exposures
# conflim = lower and upper confidence probabilities
#
# OUTPUT
#  CovProbD = Coverage probabilities of credible intervals for the difference
#             between each possible pair of values in p
#  CovProbR = Coverage probabilities of credible intervals for the
#             ratio of each possible pair of values in p
#                                       A. L. Gould  April 2013
  step1.fn <-function(lam,n,eps)
  {
    nlam <- length(lam)
    LU <- array(0,c(nlam,2))
    for (ilam in 1:nlam)
```

```
    {
      tlam <- n*lam[ilam]
      L <- max(0,qpois(eps,tlam))
      U <- qpois(1-eps,tlam)
      LU[ilam,] <- c(L,U)
    }
    return(LU)
  }

  t1 <- proc.time()[3]
  nlam <- length(lambda)
  LUx <- step1.fn(lambda,n,eps)
  LUy <- LUx
  CovProbD <- array(0,c(nlam,nlam))
  CovProbR <- CovProbD
  TrueDiff <- outer(lambda,lambda,"-")
  TrueRatio <- outer(lambda,lambda,"/")

  for (iX in 1:nlam)
  {
    X <- LUx[iX,1]:LUx[iX,2]
    fX <- dpois(X,n*lambda[iX])
    for (iY in 1:length(lambda))
    {
      Y <- LUy[iY,1]:LUy[iY,2]
      fY <- dpois(Y,n*lambda[iY])
      XY <- growarray.fn(list(X,Y))
      fXY <- apply(growarray.fn(list(fX,fY)),1,prod)
      nXY <- length(fXY)
      iXY <- (1:nXY)[fXY > eta]
      XXYY <- XY[iXY,]
      ffXY <- fXY[iXY]
      nnXY <- length(iXY)
      abcdxy <- abcd + cbind(XXYY[,1],n,XXYY[,2],n)
      for (jXY in 1:nnXY)
      {
        diffcdf <- GammaMetricCDF.fn(1,TrueDiff[iX,iY],abcdxy[jXY,])$cdf
        if ((diffcdf >= conflim[1]) & (diffcdf <= conflim[2]))
          CovProbD[iX,iY] <- CovProbD[iX,iY] + ffXY[jXY]
        ratcdf <- GammaMetricCDF.fn(2,TrueRatio[iX,iY],abcdxy[jXY,])$cdf
        if ((ratcdf >= conflim[1]) & (ratcdf <= conflim[2]))
          CovProbR[iX,iY] <- CovProbR[iX,iY] + ffXY[jXY]
      }
    }
  }
  CovProbD <- rbind(lambda,round(CovProbD,3))
  CovProbD <- cbind(c(0,lambda),CovProbD)
  CovProbR <- rbind(lambda,round(CovProbR,3))
  CovProbR <- cbind(c(0,lambda),CovProbR)
  t1 <- Elapsed.time.fn(t1)
  return(list(call=sys.call(), date=date(), Elapsed.Time=t1,
              CovProbD = CovProbD, CovProbR = CovProbR))
}

ConfFreqG.fn <- function(lambda,abcd=c(.5,1,.5,1),n=100,
                         conflim=c(0.025,0.975),eps=1e-8,eta=1e-4)
```

```
{
  step1.fn <-function(lam,n,eps)
  {
    nlam <- length(lam)
    LU <- array(0,c(nlam,2))
    for (ilam in 1:nlam)
    {
      tlam <- n*lam[ilam]
      L <- qpois(eps,tlam)
      U <- qpois(1-eps,tlam)
      LU[ilam,] <- c(L,U)
    }
    return(LU)
  }

  step2.fn <- function(diff,Lx,Ux,Ly,Uy,XYlam)
  {
    LB <- diff - sqrt((XYlam[,1]-Lx)^2 + (XYlam[,2]-Uy)^2)
    UB <- diff + sqrt((XYlam[,1]-Ux)^2 + (XYlam[,2]-Ly)^2)
    return(cbind(LB,UB))
  }

  t1 <- proc.time()[3]
  za <- qnorm(conflim[1])
  za2 <- za^2
  nlam <- length(lambda)
  LUx <- step1.fn(lambda,n,eps)
  LUy <- LUx
  CovProbD.J <- array(0,c(nlam,nlam))
  CovProbD.FT <- array(0,c(nlam,nlam))
  CovProbR <- CovProbD.J
  TrueDiff <- outer(lambda,lambda,"-")
  TrueRatio <- outer(lambda,lambda,"/")
  for (iX in 1:nlam)
  {
    X <- LUx[iX,1]:LUx[iX,2]
    fX <- dpois(X,n*lambda[iX])
    for (iY in 1:nlam)
    {
      Y <- LUy[iY,1]:LUy[iY,2]
      fY <- dpois(Y,n*lambda[iY])
      XY <- growarray.fn(list(X,Y))
      fXY <- apply(growarray.fn(list(fX,fY)),1,prod)
      nXY <- length(fXY)
      iXY <- (1:nXY)[fXY > eta]
      XXYY <- XY[iXY,]
      ffXY <- fXY[iXY]
      XYlam <- XXYY/n
      XYdiff <- XYlam[,1]-XYlam[,2]
      XYrat <- XYlam[,1]/(XYlam[,2] + eps*(XYlam[,2]==0))
      nXnY <- cbind(n,XXYY[,1],n,XXYY[,2])
      nnXY <- length(iXY)
      abcdxy <- abcd + cbind(XXYY[,1],n,XXYY[,2],n)
      LxFT <- 0.25*((sqrt(XXYY[,1]) + sqrt(XXYY[,1] + 1) + za)^2 - 1)/n
      LyFT <- 0.25*((sqrt(XXYY[,2]) + sqrt(XXYY[,2] + 1) + za)^2 - 1)/n
      UxFT <- 0.25*((sqrt(XXYY[,1]) + sqrt(XXYY[,1] + 1) - za)^2 - 1)/n
```

```
    UyFT <- 0.25*((sqrt(XXYY[,2]) + sqrt(XXYY[,2] + 1) - za)^2 - 1)/n
    LxJ <- qgamma(conflim[1],abcdxy[,1],n)
    LyJ <- qgamma(conflim[1],abcdxy[,3],n)
    UxJ <- qgamma(conflim[2],abcdxy[,1],n)
    UyJ <- qgamma(conflim[2],abcdxy[,3],n)
    LU.FT <- step2.fn(XYdiff,LxFT,UxFT,LyFT,UyFT,XYlam)
    LU.J <- step2.fn(XYdiff,LxJ,UxJ,LyJ,UyJ,XYlam)

    L.R <- array(0,nnXY)
    U.R <- array(Inf,nnXY)
    ii <- (1:nnXY)[XXYY[,2] > 0]
    if (length(ii) > 0)
    {
      xpy <- XXYY[ii,1] + XXYY[ii,2]
      xty <- XXYY[ii,1] * XXYY[ii,2]
      w1 <- 2*xty + xpy*za2
      w2 <- sqrt(xpy*za2*(4*xty + xpy*za2))
      L.R[ii] <- 0.5*(w1 - w2)/XXYY[ii,2]^2
      U.R[ii] <- 0.5*(w1 + w2)/XXYY[ii,2]^2
    }

    wFT <- (LU.FT[,1] <= TrueDiff[iX,iY]) & (TrueDiff[iX,iY] <= LU.FT[,2])
    wJ <- (LU.J[,1] <= TrueDiff[iX,iY]) & (TrueDiff[iX,iY] <= LU.J[,2])
    wR <- (L.R <= TrueRatio[iX,iY]) & (TrueRatio[iX,iY] <= U.R)
    CovProbD.FT[iX,iY] <- sum(ffXY[wFT])
    CovProbD.J[iX,iY] <- sum(ffXY[wJ])
    CovProbR[iX,iY] <- sum(ffXY[wR])
  }
}
CovProbD.FT <- rbind(lambda,round(CovProbD.FT,3))
CovProbD.FT <- cbind(c(0,lambda),CovProbD.FT)
CovProbD.J <- rbind(lambda,round(CovProbD.J,3))
CovProbD.J <- cbind(c(0,lambda),CovProbD.J)
CovProbR <- rbind(lambda,round(CovProbR,3))
CovProbR <- cbind(c(0,lambda),CovProbR)
t1 <- Elapsed.time.fn(t1)
return(list(call=sys.call(), date=date(), Elapsed.Time=t1,
            CovProbD.FT = CovProbD.FT, CovProbD.J = CovProbD.J,
            CovProbR = CovProbR))
}




AgrestiBrownLiDiff.fn <- function(nxny,conf)
{
  n1 <- nxny[,1];  x1 <- nxny[,2];  n2 <- nxny[,3];  x2 <- nxny[,4]
  pp1 <- (x1 + 0.5)/(n1 + 1)                        # B-L pseudo Jeffreys CI
  pp2 <- (x2 + 0.5)/(n2 + 1)
  dd <- pp1 - pp2
  zz <- qnorm((1+conf)/2)*sqrt(pp1*(1-pp1)/n1 + pp2*(1-pp2)/n2)
  diffL.BL.J <- dd - zz
  diffU.BL.J <- dd + zz
  pp1 <- (x1 + 1)/(n1 + 2)                          # Agresti-Caffo CI
  pp2 <- (x2 + 1)/(n2 + 2)
  dd <- pp1 - pp2
```

```
  zz <- qnorm((1+conf)/2)*sqrt(pp1*(1-pp1)/n1 + pp2*(1-pp2)/n2)
  diffL.AC <- dd - zz
  diffU.AC <- dd + zz
  n12 <- n1 + n2
  kap <- qt((1+conf)/2,n12-1)                    # B-L recentered CI
  w <- 1 + kap^2/n12
  p1 <- x1/n1
  p2 <- x2/n2
  delta <- p1 - p2
  theta <- n1/n12
  pp <- (1 - theta)*p1 + theta*p2
  pp <- pmin(pmax(pp,delta*(1-theta)),1-delta*theta)
  zz <- kap*sqrt(w*(1/n1 + 1/n2)*pp*(1-pp) - delta^2/n12)/w
  diffL.BL.rc <- delta/w - zz
  diffU.BL.rc <- delta/w  + zz
  return(round(cbind(diffL.AC,diffU.AC,diffL.BL.J,diffU.BL.J,
                     diffL.BL.rc,diffU.BL.rc),3))
}


BetaMetricCDF.fn <- function(option,metric,abcd,eps=0.0001,eta=1e-12)
{
#  If X ~ beta(a,b) and Y ~ beta(c,d) [abcd = c(a,b,c,d)], calculates cdf of
#    the difference X-Y            (option = 1)
#    the ratio X/Y                 (option = 2)
#    or the odds ratio X(1-Y)/(Y(1-X)   (option = 3)
#
#  A. L. Gould  March 2013
#
  intgD.fn <- function(x,d,abcd)
  {
    if (d >= 0) return( dbeta(x,abcd[1],abcd[2])*pbeta(x-d,abcd[3],abcd[4]))
    else return( dbeta(x,abcd[3],abcd[4])*pbeta(x+d,abcd[1],abcd[2]))
  }

  intgR.fn <- function(x,r,abcd)
    { dbeta(x,abcd[3],abcd[4])*pbeta(r*x,abcd[1],abcd[2]) }

  intgO.fn <- function(x,r,abcd)
    { dbeta(x,abcd[3],abcd[4])*pbeta(r*x/(1-x+r*x), abcd[1],abcd[2]) }

  nm <- length(metric)
  cdf <- array(0,nm)

  if (option==1)                               # Difference
    for (i in 1:nm)
      if (abs(metric[i]) < eta)
        cdf[i] <- integrate(intgR.fn,0,1,r=1,abcd=abcd)
                  $value
      else
        if (metric[i] > eta)
          if (((1-metric[i]) < eta)|(pbeta(metric[i],abcd[1],abcd[2]) < eta)
              | (pbeta(1-metric[i],abcd[3],abcd[3]) < eta))   cdf[i] <- 1
          else
              cdf[i] <- 1-integrate(intgD.fn,metric,1,d=metric[i],abcd=abcd)
                        $value
```

```
        else
          if ((((1+metric[i]) < eta) | (pbeta(1+metric[i],
          abcd[4],abcd[3]) < eta)
              | (pbeta(1+metric[i],abcd[1],abcd[2]) < eta))   cdf[i] <- 0
          else
            cdf[i] <- integrate(intgD.fn,-metric[i],1,d=metric[i],abcd=abcd)
                    $value

  if (option==2)                               # Ratio
    for (i in 1:nm)
      if (metric[i] <= 1)
        cdf[i] <- integrate(intgR.fn,0,1,r=metric[i],abcd=abcd)$value
      else
        cdf[i] <- 1-integrate(intgR.fn,0,1,r=1/metric[i],abcd=abcd[c(3,4,1,2)])
                    $value

  if (option==3)                               # Odds ratio
  for (i in 1:nm)
  {
    if (metric[i] < eta)  cdf[i] <- 0
    else if (abs(metric[i] - 1) < eta)
      cdf[i] <- integrate(intgR.fn,0,1,r=1,abcd=abcd)$value
    else
    {
      LU <- qbeta(c(eta,1-eta),abcd[3],abcd[4])
      xx <- metric[i]*LU[2]/(1+(metric[i]-1)*LU[2])
      if (pbeta(xx,abcd[1],abcd[2]) < eta)  cdf[i] <- 0
      else
        cdf[i] <- integrate(intgO.fn,LU[1],LU[2],r=metric[i],abcd=abcd)$value
    }
  }
  return(list(option=option,metric=metric,cdf=cdf))
}


BetaMetricCDFInv.fn <- function (option, targcdf, abcd, eps=0.00001)
{
#  If X ~ beta(a,b) and Y ~ beta(c,d) [abcd = c(a,b,c,d)], calculates
#  the value of the difference (option = 1), ratio (option = 2),
#  or odds ratio (option = 3)
#  at which the cdf of the metric (difference, ratio, OR)
#  takes the value(s) in targcdf.
#                               A. L. Gould   April 2013
#
  nq <- length(targcdf)
  metric <- array(0,nq)
  result <- NULL
  if (option == 1)                               # Difference
    for (i in 1:nq)
    {
      diffU <- 1
      diffL <- -1
      repeat
      {
        metric[i] <- (diffL + diffU)/2
        qq <- BetaMetricCDF.fn(1,metric[i],abcd)$cdf
```

```
        if (abs(qq - targcdf[i]) < eps) break
        if (qq < targcdf[i]) diffL <- metric[i]   else   diffU <- metric[i]
      }
    }
  else                                        # Ratio or odds ratio
  {
    zm <- BetaMetricCDF.fn(option,eps,abcd)
    for (i in 1:nq)
    {
      if (zm$cdf > targcdf[i])  metric[i] <- 0
      else
      {
        ratU <- 1
        repeat
        {
          ratU <- 10*ratU
          if (BetaMetricCDF.fn(option,ratU,abcd)$cdf > targcdf[i]) break
        }
        ratL <- 0
        repeat
        {
          metric[i] <- (ratL + ratU)/2
          z <- BetaMetricCDF.fn(option,metric[i],abcd)
          if (abs(z$cdf - targcdf[i]) < eps) break
          if (z$cdf < targcdf[i]) ratL <- metric[i]   else   ratU <- metric[i]
        }
      }
    }
  }
  return(list(option=option, abcd = abcd, targcdf=targcdf, metric=metric))
}

BPmidp.fn <- function(x,nX,nY,m,alpha=0.05,eps=0.0005)
{
#  Gets confidence limits for odds ratio using Baptista-Pike mid-p statistic
#  using the dnoncenhypergeom function from the MCMCpack package.
#  If x=0 or x=m, then a 1-sided 100(1-alpha) CI is constructed, otherwise
#  a 2-sided interval is constructed to have equal tail areas on either side
#  subject to the restriction that either tail area cannot exceed alpha/2.
#
#                                        A. L. Gould   April 2013
  nchypgeom.fn <- function(x,nX,nY,m,psi,eta=1e-14)
  {
#  Calculates density and cdf of noncentral hypergeometric distribution with
#  noncentrality psi using algorithm of Liao and Rosen,
#  AmStat 2001:55:366-369.
#  Context is 2 x 2 tables with rows x nX-x nX,
#  m-x nY-m+x nY, m nX+nY-m nX+nY.
#                                        A. L. Gould   April 2013
    mode.fn <- function(nX,nY,m,psi,L,U)
    {
      a <- psi - 1
      b <- -((nX+m+2)*psi + nY - m)
      c <- psi*(nX+1)*(m+1)
      q <- -0.5*(b+sign(b)*sqrt(b^2-4*a*c))
```

```
    mode <- trunc(c/q)
    if ((mode >= L) & (mode <= U)) return(mode)
    else return(trunc(q/a))
  }

  U <- min(nX,m)
  L <- max(0,m-nY)
  imode <- max(L,min(U,mode.fn(nX,nY,m,psi,L,U)))
  if (imode == U) crU <- NULL
  else
  {
    iU <- (imode+1):U
    crU <- cumprod(psi*(nX+1-iU)*(m+1-iU)/(iU*(nY-m+iU)))
  }
  if (imode == L) crL <- NULL
  else
  {
    iL <- (imode-1):L
    crL <- rev(cumprod((iL+1)*(nY-m+1+iL)/(psi*(nX-iL)*(m-iL))))
  }
  density <- c(crL,1,crU)
  density <- density/sum(density)
  cdf <- cumsum(density)
  result <- cbind(L:U,density,cdf)
  if (length(x) > 1) result <- result[result[,1] %in% x,]
  else if (!is.na(x)) result <- result[result[,1] %in% x,]
       else result <- result[result[,2] > eta,]
  return(result)
}

hgstep.fn <- function(x,nX,nY,m,psi)
{
  f <- nchypgeom.fn(NA,nX,nY,m,psi)
  ff <- nchypgeom.fn(x,nX,nY,m,psi)
  fff <- sum(f[f[,2]<=ff[2],2]) - ff[2]/2
  return(fff)
}

upBndsch.fn <- function(x,nX,nY,m,aa)
{
  LL <- 0;   UU <- 10
  repeat                              # Find a too-large value
  {                                   # for the upper CI bnd
    UU <- 2*UU
    hg <- hgstep.fn(x,nX,nY,m,UU)
    if (hg < aa) break
  }
  repeat                              # Find the upper CI bnd
  {                                   # by bisection
    U <- (UU + LL)/2
    if (hgstep.fn(x,nX,nY,m,U) < aa) UU <- U  else  LL <- U
```

```
      if ((UU - LL) < eps) break
    }
    return(U)
  }

  lowBndsch.fn <- function(x,nX,nY,m,aa)
  {
    LL <- 0;
    if ((x == m) | (x == nX))  UU <- 1
    else  UU <- .5*x*(nY+x-m)/((m-x)*(nX-x))
    repeat                          # Find a too-large value
    {                               # for the lower CI bnd
      UU <- 2*UU
      hg <- hgstep.fn(x,nX,nY,m,UU)
      if (hg > aa) break
    }
    repeat                          # Find the lower CI bnd
    {                               # by bisection
      L <- (UU + LL)/2
      if (hgstep.fn(x,nX,nY,m,L) < aa) LL <- L  else  UU <- L
      if ((UU - LL) < eps) break
    }
    return(L)
  }

  Lx <- max(0,m-nY)
  Ux <- min(m,nX)
  aa <- (1 + as.numeric((x==Lx)*(x==Ux)))*alpha/2
        #  Adjustment for 1- or 2-sided CI
  if (x==Lx) OR <- 0  else if (x==Ux)  OR <- Inf
  else OR <- x*(nY+x-m)/((m-x)*(nX-x))
  L <- 0
  U <- Inf
  if (Lx < Ux)
  {
    if (x < Ux)  U <- upBndsch.fn(x,nX,nY,m,aa)
    if (x > Lx)  L <- lowBndsch.fn(x,nX,nY,m,aa)
  }
  return(c(OR,L,U))
}

FagNew.fn <- function(nxny,conf,xi=c(.45,.25))
{
#  Calculates confidence bounds for the odds ratio
#  using the Fagerland-Newcombe
#  asymptotic formula (Statistics in Medicine, 2013)
#
  za <- qnorm((1+conf)/2)
  if (length(dim(nxny))==0)  nxny <- array(nxny,c(1,length(nxny)))
  x <- nxny[,2]; nmx <- nxny[,1] - x;  y <- nxny[,4];  nmy <- nxny[,3] - y
  logOR <- log((x + xi[1])*(nmy + xi[1])/((y + xi[1])*(nmx + xi[1])))
```

```
  Q <- 2*asinh(za*sqrt(1/(x+xi[2]) + 1/(nmx+xi[2])
             + 1/(y+xi[2]) + 1/(nmy+xi[2]))))
  L <- exp(logOR - Q)
  U <- exp(logOR + Q)
  return(cbind(L,U))
}
GammaMetricCDF.fn <- function(option,metric,abcd)
{
#  If X < gamma(a,b), Y ~ gamma(c,d)
#  fgamma(x,a,b) = b^a x^(a-1) exp(-bx) / Gamma(x),
#  calculates the cdf of the difference X - Y (option = 1) or the ratio X/Y
#  for each value of the metric (difference or ratio) in the vector 'metric'
#
#                                    A. L. Gould   April 2013
  intgrnd.fn <- function(x,d,abcd)
                {return(dgamma(x,abcd[1],abcd[2])*pgamma(x-d,abcd[3],
                     abcd[4]))}

  diffkern.fn <- function(d,abcd) { return(integrate(intgrnd.fn,d,Inf,
                                   d=d,abcd=abcd)$value) }

  nm <- length(metric)
  cdf <- array(1,nm)
  if (option==1)
  {
    ii <- (1:nm)[metric >= 0]
    nn <- length(ii)
    if (nn > 0) for (i in 1:nn) cdf[ii[i]] <- 1 - diffkern.fn
                   (metric[ii[i]],abcd)
    ii <- (1:nm)[metric < 0]
    nn <- length(ii)
    if (nn > 0) for (i in 1:nn) cdf[ii[i]] <- diffkern.fn
                   (-metric[ii[i]],abcd[c(3,4,1,2)])
  }
  if (option==2)                                    # cdf of ratio
  {
    w <- abcd[2]*metric/(abcd[2]*metric + abcd[4])
    cdf <- pbeta(w,abcd[1],abcd[3])
  }
  return(list(met=c("difference","ratio")[option],metric=metric,cdf=cdf))
}

GammaMetricCDFInv.fn <- function(option,metric,abcd,eps=1e-5)
{
#  Inverts the CDF of the difference (option = 1) or ratio
#  (option = 2) of two variables with gamma distributions
#
  nm <- length(metric)
  met <- array(0,nm)
  for (i in 1:nm)
  {
    metU <- 1
    repeat
    {
      metU <- 1.5*metU
```

```
      metricdf <- GammaMetricCDF.fn(option,metU,abcd)$cdf
      if (metricdf > metric[i]) break
    }
    if (option==2)  metL <- 0
    else
    {
      metL <- -1
      repeat
      {
        metL <- 1.5*metL
        metricdf <- GammaMetricCDF.fn(option,metL,abcd)$cdf
        if (metricdf < metric[i]) break
      }
    }
    repeat
    {
      met[i] <- (metL + metU)/2
      metricdf <- GammaMetricCDF.fn(option,met[i],abcd)$cdf
      if (metricdf < metric[i]) metL <- met[i]  else  metU <- met[i]
      if (metU-metL < eps) break
    }
  }
  return(list(call=sys.call(),date=date(),
             met=c("difference","ratio")[option],metric=met))
}


Newcombe.fn <- function(nxny,conf)
{
  WSbnds.fn <- function(j,pN,nxny,za,za2)
# Wilson score corrected bounds
  {
    jj <- 2*j - 1
    w <- nxny[,jj]/(za2 + nxny[,jj])
    pX <- pN[,j]*w + 0.5*(1-w)
#    v <- za*sqrt((1-w)*(pN[,j]*(1-pN[,j])*w + 0.25*(1-w)))
# corrected
    v <- 0.5*(1-w)*sqrt(za2 + 4*nxny[,jj]*pN[,j]*(1-pN[,j]))/za
# uncorrected
    LU <- cbind(pX - v, pX + v)
    return(LU)
  }

  za <- qnorm((1+conf)/2)
  za2 <- za^2
  pN <- cbind(nxny[,2]/nxny[,1],nxny[,4]/nxny[,3])
  LU1 <- WSbnds.fn(1,pN,nxny,za,za2) Newcombe hybrid
  LU2 <- WSbnds.fn(2,pN,nxny,za,za2) score intervals
  dXY <- pN[,1] - pN[,2]
  NHL <- dXY - sqrt((pN[,1] - LU1[,1])^2 + (pN[,2] - LU2[,2])^2)
  NHU <- dXY + sqrt((pN[,1] - LU1[,2])^2 + (pN[,2] - LU2[,1])^2)
  NHLU <- round(cbind(NHL,NHU),3)
  return(NHLU)
}
```

```
BayesCalcsBin.fn <- function(nxCT,ORstar,phi0,phi1,kappa,phiRopt=2,eps=1e-6,
                             numpargs=100,zeta=3,del.null=TRUE,
                             ORlist=c(seq(1,1.5,by=.1),2),cc=6)
{
# This program performs the calculations required for a Bayesian analysis
# of a collection of observed and expected drug-event report counts.
#
# Input: nxCT = matrix whose rows are (n,x) pairs -- n = no. at risk,
#               x = no. with event in the control group and the test group
#     ORstar = target value of OR indicating difference of test from control
#       phi0 = probability that odds ratio is <= ORstar if same process
#              generates control and test group event rates
#       phi1 = lower tail probability of distribution of odds ratio
#              for the event rates in the test and control groups
#              assuming the right-shifted distribution for the test group
#              evaluated at ORstar as defined for phi0
#      kappa = upper confidence level for event rate in control group
#              when parameters for prior dist'n of the control group
#              event rate are the ML estimates from the marginal count dist'n.
#    phiRopt = 1 if the value of ORstar is to be adjusted to preserve the
#                value of phi0
#            = 2 if the value of ORstar is not changed,and phi0 is allowed to
#                increase
#   numpargs = number of values p at which the posterior density is to be
#              computed
#   del.null = T if rows with zero event counts on ctl and test are omitted
#              F if not
#       zeta = parameter of prior density of p
#
#  Output: a list containing the following:
#        call = the command by which the program was invoked
#        date = the time and date when the program was run
#       pargs = a vector of the values of tau for which values of the posterior
#               density of tau was computed -- has npargs elements
# PostDen.tau = the values of the posterior density of tau evaluted for the
#               arguments given in pargs -- has npargs elements
#       ProbH0 = a vector of values of the posterior probability that the
#                parameters for the prior distribution of the rate parameter
#                in the test group are the same as for the control group
#
# A. L. Gould  June-October 2006,April 2007,December 2010,October 2011
#
  BayesCalcsBin-
Step.fn <- function(nxCT,ORstar,phi0,phi1,kappa,phiRopt=2,eps=1e-6,
                             numpargs=100,zeta=3,
                             ORlist=c(seq(1,1.5,by=.1),2),cc=6)
  {
    t1 <- proc.time()[3]
    M <- dim(nxCT)[1]
    zz <- GetBayesCalcsBinPrior.fn(phi0,ORstar,kappa,nxCT[,1:2])
    CtlPriorParams <- zz$CtlPriorParams
    pXU <- zz$pXU
    z <- AltPriorParams.fn(nxCT[,1:2],CtlPriorParams,phi0,phi1,ORstar,
                           phiRopt=phiRopt,eps=eps)
    abcd <- as.matrix(cbind(z$ai,z$di,z$ci,z$di))
    TestPriorParam1 <- z$TestPriorParam1
```

```
    y <- GetModetau.Bin.fn(nxCT[,3:4],abcd,cc=cc)            # mode of tau distn
    tau <- seq(y$tauL,y$tauU,length.out=numpargs+1)          # limits for tau
    taurat <- (1-tau)/tau
    frat <- y$fTC
    taufrat <- 1 + taurat%o%frat
    dim(taufrat) <- dim(taufrat)[1:2]
    taufratprod <- apply(taufrat,1,prod)
    ftau <- exp((zeta+M)*log(tau))
    ftaufratprod <- ftau*taufratprod                # Simpson Rule integrand
    normconst <- SimpRule.fn(tau,ftaufratprod)      # for PostDen.tau
    PostDen.tau <- ftaufratprod/normconst
    ftaufrat <- PostDen.tau/taufrat                 # Simpson Rule integrand
    ProbH0 <- SimpRule.fn(tau,ftaufrat)             # for ProbH0
    abcd1 <- cbind(abcd[,3:4]+cbind(nxCT[,2],nxCT[,1]-nxCT[,2]),abcd[,3:4])
    abcd2 <- cbind(abcd[,1:2]+cbind(nxCT[,2],nxCT[,1]-nxCT[,2]),abcd[,3:4])
    cdf1 <- run.PostORCDFDen.fn(ORlist,abcd1)$cdf
# Posterior cdf of odds ratio
    cdf2 <- run.PostORCDFDen.fn(ORlist,abcd2)$cdf    # under each model
    PostCDFOR <- 0*cdf1
    for (j in 1:length(ORlist))
      PostCDFOR[,j] <- ProbH0*cdf1[,j] + (1 - ProbH0)*cdf2[,j]
    dimnames(PostCDFOR)[[2]]<-paste("OR=",ORlist,sep="")
    t2 <- Elapsed.time.fn(t1)
    list(call=sys.call(),date=date(),Elapsed.Time=t2,true.phi0=z$true.phi0,
        phi0=phi0,ORstar=ORstar,kappa=kappa,phi1=phi1,pargs=tau,pXU=pXU,
        CtlPriorParams=CtlPriorParams,TestPriorParam1=TestPriorParam1,
        PostDen.tau=PostDen.tau,ProbH0=ProbH0,PostCDFOR=round(PostCDFOR,3))
  }


  AltPriorParams.fn <- func-
tion (nxC,CtlPriorParams,phi0,phi1,ORstar,phiRopt = 2,
                          eps = 1e-04)
  {
    a <- PostORCDFInv1.fn(phi1,ORstar,CtlPriorParams,eps = eps)$ab[1]
    nxC <- as.matrix(nxC)
    if (dim(nxC)[2] < 2)    nxC <- t(as.matrix(nxC))
    NN <- dim(nxC)[1]
    cdi <- cbind(CtlPriorParams[1] + nxC[,2],CtlPriorParams[2] +
                nxC[,1] - nxC[,2])
    if (phiRopt == 1)
    {
      true.phi0 <- phi0
      ai <- NULL
      ORlist <- NULL
      for (i in 1:NN)
      {
        ORi <- PostORCDFInv.fn(phi0,c(cdi[i,],cdi[i,]))$r
        ai <- c(ai,PostORCDFInv1.fn(phi1,ORi,c(cdi[i,]),eps=eps)$ab[1])
        ORlist <- c(ORlist,ORi)
      }
    }
    else
    {
      ai <- a + nxC[,2]
      true.phi0 <- NULL
      ORlist <- ORstar
```

```
    for(i in 1:NN)
      true.phi0 <- c(true.phi0,PostORCDFDen.fn
                  (ORstar,c(cdi[i,],cdi[i,]))$cdf)
  }
  return(list(TestPriorParam1 = a,true.phi0 = true.phi0,ai = ai,
            ci = cdi[,1],di = cdi[,2],ORlist = ORlist))
}


GetBayesCalcsBinPrior.fn <- function (phi0,ORstar,kappa,nx,eps = 1e-06)
{
  ab <- betabinML.fn(nx)
  pXU <- qbeta(kappa,ab$a,ab$b)
  aL <- 0
  aU <- ab$a
  repeat
  {
    ab <- c(aU,Get2ndParam.fn(aU,kappa,pXU,eps = eps))
    cdf <- PostORCDFDen.fn(ORstar,c(ab,ab))$cdf
    if (cdf > phi0) break
    aU <- 1.5 * aU
  }
  repeat
  {
    a <- (aL + aU)/2
    ab <- c(a,Get2ndParam.fn(a,kappa,pXU,eps = eps))
    f <- PostORCDFDen.fn(ORstar,c(ab,ab))$cdf
    if (abs(f - phi0) < eps) break
    if (f < phi0)  aL <- a  else  aU <- a
  }
  return(list(CtlPriorParams = ab,pXU = pXU))
}


GetModetau.Bin.fn <- function(nx,abcd,lims=c(-1e12,1e12),zeta=3,cc=6)
{
#  This program calculates the mode of the posterior density of tau,
#  the probability that the binomial event rates in a test and in a control
#  group are generated by (beta) distributions with parameters (c,d) and
#  (c,d) as opposed to (a,d) and (c,d). It also calculates the lower and
#  upper limits of the range of values for which the posterior density
#  of tau is 'nonzero'.
#
#  Input:
#        nx = a matrix whose rows are observed (at risk,event count) pairs
#      abcd = an M x 4 matrix whose first two columns are values (a,b) of
#             the parameter of a beta distribution for the rate parameter
#             in the test group and whose last two columns are values (c,d)
#             of the parameter of a beta distribution for the rate
#             parameter in the control group
#      lims = initial proposals for the limits on logit(tau)
#      zeta = parameter of prior for tau (beta(zeta+1,1))
#        cc = smallest number of log units such that if the difference
#             between the logarithm of the posterior density of tau
#             evalated at the mode and at tauL and tauU is exceeds cc,then
#             the limits for the range of tau values for which
```

```
#             the posterior density is "nonzero" is (tauL,tauU)
#
#  Output: a list containing the following:
#
#      call = command invoking the function
#      tauL = lower limit of range of useful tau values
#      tauU = upper limit of range of useful tau values
#       fTC = ratio of beta-binomial density values corresponding to
#             observed (at-risk,with event) pairs assuming (a,b) and (c,d)
#             parameter values (use normal approx.
#                           if param values are large)
#
#  A. L. Gould  June-October 2006,April 2007,October 2011
#
  M <- dim(nx)[1]
  abC <- abcd[,3] + abcd[,4]
  abT <- abcd[,1] + abcd[,2]
  if (max(outer(abcd,nx[,1],"+")) > 1000)
  {
    mnC <- nx[,1]*abcd[,3]/abC
    mnT <- nx[,1]*abcd[,1]/abT
    vC <- nx[,1]*abcd[,3]*abcd[,4]*(1 + (nx[,1]-1)/(abC+1))/(abC*abC)
    vT <- nx[,1]*abcd[,1]*abcd[,2]*(1 + (nx[,1]-1)/(abT+1))/(abT*abT)
    sdC <- sqrt(vC)
    sdT <- sqrt(vT)
    fC <- dnorm(nx[,2],mnC,sdC,log=T)
    fT <- dnorm(nx[,2],mnT,sdT,log=T)
    fTC <- fT - fC
  }
  else
  {
    fC <- dghyper(nx[,2],-abcd[,3],nx[,1],-abC,log=T)
    fT <- dghyper(nx[,2],-abcd[,1],nx[,1],-abT,log=T)
    xnx <- as.matrix(nx)%*%array(c(0,1,1,-1),c(2,2))
    w1<- lgamma(cbind(xnx,xnx)+abcd)%*%c(1,1,-1,-1)
    w2 <- abcd%*%array(c(1,1,rep(0,4)),c(4,2))
    w3 <- lgamma(w2+as.matrix(nx[,c(1,1)]))%*%c(-1,1)
    w2 <- lgamma(w2)%*%c(1,-1) + lgamma(abcd)%*%c(-1,-1,1,1)
    fTC <- w1 + w2 + w3
  }
  fTC <- exp(fTC)

  test.fn <- function(z,x,a) {sum((x-1)/(1 + x*exp(-z)))-a}
  fden.fn <- function(tau,fTC,aM){(aM)*log(tau)
                    + sum(log(1+fTC*(1-tau)/tau))}

  yL <- log(1E-50)
  yU <- log(1E50)
  zL <- test.fn(yL,fTC,zeta)
  zU <- test.fn(yU,fTC,zeta)
  if (sign(zL) == sign(zU))            # Mode is at zero or 1
  {
    zL <- fden.fn(1E-12,fTC,(zeta+M))
    zU <- fden.fn((1-1E-12),fTC,(zeta+M))
```

```
    if (zL < zU)
    {
      tauU <- 1
      mode <- 1
      fmode <- zU
      tauL <- 0.95*tauU
      while(fmode - fden.fn(tauL,fTC,(zeta+M)) < cc) {tauL <- 0.95*tauL}
    }
    else
    {
      tauL <- 0
      mode <- 0
      fmode <- zL
      tauU <- 0.95*(1-tauL)
      while(fmode - fden.fn(tauU,fTC,(zeta+M)) < cc) {tauU <- 1-0.95
                                                          (1-tauU)}

    }
  }
  else                               # Mode is between 0 & 1
  {
    y <- exp(-uniroot(test.fn,lims,x=fTC,a=zeta)$root)
    mode <- 1/(1 + y)                              # this is the mode
    fmode <- fden.fn(mode,fTC,(zeta+M))
    tauL <- 0.95*mode
    while((fmode - fden.fn(tauL,fTC,(zeta+M))) < cc) {tauL <- 0.95*tauL}
    tauU <- 1
  }
  return(list(call=sys.call(),tauL=tauL,tauU=tauU,fTC=fTC))
}

Get2ndParam.fn <- function(a,kappa,pU,eps=0.001)
{
#  This program finds the value of b such that the cdf of a beta
#  distribution with parameters (a,b) evaluated at pU equals kappa.

  bL <- 0
  bU <- 10
  repeat { if (pbeta(pU,a,bU) < kappa) bU <- 2*bU else break }
  repeat
  {
    b <- (bL + bU)/2
    dp <- pbeta(pU,a,b)
    if (abs(dp-kappa) < eps) break
    else if (dp > kappa) bU <- b else bL <- b
  }
  return(b)
}

nnxCT <- nxCT
if (del.null)  nnxCT <- nnxCT[(nnxCT[,2] + nnxCT[,4]) > 0,]
nphi0 <- length(phi0)
nORstar <- length(ORstar)
nkap <- length(kappa)
nphi1 <- length(phi1)
ncases <- nphi0*nORstar*nkap*nphi1
```

```
result <- vector("list",ncases)
icase <- 0
t1 <- proc.time()[3]
for (iphi0 in 1:nphi0)
  for (iORstar in 1:nORstar)
    for (ikap in 1:nkap)
      for (iphi1 in 1:nphi1)
      {
        icase <- icase + 1
        z <- BayesCalcsBinStep.fn(nnxCT,ORstar[iORstar],phi0[iphi0],
            phi1[iphi1],kappa[ikap],phiRopt=phiRopt,eps=eps,
            numpargs=numpargs,zeta=zeta,ORlist=ORlist,cc=cc)
        result[[icase]] <- c(kappa[ikap],z$pXU,phi0[iphi0],ORstar[iORstar],
                              phi1[iphi1],z)
        names(result[[icase]])[1:5] <- c("kappa","pXU","phi0",
                                          "ORstar","phi1")
      }
t2 <- Elapsed.time.fn(t1)
return(list(call=sys.call(),date=date(),Elapsed.Time=t2,result=result))
```

# References

[1] Agresti, A. and Min, Y. (2005) Frequentist performance of Bayesian confidence intervals for comparing proportions in 2 × 2 contingency tables. *Biometrics*, **61**, 515–523.

[2] Brown, L. and Li, X. (2005) Confidence intervals for two sample binomial distributions. *Journal of Statistical Planning and Inference*, **130**, 359–375.

[3] Fagerland, M.W., Lydersen, S. and Laake, P. (2011) Recommended confidence intervals for two independent binomial proportions. *Statistical Methods in Medical Research*. doi: 10.1177/0962280211415469

[4] Fagerland, M.W. and Newcombe, R.G. (2013) Confidence intervals for odds ratio and relative risk based on the inverse hyperbolic sine transformation. *Statistics in Medicine*, **32**, 2823–2836.

[5] Farrington, C.P. and Manning, G. (1990) Test statistics and sample size formulae for comparative binomial trials with null hypothesis of non-zero risk difference or non-unity relative risk. *Statistics in Medicine*, **9**, 1454.

[6] Newcombe, R. G. Interval estimation for the difference between independent proportions: Comparison of eleven methods, *Statistics in Medicine*, **17**, 873–890 (1998). Corrigendum 18, 1293 (1989)

[7] Newcombe, R.G. and Nurminen, M. (2011) In defence of score intervals for proportions and their differences. *Communications in Statistics – Theory and Methods*, **40**, 1271–1282.

[8] Santner, T.J., Pradhan, V., Senchaudhuri, P. *et al.* (2007) Small-sample comparisons of confidence intervals for the difference of two independent binomial proportions. *Computational Statistics and Data Analysis*, **51**, 5791–5799.

[9] Zhang, H., Gutiérrez Rojas, H.A. and Cepeda Cuervo, E. (2010) Confidence and credibility intervals for the difference of two proportions. *Revista Colombiana de Estadística*, **33**, 63–88.

[10] Hamilton, M.A. (1979) Choosing the parameter for a 2 × 2 table or a 2 × 2 × 2 table analysis. *American Journal of Epidemiology*, **109**, 362–375.

[11] Agresti, A. and Min, Y.Y. (2002) Unconditional small-sample confidence intervals for the odds ratio. *Biostatistics*, **3**, 379–386.

[12] Lydersen, S., Fagerland, M.W. and Laake, P. (2009) Recommended tests for association in $2 \times 2$ tables. *Statistics in Medicine*, **28**, 1159–1175.

[13] Mehrotra, D.V., Chan, I.S.F. and Berger, R.L. (2003) A cautionary note on exact unconditional inference for a difference between two independent binomial proportions. *Biometrics*, **59**, 441–450.

[14] Krishnamoorthy, K. and Lee, M. (2010) Inference for functions of parameters in discrete distributions based on fiducial approach: binomial and Poisson cases. *Journal of Statistical Planning and Inference*, **140**, 1182–1192.

[15] Mee, R.W. (1984) Confidence bounds for the difference between two probabilities (letter). *Biometrics*, **40**, 1175–1176.

[16] Miettinen, O. and Nurminen, M. (1985) Comparative analysis of two rates. *Statistics in Medicine*, **4**, 213–226.

[17] R Development Core Team. *R: A Language and Environment for Statistical Computing*, R Development Core Team, Vienna, http://www.R-project.org (accessed 24 June 2014).

[18] Wilson, E.B. (1927) Probable inference, the law of succession, and statistical inference. *Journal of the American Statistical Association*, **22**, 209–212.

[19] Agresti, A. and Caffo, B. (2000) Simple and effective confidence intervals for proportions and differences of proportions result from adding two success and two failures. *Annals of Statistics*, **54**, 280–288.

[20] Koopman, P.A.R. (1984) Confidence limits for the ratio of two binomial proportions. *Biometrics*, **40**, 513–517.

[21] Nam, J. (1995) Confidence limits for the ratio of two binomial proportions based on likelihood scores. *Biometrical Journal*, **37**, 375–379.

[22] Gart, J.J. and Nam, J. (1988) Approximate interval estimation of the ratio of binomial parameters: a review and correction for skewness. *Biometrics*, **44**, 323–338.

[23] Aitchison, J. and Bacon-Shone, J. (1981) Bayesian risk ratio analysis. *American Statistician*, **35**, 254–257.

[24] Gould, A.L. (1988) Applications of interval inference, in *Biopharmaceutical Statistics for Drug Development* (ed K.E. Peace), Marcel Dekker, New York, pp. 509–541.

[25] Baptista, J. and Pike, M.C. (1977) Exact two-sided confidence limits for the odds ratio in a 2 x 2 table. *Applied Statistics*, **26**, 214–220.

[26] Liao, J.G. and Rosen, O. (2001) Fast and stable algorithms for computing and sampling from the noncentral hypergeometric distribution. *American Statistician*, **55**, 366–369.

[27] Mehrotra, D.V. and Heyse, J.F. (2004) Use of the false discovery rate for evaluating clinical safety data. *Statistical Methods in Medical Research*, **13**, 227–238.

[28] Li, H.-Q., Tang, M.L., Poon, W.-Y. and Tang, N.-S. (2011) Confidence intervals for difference between two Poisson rates. *Communications in Statistics – Simulation and Computation*, **40**, 1478–1493.

[29] Zou, G.Y. and Donner, A. (2008) Construction of confidence limits about effect measures. A general approach. *Statistics in Medicine*, **27**, 1693–1702.

[30] Byrne, J. and Kabila, P. (2005) Comparison of Poisson confidence intervals. *Communications in Statistics-Theory and Methods*, **34**, 545–556.

[31] Brown, L.D., Cai, T. and DasGupta, A. (2001) Interval estimation for a binomial proportion (with discussion). *Statistical Science*, **16**, 101–133.

[32] Graham, P.L., Mengersen, K. and Morton, A.P. (2003) Confidence limits for the ratio of two rates based on likelihood scores: non-iterative method. *Statistics in Medicine*, **22**, 2071–2083.

[33] Berry, S.M. and Berry, D.A. (2004) Accounting for multiplicities in assessing drug safety: a three-level hierarchical mixture model. *Biometrics*, **60**, 418–426.

[34] Gould, A.L. (2008) Detecting potential safety issues in clinical trials by Bayesian screening. *Biometrical Journal*, **50**, 837–851.

[35] Gould, A.L. (2013) Detecting potential safety issues in large clinical or observational trials by Bayesian screening when event counts arise from Poisson distributions. *Journal of Biopharmaceutical Statistics*, **23**, 829–847.

[36] ICH Expert Working Group (1998) Statistical Principles for Clinical Trials E9, http://www.ich.org/fileadmin/Public_Web_Site/ICH_Products/Guidelines/Efficacy/E9/Step4/E9_Guideline.pdf (accessed 29 October 2007).

[37] Scott, J.G. and Berger, J.O. (2010) Bayes and empirical-Bayes multiplicity adjustment in the variable-selection problem. *Annals of Statistics*, **38**, 2587–2619.

# 7

# Statistical analysis of recurrent adverse events

**Liqun Diao, Richard J. Cook and Ker-Ai Lee**

*Department of Statistics and Actuarial Science, University of Waterloo,*
*200 University Avenue West, Waterloo, ON, Canada N2L 3G1*

## 7.1 Introduction

In many clinical trials, adverse events may occur repeatedly over the course of treatment and follow-up. Adverse events may be quick to resolve and hence transient in nature, may lead to permanent morbidity or disability, and may be terminal (i.e., death). In trials of testosterone supplementation in older men, adverse events can be cardiovascular, respiratory, or cutaneous [1] and within the cardiovascular adverse events, they vary in severity from peripheral edema to myocardial infarction and death. Cancer patients in trials of chemotherapies experience a wide range of adverse events including acute episodes of pain, nausea, and rash [2]. Patients undergoing transplant may receive medications designed to compromise the immune system to reduce the rate of graft versus host disease. Such medications put patients at elevated risk of infection and so careful examination of the incidence, duration, and severity of infections is essential [3].

We focus here primarily on the setting of transient adverse events for which it may be sensible to count the number of occurrences and make comparisons between groups on the basis of these counts. This is often reasonable when individuals are followed for the same length of time and there is little interest in when the events occur. In settings where the duration of follow-up varies between individuals or when interest lies in the timing of adverse events, analyses based on rate or mean functions are appealing, and these are readily adapted to deal with censoring due to incomplete follow-up. Even in this setting, there are often multiple types

*Statistical Methods for Evaluating Safety in Medical Product Development*, First Edition.
Edited by A. Lawrence Gould.
© 2015 John Wiley & Sons, Ltd. Published 2015 by John Wiley & Sons, Ltd.

of events that can arise, and they may vary in their severity. Separate analyses of the different types or severities of adverse events are often useful to understand the incidences of different types of events within groups and to facilitate comparisons between groups.

Challenges arise when the adverse events may vary dramatically in their severity, the greatest of which arises when one or more adverse events may be fatal. In this setting it is less appealing to simply count events since the occurrence of a fatal event is not equivalent to a non-fatal transient event. Moreover, the occurrence of the fatal event precludes the future occurrence of other events and so a competing-risk problem arises [4]. In this setting it is necessary to consider the incidence of non-fatal and fatal adverse events together.

We begin the next section by defining notation and discussing general models for recurrent events.

## 7.2 Recurrent adverse event analysis

### 7.2.1 Statistical methods for a single sample

We begin the discussion with consideration of data from one treatment group. The time of randomization is denoted by $T_0 = 0$ and we let $0 < T_1 < T_2 < \cdots < T_k < \cdots$ denote the times of events, where $T_k$ is the time of the $k$th adverse event. Let $N(t) = \sum_{k=1}^{\infty} I(T_k \leq t)$ record the number of events over $(0, t]$, where $I(\cdot)$ is the indicator function such that $I(A) = 1$ if $A$ is true and $I(A) = 0$ otherwise. Let $\Delta N(t) = N((t + \Delta t)^-) - N(t^-)$ denote the number of events over $[t, t + \Delta t)$. Let $dN(t) = \lim_{\Delta t \to 0} \Delta N(t) = 1$ indicate whether an event occurs at time $t$, and let $dN(t) = 0$ otherwise. The associated right-continuous counting process is $\{N(s), 0 < s\}$, and $H(t) = \{N(s), 0 < s < t\}$ denotes the history of the event process which records the number and times of events over $(0, t)$. Figure 7.1 contains a schematic relating the times of the events to the counting process. Each individual in a sample will contribute one such sample path, and statistical analyses are typically directed at modeling the event generating

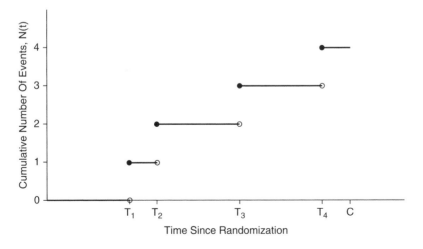

**Figure 7.1** Schematic diagram relating the times of recurrent events and the counting process $\{N(s), 0 < s\}$.

process or summarizing different aspects of the data in simple but informative ways. We turn to a discussion about models.

The intensity function of the recurrent event process is the instantaneous conditional probability of an event occurring at $t$ given the history of the process at $t$, and is written as

$$\lambda\,(t \mid H(t)) = \lim_{\Delta \to 0} \frac{P(\Delta N(t) = 1 \mid H(t))}{\Delta t}.$$

If two events cannot occur at the same time, then this intensity completely specifies the event process and a likelihood can be constructed on which to base inference. To be useful, however, such a likelihood must accommodate random right censoring.

Let $[0, C_A]$ denote the planned period of observation, where $C_A > 0$ is an administrative censoring time of the trial and hence common across all individuals. Suppose further that $C_R > 0$ is a random right-censoring time [5, 6] which may represent the time of withdrawal from a study; the net duration of follow-up is then

$$C = \min(C_A, C_R).$$

We let $Y(s) = I(s \leq C)$ indicate whether an individual is under observation at time $s$. Then if $d\overline{N}(t) = Y(t)dN(t)$, $d\overline{N}(t) = 1$ implies that an event occurred and was observed at $t$; we define $\overline{N}(t) = \int_0^t d\overline{N}(s)$.

Under the assumption of conditionally independent and non-informative censoring, the conditional probability for the outcome that "$n$ events occur at times $t_1 < \cdots < t_n$" over $(0, C]$ is

$$\prod_{j=1}^{n} \lambda(t_j \mid H(t_j)) \times \exp\left\{ -\int_0^\infty Y(u)\,\lambda(u \mid H(u))\,du \right\},$$

and the likelihood from a group of $m$ independent individuals processes is a product of such terms. This is technically a "partial" likelihood since we have ignored the component of the full likelihood pertaining to the random censoring time, but it can be treated as an ordinary likelihood function for estimating or testing model parameters of interest [7].

In clinical trials it is inappropriate to formulate models which involve basing treatment comparisons conditionally on information obtained post-randomization since it may be responsive to treatment [5], and in any event interest usually lies in estimates of simple marginal quantities. Because of this, treatment comparisons are frequently made on the basis of the mean function $\mu(t) = E\{N(t)\}$ or the rate function $\rho(t) = d\mu(t)/dt$. Mean and rate functions arise from Poisson processes, for which the intensity function is a rate function (i.e., $\lambda(t \mid H(t)) = \rho(t)$), but they are interpretable summary features of any processes and play a useful role in clinical trials.

When dealing with a sample of size $m$ we introduce a subscript $i$ to index individuals, and the likelihood under a Poisson model with rate $\rho(s; \theta)$ becomes $L(\theta) = \prod_{i=1}^{m} L_i(\theta)$, where

$$L_i(\theta) \propto \left\{ \prod_{j=1}^{n_i} \rho\left(t_{ij}; \theta\right) \right\} \exp\left( -\int_0^\infty Y_i(s)\,\rho(s; \theta)ds \right). \qquad (7.1)$$

The maximum likelihood estimate $\hat{\theta}$ is the solution to the score equation

$$U(\theta) = \sum_{i=1}^{m} U_i(\theta) = 0\,,$$

where
$$U_i(\boldsymbol{\theta}) = \frac{\partial \log L_i(\boldsymbol{\theta})}{\partial \boldsymbol{\theta}} = \int_0^\infty Y_i(s) \frac{\partial \log \rho_0(s;\ \boldsymbol{\theta})}{\partial \boldsymbol{\theta}} \{dN_i(s) - \rho(s;\ \boldsymbol{\theta})ds\}\ .$$

Moreover,
$$\sqrt{m}(\hat{\boldsymbol{\theta}} - \boldsymbol{\theta}) \xrightarrow{D} N(0,\ \mathbf{A}^{-1}(\boldsymbol{\theta})\mathbf{B}(\boldsymbol{\theta})\mathbf{A}^{-1}(\boldsymbol{\theta})),$$

as $m \to \infty$, where $\mathbf{A}(\boldsymbol{\theta}) = -E[(\partial U_i(\boldsymbol{\theta})/\partial \boldsymbol{\theta})']$ and $\mathbf{B}(\theta) = E[U_i(\boldsymbol{\theta})U_i'(\boldsymbol{\theta})]$. If the model is correctly specified, $\mathbf{A}(\boldsymbol{\theta}) = \mathbf{B}(\boldsymbol{\theta})$ and asvar $(\sqrt{m}(\hat{\boldsymbol{\theta}} - \boldsymbol{\theta})) = \mathbf{A}^{-1}(\boldsymbol{\theta})$. If the model is misspecified, the asymptotic covariance matrix has the more complex form $\mathbf{A}^{-1}(\boldsymbol{\theta})\mathbf{B}(\boldsymbol{\theta})\mathbf{A}^{-1}(\boldsymbol{\theta})$, which is the robust asymptotic covariance matrix that can provide protection from some forms of model misspecification [8]. The robust covariance matrix is estimated in practice by

$$\hat{\mathbf{A}}^{-1}(\hat{\boldsymbol{\theta}})\hat{\mathbf{B}}(\hat{\boldsymbol{\theta}})\hat{\mathbf{A}}^{-1}(\hat{\boldsymbol{\theta}})\ ,$$

where

$$\hat{\mathbf{A}}(\hat{\boldsymbol{\theta}}) = -m^{-1}\sum_{i=1}^m \partial U_i(\boldsymbol{\theta})/\partial \boldsymbol{\theta}'|_{\boldsymbol{\theta}=\hat{\boldsymbol{\theta}}} \quad \text{and} \quad \hat{\mathbf{B}}(\hat{\boldsymbol{\theta}}) = m^{-1}\sum_{i=1}^m U_i(\boldsymbol{\theta})U_i'(\boldsymbol{\theta})|_{\boldsymbol{\theta}=\hat{\boldsymbol{\theta}}}.$$

The former is easily obtained from the observed information matrix of a Poisson likelihood and the latter can be relatively easily computed based on the score contributions.

Nonparametric analyses can be carried out when one wants to avoid parametric assumptions about the rate or mean functions. In this case we treat $d\mu(t) = \rho(t)dt$ as a parameter, so we obtain

$$U_i(s) = Y_i(s)\{dN_i(s) - d\mu(s)\} = 0,\ s \geq 0,$$

which renders $d\hat{\mu}(s) = d\overline{N}_\bullet(s)/Y_\bullet(s)$, where $d\overline{N}_\bullet(s) = \sum_{i=1}^m Y_i(s)dN_i(s)$ and $Y_\bullet(s) = \sum_{i=1}^m Y_i(s)$. Note that the estimated rate of events is zero except at times when one or more events have occurred. The Nelson–Aalen estimate [9–11] of the mean function is given by

$$\hat{\mu}(t) = \int_0^t d\hat{\mu}(s). \tag{7.2}$$

Lawless and Nadeau [8] describe how to compute robust variance estimates that remain valid for any processes subject to independent censoring.

## 7.2.2    Recurrent event analysis and death

A challenge that has received some attention in recent years is the summary of the incidence of recurrent events when mortality rates are non-negligible. Simple summary measures such as event counts can be low due to a better adverse event profile from a superior treatment, or because of a higher mortality rate. The issue is that individuals experience a competing risk of death, following which no adverse events will be experienced. Counts of events, or even reports on the proportion of individuals experiencing an adverse event, are largely meaningless in this situation. Analyses based on events in time are preferable since they address the temporal ordering of the adverse events and death. Analyses directed at joint consideration of adverse events and death are warranted. In this case, it is natural to estimate the expected number of adverse events over time using a modification of the Nelson–Aalen mean function estimate. Let $D$ denote the time from randomization to death for an individual, and $\mathcal{F}(t) = P(D \geq t)$ denote the corresponding survival function. Let $d\mu^\dagger(t) = E(dN(t) \mid D \geq t)$ denote the rate of events at $t$ among individuals who survived to time $t$. The quantity

$$\mu^\dagger(t) = \int_0^t \mathcal{F}(s) d\mu^\dagger(s) \tag{7.3}$$

is the expected number of events over the interval $(0, t]$ accounting for the possibility of death and the fact that death precludes the occurrence of future events [10]. This can be estimated by noting that if $\overline{Y}_i(s) = Y_i(s)I(D_i \geq s)$, then an estimate of the rate is

$$d\widehat{\mu}^\dagger(s) = \frac{\sum_{i=1}^m \overline{Y}_i(s) \, dN_i(s)}{\sum_{i=1}^m \overline{Y}_i(s)},$$

and if $\widehat{\mathcal{F}}(t)$ is the Kaplan–Meier estimate of the survival function, an estimate of the cumulative mean function in equation (7.3) is

$$\widehat{\mu}^\dagger(t) = \int_0^t \widehat{\mathcal{F}}(s) d\widehat{\mu}^\dagger(s). \tag{7.4}$$

Ghosh and Lin [12] describe a multivariate test for treatment effects on the mean function in equation (7.4) and the survival distribution.

### 7.2.3  Summary statistics for recurrent adverse events

When interest lies in descriptive summary statistics for adverse events, counts are often used. Perhaps the crudest summary is the number of patients experiencing at least one adverse event, given by $\sum_{i=1}^m I(n_i > 0)$; the corresponding percentage of patients affected is also a natural summary. This of course does not convey information about the overall burden of adverse events, and it is important to record and report information of this nature. A simple count of the total number of adverse events is often reported for each treatment group, which we write as $n = \sum_{i=1}^m n_i$, and the mean number of events is $n/m$. These summaries, however, do not account for the duration of time individuals were exposed to drug or at risk of experiencing adverse events. A crude event rate analysis, based on the assumption that the adverse events are governed by a time homogeneous Poisson process (i.e., $\lambda(t \mid H(t)) = \rho(t) = \rho$), leads to the estimate $\widehat{\rho} = n/C$, where $C = \sum_{i=1}^m C_i$ is the total person-time at risk in the particular treatment group. This is sometimes referred to as an "events per person-years" analysis [13], or an "exposure-adjusted incidence rate" [14]. While this is a simple and seemingly easy-to-interpret summary measure, it is important to note that its interpretation depends on the validity of the assumption that the rate is constant in time and that individuals' follow-up times are independent of the occurrence of adverse events (i.e., experiencing an adverse event at time $t$ does not alter the risk of censoring in the future) [15]. The computation of a standard error for this estimate should not be based on the Poisson assumption since this implicitly assumes that the events are independent [16]. There often is an association between events in the sense that the occurrence of one event increases the risks of another event. This arises when there is heterogeneity in the event rate between individuals, and can be dealt with by using a robust variance estimate [17] or more general models for counts which allow for heterogeneity between individuals in the propensity for events [10, 18]. Such summary statistics are then often reported by the severity of the events, by the affected organ system, and by their relation to the treatment received [19].

A more detailed display of the incidence of adverse events is often appealing based on event charts [20–22]. Different symbols can be used to represent different types of adverse events to shed light on the risks of different events and the temporal relationships between them [23].

## 7.3   Comparisons of adverse event rates

Simple regression models are appealing when comparing treatment groups and we describe one such regression approach here. Let $X = 1$ if an individual is treated and $X = 0$ if they are randomized to the control arm. A proportional rate model is specified as

$$\lambda(t|H(t), X) = \rho_0(t) \exp(\beta X),$$ (7.5)

where $\rho_0(t)$ is the rate function for individuals in the control arm and $\exp(\beta)$ is a relative rate, such that if $\exp(\beta) > 1$ then events occur at a higher rate in the treatment group compared to the control group. When $\rho_0(t) \geq 0$ is of an unspecified form (analogous to the way the baseline hazard is of an unspecified form in Cox regression) then this is called the Andersen–Gill model [24]. Robust variance estimation provides protection against departures from a Poisson model and has led to widespread use of this model in clinical trials [8, 10, 25].

Statistics directed at testing the null hypothesis that the event rates are the same in the two treatment groups can also be considered, in much the same way (generalized) log-rank statistics can be used in survival analyses in concert with Kaplan–Meier estimation of survival distributions and Cox regression. Here we introduce a subscript to denote treatment group and we let $C_{ki}$ denote the right-censoring time for individual $i$ in treatment group $k$, $Y_{ki}(s) = I(s \leq C_{ki})$, and $dN_{ki}(s) = 1$ if individual $i$ in treatment group $k$ has an event at time $s$, with $dN_{ki}(s) = 0$ otherwise. If $\mu_k(t) = E\{N_{ki}(s)\}$ is the mean function for treatment group $k$, $\widehat{\mu}_k(t) = \int_0^t d\widehat{\mu}_k(s)$ where $d\widehat{\mu}_k(s) = d\overline{N}_{k\bullet}(s)/Y_{k\bullet}(s)$, with $d\overline{N}_{k\bullet}(s) = \sum_{i=1}^{m_k} Y_{ki}(s)dN_{ki}(s)$ and $Y_{k\bullet}(s) = \sum_{i=1}^{m_k} Y_{ki}(s)$. The two-sample test statistics have the form

$$U = \int_0^\infty w(s)\{d\widehat{\mu}_2(s) - d\widehat{\mu}_1(s)\},$$ (7.6)

where $w(s)$ is a weight function. If $w(s) = Y_{1\bullet}(s)Y_{2\bullet}(s)a(s)/Y_{\bullet\bullet}(s)$ then a log-rank type test is obtained when we set $a(s) = 1$. A consistent variance estimator for $U/\sqrt{m}$ is given by

$$\widehat{\text{var}}_R\{U\}/m = \frac{1}{m}\sum_{k=1}^2 \sum_{i=1}^{m_k} \left[\int_0^\infty w(s)\frac{Y_{ki}(s)}{Y_{k\bullet}(s)}\{dN_{ki}(s) - d\widehat{\mu}_k(s)\}\right]^2.$$ (7.7)

This variance estimator is robust to departure from Poisson assumptions and as $Y_{1\bullet}(s)$ and $Y_{2\bullet}(s)$ become large over $[0, C_A]$, the pseudo-score statistic $T^2 = U^2/\widehat{\text{var}}_R\{U\}$ approaches a $\chi_1^2$ random variable under $H_0$ for a wide class of underlying point processes. Large observed values of $T^2$ provide evidence against $H_0$. When samples are small or events are rare, one can alternatively consider randomization tests in which $p$-values are computed by computing the probability of observing a test statistic as large as the observed statistic based on the randomization distribution [13].

## 7.4    Remarks on computing and an application

### 7.4.1    Computing and software

Therneau and Hamilton [26], Therneau and Grambsch [27], and Cook and Lawless [10] provide detailed discussions on how to construct data frames and carry out recurrent-event analyses using functions for survival analysis in R (http://www.R-project.org/) or TIBCO Spotfire S+ (http://www.tibco.com/). In R or S-PLUS the key function is coxph, and PROC PHREG in SAS plays a central role. The webpage http://www.math.uwaterloo.ca/~rjcook /book.html contains freely available sample code in S-PLUS and SAS.

To see why survival analysis software can be helpful, consider a data set where $0 < t_{i1} < t_{i2} < \cdots < t_{i,n_i} < C_i$ denote the times of $n_i$ events observed for individual $i$ over $[0, C_i]$ with treatment covariate $X_i$. Expression (7.1) can be generalized to include the covariate under a multiplicative Poisson regression model and the integral in the exponent can be decomposed so the analog of (7.1) can be written as

$$L_i(\boldsymbol{\theta}) \propto \prod_{j=1}^{n_i} \left\{ \rho\left(t_{ij}|x_i; \boldsymbol{\theta}\right) \exp\left(-\int_{t_{i,j-1}}^{t_{ij}} \rho\left(s|x_i; \boldsymbol{\theta}\right) ds \right) \right\} \exp\left(-\int_{t_{i,n_i}}^{C_i} \rho\left(s|x_i; \boldsymbol{\theta}\right) ds \right).$$

Each of the terms in this product has the form of a density for a left-truncated (at $t_{i,j-1}$) survival time ($t_{ij}$), and the last term has the form of a right-censored observation (at $C_i$) of a left-truncated survival time (left-truncated at $t_{i,n_i}$). Because we can express the likelihood for such a recurrent event analysis as a product of terms that arise in likelihoods for left-truncated right-censored survival data, survival analysis software can be exploited for recurrent event analysis of this type.

As an illustration we consider a simulated data set of $m = 100$ individuals randomized to receive either an experimental intervention ($X = 1$) or a control treatment ($X = 0$) with recurrent events generated from a time homogeneous Poisson process with rate $\rho(t \mid x) = \rho_0 \exp(\beta x)$, where $\rho_0 = 1$ and $\exp(\beta) = 0.75$. Without loss of generality, suppose individuals are to be followed over the interval $[0, 1]$ so the expected number of events in the control group is $E(N(1) \mid X = 0) = 1$, and $E(N(1) \mid X = 1) = 0.75$. We suppose further that individuals may withdraw from the study early and consider a random censoring time $C$ which is exponentially distributed such that $P(C > 1) = 0.6$, so we observe individuals over $[0, \min(C, 1)]$.

The simulated data are recorded in a data frame recurrent.dat and the contents pertaining to five individuals are displayed in the counting process format [27] in what follows (Table 7.1). The variables include a subject identifier (id), the times of the beginning (start, representing $t_{i,j-1}$) and end (stop, representing $t_{ij}$ or $C_i$) of each period at risk, an indicator of whether the period ended with the occurrence of an event or not (status), a treatment indicator (treat), and a variable which simply records the line number within each individual contribution (enum). The first individual (id $= 1$) completed the planned period of observation without experiencing an event. The second individual (id $= 2$) experienced an event at $t_{21} = 0.17$ and withdrew from the study at $C_2 = 0.93$.

**Table 7.1**  Simulated data.

| id | start | stop | status | treat | enum |
|----|-------|------|--------|-------|------|
| 1 | 0 | 1 | 0 | 0 | 1 |
| 2 | 0 | 0.17 | 1 | 0 | 1 |
| 2 | 0.17 | 0.93 | 0 | 0 | 2 |
| 3 | 0 | 0.27 | 1 | 1 | 1 |
| 3 | 0.27 | 0.57 | 1 | 1 | 2 |
| 3 | 0.57 | 0.96 | 0 | 1 | 3 |
| 4 | 0 | 0.56 | 1 | 0 | 1 |
| 4 | 0.56 | 0.92 | 1 | 0 | 2 |
| 4 | 0.92 | 1 | 0 | 0 | 3 |
| 5 | 0 | 0.64 | 1 | 1 | 1 |
| 5 | 0.64 | 0.65 | 1 | 1 | 2 |
| 5 | 0.65 | 0.7 | 1 | 1 | 3 |
| 5 | 0.7 | 1 | 0 | 1 | 4 |
| ⋮ | ⋮ | ⋮ | ⋮ | ⋮ | ⋮ |

To obtain the Nelson–Aalen estimate (equation (7.2)) for the control group, in R we proceed as follows:

```
> simdata <- read.table("recurrent.dat", header=T)
> library(survival)
> fit0 <- coxph(Surv(start, stop, status) ~ 1, data=simdata,
              subset=(treat == 0), method="breslow")
> na0 <- survfit(fit0, type="aalen")
> plot(na0, fun="cumhaz", xlab="YEARS SINCE RANDOMIZATION",
              ylab="NELSON-AALEN ESTIMATE")
```

The so-called counting process style of preparing the data means the coxph function can be called immediately with the subset option used to restrict attention to control subjects. The survfit function is normally used to provide an estimate of a survival distribution. Here, however, we use it to obtain an estimate of the cumulative mean function by specifying the aalen method and selecting the cumhaz function in the plotting statement.

An estimate of the regression coefficient in equation (7.5) is obtained by the call

```
> fit <- coxph(Surv(start, stop, status) ~ treat + cluster(id),
              data=simdata, method="breslow")
```

and the contents of the fit object are obtained using the summary statement:

```
> summary(fit)
  n= 169, number of events= 69

              coef  exp(coef)  se(coef)  robust se        z  Pr(>|z|)
  treat  -0.22738    0.79662   0.24172    0.25132  -0.9048    0.3656
```

```
           exp(coef)     exp(-coef)     lower .95     upper .95
treat      0.79662          1.2553        0.48677        1.3037


Concordance= 0.535    (se = 0.031 )
Rsquare= 0.005    (max possible= 0.97 )
Likelihood ratio test= 0.89 on 1 df, p=0.34606
Wald test              = 0.82 on 1 df, p=0.3656
Score (logrank) test = 0.89 on 1 df, p=0.34584,
Robust = 0.76 p=0.38272


(Note: the likelihood ratio and score tests assume
 independence of observations within a cluster, the Wald
 and robust score tests do not.)
```

The cluster(id) specification ensures that robust variance estimates are computed and that we are protected against extra-Poisson variation or other forms of misspecification provided the proportional rate specification in equation (7.5) is correct. Here we find $\exp(\hat{\beta}) = 0.80$, corresponding to a 20% reduction in the rate of events in the treatment arm (95% confidence interval (0.49, 1.30); $p -$ value $= 0.366$). The log-rank test reported under the output for the estimate is the robust log-rank test based on equation (7.7) and so is also valid for the non-Poisson processes. It gives a $p$-value of 0.383, in close agreement with the Wald-based $p$-value.

Another approach for dealing with extra-Poisson variation is to consider mixed Poisson models. Under this framework each individual generates events according to a Poisson process but with their own rate. Parsimonious models are obtained by constraining these individuals' rate functions to be proportional to one another. A multiplicative random effect (often called a "frailty") acting on a baseline rate function can then be introduced such that the variation in the random effect reflects the extent of heterogeneity in the event rates across the population. In R/S-PLUS the frailty(id) option in the coxph function enables one to fit semi-parametric mixed Poisson models, and other packages (e.g., frailtypack [28]) offer more complex random effect structures. Details on how to fit recurrent event models in STATA are found in [29].

## 7.4.2   Illustration: Analyses of bleeding in a transfusion trial

As an illustration, we consider here data from a transfusion trial in which bleeding is an adverse event of interest. Bleeding is classified according to the World Health Organization (WHO) Bleeding scale which includes grades of 0 for no bleeding, 1 for petechial bleeding, 2 for mild blood loss (clinically significant bleeding), 3 for gross blood loss requiring transfusion (severe), and 4 for debilitating blood loss, retinal bleeding, or cerebral bleeding associated with death [30]. In Table 7.2 the number of individuals affected with bleeding of each type is indicated by treatment group along with the associated percentages. It can be seen that there is generally a higher percentage of individuals affected by bleeding in the reference group; the analyses with ranges of bleeding grades are more suitable since they look at all bleeding and progressively more severe forms of bleeding. When aggregated in this way the reference arm always led to higher bleeding rates.

Also reported are the number of bleeding days by grade of bleeding, across individuals within treatment groups; the numbers under the column headed "Rate" are the "events per person-day" estimated bleeding rates, obtained by dividing the number of days with the

**Table 7.2**  Tabulation of the number of individuals experiencing bleeding overall and by WHO grade of bleeding as well as the total number of events occuring by group.

| | Experimental | | | | Reference | | | |
|---|---|---|---|---|---|---|---|---|
| | Affected individuals | | Events | | Affected individuals | | Events | |
| Bleeding grade | N | % | N | Rate | N | % | N | Rate |
| Grade 1–4 | 58 | 48.7 | 237 | 0.08 | 87 | 66.4 | 379 | 0.122 |
| Grade 2–4 | 22 | 18.5 | 54 | 0.02 | 27 | 20.6 | 117 | 0.038 |
| Grade 3–4 | 10 | 8.4 | 19 | 0.01 | 15 | 11.5 | 49 | 0.016 |
| Grade 1 | 51 | 42.9 | 183 | 0.06 | 72 | 55 | 262 | 0.084 |
| Grade 2 | 14 | 11.8 | 35 | 0.01 | 15 | 11.5 | 68 | 0.022 |
| Grade 3 | 8 | 6.7 | 16 | 0.01 | 13 | 9.9 | 29 | 0.009 |
| Grade 4 | 2 | 1.7 | 3 | 0 | 3 | 2.3 | 20 | 0.006 |

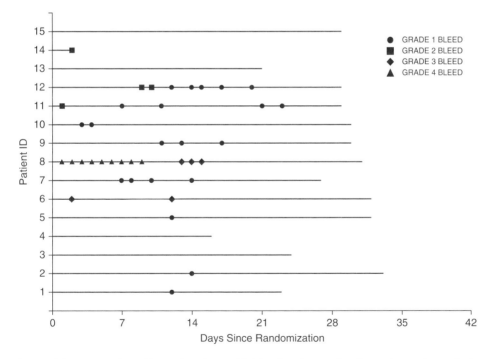

**Figure 7.2**  Event chart displaying days with bleeding by grade of severity and transfusion interventions.

indicated grade(s) of bleeding, by the number of person-days of observation. Here we also find that the bleeding rates are higher in the reference group.

Figure 7.2 shows an event chart for a sample of 15 individuals from [31]. The chart uses different symbols for the different grades of bleeding as indicated by the legend, and it can

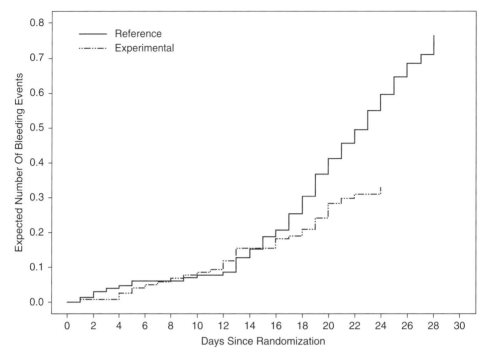

**Figure 7.3**   Nelson–Aalen estimates of the expected number of bleeding events by treatment arm.

be seen that there is considerable variation in the rate of bleeding; individuals 3, 4, 13, and 15 do not experience any bleeding, but individual 8 experiences multiple consecutive days of bleeding. This is suggestive of a type of heterogeneity which warrants use of a permutation test or robust variance estimates to provide protection against extra-Poisson variation.

Figure 7.3 gives the Nelson–Aalen estimates of the mean functions for the expected number of days with bleeding as a function of time since randomization. A test of the null hypothesis of common bleeding rates between treatment arms based on equation (7.6) gives a test statistic $T = 1.33$ and a $p$-value of 0.250, so there is insufficient evidence to reject the null hypothesis of a common bleeding rate between the two groups.

## 7.5   Discussion

Adverse events often are infrequent. As a result, analyses often are descriptive in nature and amount to a tabulation of the number of events and the number of affected individuals by treatment group. A further breakdown of the data by the severity of the adverse event, the affected organ system, and the relation to the treatment received, means that cell counts in contingency tables are often very small. Statistical tests in such settings are most suitably based on exact methods or randomization tests. With relatively rare events, the power to detect significant increases in adverse events is therefore much lower than it is for the primary outcome on which the sample size was based, so it is best to emphasize estimates and confidence intervals rather than the decision-theoretic interpretation of hypothesis tests. It is increasingly common for the Food and Drug Administration to recommend conduct of large Phase 4 trials to facilitate the collection of more extensive adverse event data in a sample of individuals treated under the standard of care. The larger samples are typically both larger and more representative of the target population. Formal surveillance can ensure good-quality data are collected and more meaningful analyses can be carried out on the incidence of rare, but clinically important, events. This is particularly important when the adverse events have long sequelae, as is the case in the development of adult sarcomas among individuals surviving childhood cancers treated with radiotherapy [32]. In settings with very strong therapeutic interventions adverse events may be frequent and sufficiently serious that they may be comparable in importance to the outcomes of primary interest. This was the case in early trials of treatments for individuals with HIV infection, and is often the case in studies of high-dose chemotherapies. In Phase 3 trials of this setting it is important to monitor treatment effects for both the primary outcomes and adverse events so that trials can be terminated when evidence emerges about the impact of treatment on these outcomes [33, 34].

# References

[1] Basaria, S., Coviello, A.D., Travison, T.G. *et al.* (2010) Adverse events associated with testosterone administration. *New England Journal of Medicine*, **363**, 109–122.

[2] Cobleigh, M.A., Vogel, C.L., Tripaty, D. *et al.* (1999) Multinational study of efficacy and safety of humanized anti-HER2 monoclonal antibody in women who have HER2-overexpressing metastatic breast cancer that has progressed after chemotherapy for metastatic disease. *Journal of Clinical Oncology*, **17**, 2639–2648.

[3] Cole, E.H., Cattran, D.C., Farewell, V.T. *et al.* (1994) A comparison of rabbit antithymocyte serum and OKT3 as prophylaxis against renal allograft rejection. *Transplantation*, **57**, 60–67.

[4] Crowder, M.J. (2001) *Classical Competing Risks*, Chapman & Hall/CRC Press, Boca Raton, FL.

[5] Kalbfleisch, J.D. and Prentice, R.L. (2002) *The Statistical Analysis of Failure Time Data*, John Wiley & Sons, Inc., New York.

[6] Lawless, J.F. (2003) *Statistical Models and Methods for Lifetime Data*, John Wiley & Sons, Inc., Hoboken, NJ.

[7] Andersen, P.K., Borgan, Ø., Gill, R.D. and Keiding, N. (1993) *Statistical Models Based on Counting Processes*, Springer-Verlag, New York.

[8] Lawless, J.F. and Nadeau, J.C. (1995) Nonparametric estimation of cumulative mean functions for recurrent events. *Technometrics*, **37**, 158–168.

[9] Aalen, O.O. (1978) Nonparametric inference for a family of counting processes. *Annals of Statistics*, **6**, 701–726.

[10] Cook, R.J. and Lawless, J.F. (2007) *Statistical Analysis of Recurrent Events*, Springer, New York.

[11] Nelson, W. (1969) Hazard plotting for incomplete failure data. *Journal of Quality Technology*, **1**, 27–52.

[12] Ghosh, D. and Lin, D.Y. (2000) Nonparametric analysis of recurrent events and death. *Biometrics*, **56**, 554–562.

[13] Freedman, L., Sylvester, R. and Byar, D.P. (1989) Using permutation tests and bootstrap confidence intervals to analyse repeated events data from clinical trials. *Controlled Clinical Trials*, **10**, 129–141.

[14] Siddiqui, O. (2009) Statistical methods to analyze adverse events data of randomized clinical trials. *Journal of Biopharmaceutical Statistics*, **19**, 889–899.

[15] Cook, R.J. and Major, P. (2001) Methodology for treatment evaluation in patients with cancer metastatic to the bone. *Journal of the National Cancer Institute*, **93**, 534–538.

[16] Glynn, R.J. and Buring, J.E. (2001) Coutning recurrent events in cancer research. *Journal of the National Cancer Institute*, **93**, 486–489.

[17] McCullagh, P. and Nelder, J.A. (1989) *Generalized Linear Models*, 2nd edn, Chapman & Hall, London.

[18] Lawless, J.F. (1987) Negative binomial and mixed Poisson regression. *Canadian Journal of Statistics/Revue Canadienne de Statistique*, **15**, 209–225.

[19] Goldberg-Alberts, R. and Page, S. (2006) Multivariate analysis of adverse events. *Drug Information Journal*, **40**, 99–110.

[20] Dubin, J.A. and O'Malley, S.S. (2010) Event charts for the analysis of adverse events in longitudinal studies: an example from a smoking cessation pharmacotherapy trial. *Open Epidemiology Journal*, **3**, 34–41.

[21] Hsu, C., Zhou, Z., and Hardin, J.M. (2002) A useful chart to display adverse event occurrences in clinical trials. *Proceedings of the 27th Annual SAS Users Group International Conference*, pp. 119–127.

[22] Lee, J.J., Hess, K.R. and Dubin, J.A. (2000) Extensions and applications of event charts. *American Statistician*, **54**, 63–70.

[23] Guttner, A., Kubler, J. and Pigeot, I. (2007) Multivariate time-to-event analysis of multiple adverse events of drugs in integrated analyses. *Statistics in Medicine*, **26**, 1518–1531.

[24] Andersen, P.K. and Gill, R.D. (1982) Cox's regression model for counting processes: a large sample study. *Annals of Statistics*, **10**, 1100–1120.

[25] Lin, D.Y., Wei, L.J., Yang, I. and Ying, Z. (2000) Semiparametric regression for the mean and rate functions of recurrent events. *Journal of the Royal Statistical Society, Series B*, **62**, 711–730.

[26] Therneau, T.A. and Hamilton, S.A. (1997) rhDNase as an example of recurrent event analysis. *Statistics in Medicine*, **16**, 2029–2047.

[27] Therneau, T.A. and Grambsch, P.M. (2000) *Modeling Survival Data: Extending the Cox Model*, Springer, New York.

[28] Rondeau, V., Mazroui, Y. and Gonzalez, J.R. (2012) frailtypack: an R package for the analysis of correlated survival data with frailty models using penalized likelihood estimation or parametrical estimation. *Journal of Statistical Software*, **47**, 1–28.

[29] Cleves, M. (1999) Analysis of Multiple Failure-Time Survival Data, Stata Technical Bulletin STB-49, pp. 30–39, http://www.stata.com/support/faqs/statistics/multiple-failure-time-data/ (accessed 25 June 2014).

[30] Webert, K.E., Cook, R.J., Sigouin, C. *et al.* (2006) The risk of bleeding in thrombocytopenic patients with acute myeloid leukemia. *Heematologica*, **91**, 1530–1537.

[31] Rebulla, P., Finazzi, R., Marangoni, F. *et al.* (1997) The threshold for prophylactic platelet transfusions in adults with acute myeloid leukemia. *New England Journal of Medicine*, **337**, 1870–1875.

[32] Henderson, T.O., Whitton, J., Stovall, M. *et al.* (2007) Secondary sarcomas in childhood cancer survivors: a report from the childhood cancer survivor study. *Journal of the National Cancer Institute*, **99**, 300–308.

[33] Cook, R.J. and Farewell, V.T. (1994) Guidelines for monitoring efficacy and toxicity responses in clinical-trials. *Biometrics*, **50**, 1146–1152.

[34] Jennison, C. and Turnbull, B.W. (1993) Group sequential tests for bivariate response: interim analyses of clinical trials with both efficacy and safety endpoints. *Biometrics*, **49**, 741–752.

# 8

# Cardiovascular toxicity, especially QT/QTc prolongation

## Arne Ring[1,2] and Robert Schall[2,3]

[1]*Leicester Clinical Trials Unit, University of Leicester, LE5 4PW, UK*

[2]*Department of Mathematical Statistics and Actuarial Science, University of the Free State, 205 Nelson Mandela Drive, Bloemfontein 9301, South Africa*

[3]*Quintiles Biostatistics, Bloemfontein 9301, South Africa*

## 8.1 Introduction

### 8.1.1 The QT interval as a biomarker of cardiovascular risk

The cardiovascular safety of drugs has always been an important aspect of drug development. However, during the last 15 years a major new focus has emerged following the discovery that some drugs have the potential to alter the electrocardiogram (ECG) in a proarrhythmic way. This phenomenon can lead to so-called "torsade de pointes" (TdP) and subsequently to sudden death.

Normal electric action causes the heart to contract its muscles, typically about once per second. During TdP the electrical action becomes too frequent (Figure 8.1) so that the heart muscle can no longer relax and blood is no longer pushed into the circulation. Sometimes the electrical action normalizes spontaneously but, if it does not, TdP becomes fatal as the body is deprived of oxygen. However, sudden death due to TdP is such a rare event that its risk cannot be assessed adequately in clinical outcome trials. At any rate, such outcome trials would have to be large, expensive, and would require long follow-up times.

An alternate pattern of prolonged and shortened QT intervals typically occurs before the ECG is changed toward TdP (Figure 8.1). TdP, therefore, is associated with a prolongation of

*Statistical Methods for Evaluating Safety in Medical Product Development*, First Edition.
Edited by A. Lawrence Gould.
© 2015 John Wiley & Sons, Ltd. Published 2015 by John Wiley & Sons, Ltd.

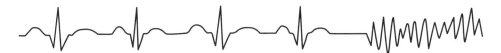

**Figure 8.1**    Torsade de pointes following long and short QT intervals.

the QT interval and hence the QT interval has been identified as a safety biomarker for the assessment of the risk of TdP in general populations. However, prolongation of the QT interval is not always pro-arrhythmic; the clinical conditions for pro-arrhythmia are described in [1].

It is well known that the QT interval may be changed by various mechanisms. The discovery that drugs, too, may prolong the QT interval has raised concerns that such drugs might cause TdP [2]. These concerns led to the development of regulatory guidance on how to evaluate the potential of drugs to prolong the QT interval, in an effort to assure the cardiovascular safety of drugs. The relevant Committee for Medicinal Products for Human Use guideline was first released in 1997 [3], followed by a more detailed guidance drafted by the Canadian authority [4]. Finally, the international guidances ICH S7B [5] (Safety Pharmacology) and ICH E14 [6] (Clinical Evaluation of QT Prolongation) were discussed and agreed upon.

In summary, the QT interval is an imperfect biomarker with high sensitivity but relatively low specificity for TdP. Although other markers for the antiarrhythmic potential of a drug have been proposed, today the QT interval is the most widely used biomarker for the assessment of the risk of TdP.

### 8.1.2    Association of the QT interval with the heart rate

The length of a normal QT interval ranges between 350 and 450 ms, depending on heart rate and gender [7]. Drug induced prolongation beyond 5–10 ms has been considered to be clinically relevant [8], which equates to only 1.25–2.5% of an absolute length of 400 ms. Therefore, it is important to measure the QT interval with high precision and reproducibility, and to evaluate changes in QT interval independent of any confounding variables.

Because the QT interval is a major portion of the heart beat (Figure 8.1), the QT interval varies inversely with changes in the heart rate. The heart rate itself is subject to substantial random fluctuation as well as to systematic changes, for example, through physical action or food intake. In the assessment of QT interval prolongation, an effect of the drug on the QT interval as such must be distinguished from an effect of the drug on the QT interval that is explained by the drug's effect on the heart rate. The statistical methods that can make this distinction will be detailed in Section 8.4 below.

In Section 8.2 we will outline how assessments of QT prolongation can be implemented in clinical drug development. Then, in Section 8.3, we describe the design of "thorough QT" (TQT) trials, and in Section 8.4 we describe the analysis of confirmatory TQT trials.

## 8.2    Implementation in preclinical and clinical drug development

### 8.2.1    Evaluations from sponsor perspective

The international guidelines ICH S7B [5] and ICH E14 [6] provide a general framework for the evaluation of QT prolongation. The ICH S7B guideline recommends that, prior to the first clinical trial in humans, three *in vitro* and *in vivo* evaluations should be performed to assess a drug's potential to delay ventricular depolarization. If all three tests fail to suggest such a potential, the risk of QT prolongation in humans is deemed low.

Otherwise, if at least one of the prior evaluations suggests a potential of the drug to delay ventricular depolarization, a risk–benefit assessment needs to be made in order to select a suitable candidate drug for development, based on efficacy, safety, and pharmacology properties. If it is otherwise acceptable, candidate drugs with moderate pre-clinical QT liability might still progress to clinical development. However, usually such a drug would require more thorough ECG evaluations.

The ICH E14 guideline for clinical evaluation specifies a requirement for so-called "thorough QT" trials early in drug development. The primary objective of such trials is to demonstrate the absence of QT effects, in terms of a non-inferiority test of the drug against placebo with a non-inferiority margin of 10 ms (that is, the mean QT prolongation must be shown to be less than 10 ms). In agreement with other guidelines (ICH E9/E10), such a trial should also include a positive control to demonstrate assay sensitivity.

Because TQT studies are among the most expensive clinical pharmacological trials within a drug development program, the timing of a TQT trial should be based on an evaluation of the risk that the drug prolongs the QT interval. Most pharmaceutical companies apply the general "learn and confirm" concept to the investigation of QT prolongation for new drug candidates [9, 10], starting with pre-clinical evaluations and subsequently incorporating new knowledge obtained during the development of the drug. Figure 8.2 provides an overview of the possible pathways for QT evaluation in drug development programs.

In early development, typically, two to four dose escalation trials will be performed until proof of concept is established. All ECG and drug concentration data obtained up to this point should then be included in a pooled pharmacometric evaluation. This evaluation could increase or decrease the evidence for potential of QT prolongation that had previously been established. However, most regulatory bodies will not (yet) accept data from early dose-escalation trials alone as formal proof of absence of QT liability.

In most cases it is strongly recommended to use high-quality ECG recordings during dose-escalation trials in the early phase of clinical pharmacological development. However,

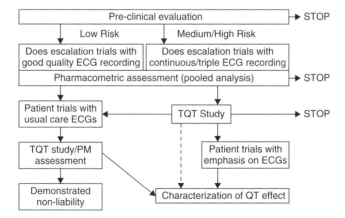

**Figure 8.2** Role of cardiac safety investigations in drug development for decision of timing and objective of the thorough QT study. Drugs which are deemed with to have low QT(c) liability would follow a path at the left-hand side.

for drugs without pre-clinical QT liability, recording of standard 10-second ECGs might suffice. In contrast, for drugs with pre-clinical QT liability, continuous ECGs or triple ECGs are recommended at this stage, to provide the most thorough evaluation of the potential for QT prolongation.

Confirmation of low QT liability before initiation of large patient trials would decrease both the need for early TQT trials and the burden of substantial QT evaluations in Phase 2b/3. On the other hand, if some QT liability is likely, it is recommended to perform a TQT trial before starting costly patient trials, to quantify the effect size.

Before submitting the final drug package for market approval, an updated pharmacometric assessment should be carried out. In future, this might suffice as evidence for the absence of a QT liability, while at present some regulatory authorities might still require a TQT study.

The timing of the TQT trial should not be guided only by a drug's potential liability for QT interval prolongation. Other changes observed in the ECG might also raise concerns or trigger the need for additional safety investigations. Specifically a drug's potential to change the heart rate should be included in the safety evaluation because the length of the QT interval is closely related to the length of the heartbeat. Drug-induced changes in heart rate will usually create the need for appropriate statistical methods during the evaluation of QT prolongation (see sections below), and could imply that the magnitude of "heart rate corrected" changes in the QT interval (QTc) would be estimated with less precision.

Figure 8.3 indicates the outcome areas for both heart rate and QTc interval, based on cumulative pooled analyses of early phase data of drug exposure and ECG recordings, at relevant supra-therapeutic doses. The actual values of the limits might depend on the therapeutic area and a general risk–benefit evaluation, but the general framework would be similar.

The different areas in Figure 8.3 indicate different risk conclusions. In the unshaded (central) area, early phase data do not suggest a potential of the drug to alter either the heart rate or the QT(c) interval to a clinically relevant extent. The aim of the TQT study would be to confirm these early findings. Because of the small risk of failing to confirm lack of QT prolongation and lack of changes in heart rate the TQT trial could be performed with a straightforward study design and in parallel with Phase 3 trials. The light shaded areas above and below the central area indicate potential alterations of the heart rate but not of QTc. Again, the TQT study could be done in parallel with Phase 3 trials, although more detailed ECG data might be collected and there should be a strong focus on appropriate heart rate correction methods. For drugs in which the HR (heart rate)/QTc parameter estimation overlaps with the medium shaded area, the data indicate the potential to impact slightly on the QT interval but not on heart rate and it is advised to perform a TQT study rather early (during Phase 2) with major emphasis on the characterization of the potential QT liability. The dark shaded area would indicate drugs that might alter QT intervals to a clinically relevant extent. In this case, a thorough risk–benefit investigation is required. If drug development is continued the TQT study needs to be performed rather early, with major emphasis on the characterization of the potential QT liability.

## 8.2.2   Regulatory considerations on TQT trials

Initially after the release of ICH E14 it was generally understood that performance of a TQT study was a requirement for all new drug applications (NDAs). Although the guideline encouraged exploring alternative assessments of QT effect of a drug, the recommendations were vague in this respect so that most sponsors chose to undertake at least one dedicated ECG

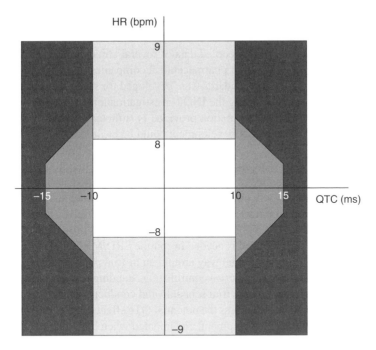

**Figure 8.3**    Schematic view of limits for changes in heart rate (HR) and heart rate corrected QTc interval for the categorization of potential risks during early drug development. A drug would fall into one of the categories if the confidence intervals for the parameter changes (not only the mean estimates) are included in the range. Unshaded areas: no change of heart rate or QT(c) to a clinically relevant extent. Light shaded areas: data indicate potential to alter heart rate but not QTc. Medium shaded areas: data indicate potential to impact slightly on the QT interval but not on heart rate. Dark shaded areas: data indicate potential to prolong QT interval to a clinically relevant extent.

trial. Therefore, by now a large number of TQT trials have been performed, and over 200 such trials have been submitted to the FDA between Nov 2005 and Mar 2013 as part of an NDA [11]. About a quarter of the drugs investigated were considered to be "QT prolongers", of which the majority had a $\Delta\Delta$QTc prolongation between 10 and 20 ms.

In contrast to a general belief in the pharmaceutical industry, a large percentage (89%) of drugs with QT liability was in fact approved by the FDA, based on a generally favorable risk benefit profile [11]. Although the majority of these drugs will have contraindications, warnings or precautions in their label, overall the development of those drugs was successful. This experience shows that stopping drug development solely on the basis of QT liability is not warranted, although a thorough investigation of ECG effects is advocated for all drugs.

As outlined in section 8.2.1, the TQT study is only one element of the assessment of the cardiovascular risk of a drug. It has recently been discussed [12,13] whether a robust investigation of ECG intervals during early clinical development could fully replace the need for a TQT trial, both with regard to demonstrating the absence of a QTc effect and with regard to the quantification of such an effect if it exists. Nowadays, most Single-Rising-Dose (SRD) trials and Multiple-Rising Dose (MRD) trials record ECGs regularly (Figure 8.2) – and an extension of such trials to record triple ECGs to increase the precision of ECG measurements would cause only a minor cost increase. Furthermore, appropriate statistical and pharmaco-metric evaluation methods based on pooled data of several clinical pharmacology trials have already been used internally by major pharmaceutical companies in order to quantify the risk of QT prolongation. If regulatory standards were developed for such analyses, sponsors could submit their data early, namely during the IND (investigational new drug) process, and could receive a decision whether the information provided is sufficient. Based on such a decision the need for a TQT trial during later development could be evaluated.

Kleiman *et al.* [13] strongly argue in favour of this alternative procedure for QTc assessment, and for a waver of the requirement for a TQT trial, in particular in order to reduce costs while maintaining a high quality of risk evaluation. However, the Cardiac Safety Research Consortium (CSRC) has recently published a white paper [12] which takes a more conservative viewpoint. In agreement with Kleiman *et al.* [13] the CSRC advocates the investigation of the drug concentration-QT response relationship early during drug development, while it questions whether a positive control is needed in routine SRD/MRD trials to address the E14 request of assay sensitivity. A potential way around an in-trial positive control arm would be to investigate non-pharmacologic positive controls (e.g. standing response [14]), which could be performed with less impact on the trial schedule and conduct.

In summary, a detailed plan to assess the potential QTc effect of new compounds should be created during the pre-clinical development, and updated when high quality clinical trial data are obtained. If thorough investigations lead to the conclusion that a drug has low potential for QTc prolongation, sponsors might attempt to obtain a waiver for the TQT trial; such an attempt is certainly worth a try.

# 8.3    Design considerations for "Thorough QT trials"

In this section we present design options for TQT trials and discuss practical examples from the literature. We focus on healthy volunteer trials with non-cytotoxic drugs.

TQT trials constitute a large investment during drug development, and often are the largest clinical pharmacology studies within a clinical development program. Thoughtful planning and design will help to increase the success rate of these studies and to reduce their cost. Numerous investigations have been performed to find optimal design elements for TQT trials. Specifically, design options have been investigated and discussed in the literature to optimize the power and to reduce the sample size of TQT trials, although the results of relevant investigations do not always agree with each other because of the complexity of the issues. Beside those elements which are dictated by the efficacy and safety profile of the drug, such as the selection of the dose and the timing of ECG recordings and blood samples, other design features could be adjusted based on the statistical efficiency of the methods.

## 8.3.1    Selection of therapeutic and supra-therapeutic exposure

TQT trials are performed to compare (heart rate corrected) QT intervals following the administration of at least two dose levels of the investigational drug and of placebo; here the active is usually administered at both a therapeutic and a supra-therapeutic dose intended to represent a worst-case scenario for drug exposure. (The option to omit the therapeutic dose level and instead to interpolate the QT effect from an exposure response analysis has been discussed in the literature [15]; this approach is seldom used, however, and is beyond the scope of this chapter.) Because of the non-inferiority objective of a TQT trial, assay sensitivity must be confirmed using the active control treatment moxifloxacin 400 mg, which is known to prolong the QT interval between 8 and 12 ms without causing major changes in the heart rate. In summary, a typical TQT trial will investigate four treatments, namely placebo, a therapeutic and a supra-therapeutic dose of the drug under investigation, and the active control treatment, usually moxifloxacin 400 mg.

A TQT trial for a drug that does not affect the heart rate will be simpler. In this case the only aim is to demonstrate the absence of the QT(c) effect, and the choice of a heart rate correction method is not crucial (although it is important to choose at least a simple one, such as the Fridericia correction – see Sections 8.4.2.9 and 8.4.2.10 below – to reduce the impact of natural heart rate variability).

## 8.3.2    Single-versus multiple-dose studies; co-administration of interacting drugs

Single-dose designs are the preferred option if there are no major metabolites of the drug under investigation, if there is no accumulation of the drug over time, and if there are no pharmacokinetic interactions with other drugs that would increase drug exposure. The choice of the supra-therapeutic dose – a multiple of the therapeutic dose – should predominantly be determined by the safety profile of the drug. Up to 10-fold and larger multiples have been recommended [16] and implemented for drugs such as sitagliptin [17] and linagliptin [18]. Although sitagliptin showed a minor QTc effect of about 8 ms with eightfold therapeutic dose (and no QT effect on the therapeutic dose), the characterization of the QT effect over this wide dose range was welcomed by regulatory authorities and did not lead to any restrictions and warnings, as an eightfold exposure is very unlikely to be reached in patient populations (see Section 8.5).

If there is significant accumulation of the drug or of a metabolite, the design of the QT trial should include and evaluate multiple doses over the accumulation interval. This will also be the case if (supra-)therapeutic doses can be reached only by using up-titration of doses [19].

Drug interactions might be used to reach supra-therapeutic exposure if administration of larger doses is not feasible. However, this option can only be recommended if the interacting drug has been shown to have no QT liability, or if the interacting drug will routinely be co-administered with the new drug. An example is ritonavir, which is a strong CYP3A4 inhibitor and acts typically as HIV base therapy [20]. Combinations with ritonavir have been investigated in TQT trials [21, 22]. In contrast, some ketaconazole (CYP3A4/5) interaction studies have not been successful, as ketaconazole causes QT prolongation [23], and pharmacodynamic interactions have also been observed [24, 25].

## 8.3.3    Baseline measurements

Another major design consideration is the selection of appropriate baseline measures of heart rate and QT interval. Although the major objective of a clinical trial is the comparison of randomized treatments with each other, the choice of baseline measurements can affect the size of the standard error of the between-treatment estimates of the QTc effects. For single-dose cross-over trials, the choice of a pre-dose ECG in each study period was demonstrated to lead to the smallest standard errors in several investigations (e.g., [26, 27]). For single-dose parallel trials, some authors recommend performing full 24-hour baseline profiles to account for the individual circadian rhythm, while others found pre-dose baselines to be sufficient. For multiple dose trials, baselines appeared not to reduce the standard error of interest [19, 21, 26].

### 8.3.4   Parallel versus cross-over design

The decision for parallel vs. cross-over designs often follows practical considerations, specifically with regard to the time required to conduct the study and the availability of the results. When timing is not critical, cross-over designs might be preferred, because studies in healthy volunteers generally benefit from low drop-out rates. For example, in a four-period cross-over TQT trial with washout periods of 6 weeks between treatments only one of the 44 subjects discontinued the study prematurely [18].

### 8.3.5   Timing of ECG measurements

The timing of ECG measurements should correspond to the pharmacokinetic disposition of the drug. Several measurements should be taken around the maximum concentration of the drug (and potentially of a metabolite), but the declining phase of the exposure, too, should be adequately covered by ECG measurements. Because a TQT trial is conducted to assess drug safety, all time points for measurement are considered with equal importance. The estimate of QTc prolongation under active treatment, relative to placebo, will be compared against the non-inferiority margin of 10 ms at each measurement time. In other words, all repeated QTc measurements for the primary endpoints will be tested through an intersection–union test (IUT). This conservative approach has been discussed in the literature (e.g., [28, 29]); it implies that the estimate of maximum QTc prolongation over time is biased upward and hence overestimates the potential of a drug to prolong QT. A number of approaches have been proposed to account for this bias [30]. On the other hand, the aim of the ICH E14 guidance is to rule out an effect of about 5 ms, so that the draft version (Step 2) of this guideline proposed a non-inferiority margin of 8 ms for the 90% confidence interval (CI) of the placebo-corrected QTc interval. During the consultation period, this level was raised to the current 10 ms limit, and the difference of 2 ms can be viewed as a correction for the bias (this magnitude is often found for the maximum QTc effect for TQT trials with drugs that do not cause QT prolongation).

### 8.3.6   Sample size

Because of the complex primary endpoint in TQT studies, sample size calculations are often quite challenging as they have to account for potential drug effects as well as for correlation between the endpoints. Several authors have examined various scenarios [31–33], and many TQT trials have been performed with about 40 subjects (either with cross-over designs or with 40 subjects per treatment group in parallel designs), based on high-quality determination of the ECG intervals from triple ECGs [34]. Recently, a fully powered TQT trial was successfully performed with only 30 subjects using a double-placebo design [35, 36], which can save costs [37].

### 8.3.7   Complex situations

Design considerations become more complex if the investigational drug has shown a potential to prolong the QT interval or change the heart rate, either pre-clinically or clinically, as indicated in the previous section. In this case it must be decided first whether it will be feasible to demonstrate that the effect is not clinically relevant (the 90% CI for the QT effect does not exceed the 10 ms limit). This approach might be an option if the drug alters only the heart rate, under the assumption that the heart rate corrected QT interval is not prolonged. Otherwise the aim of the TQT study will be to characterize and quantify the magnitude of the QT prolongation with sufficient precision. In both cases, the choice of an adequate method or heart rate correction is crucial for the success of the trial and the interpretability of the results (see Section 8.5 below).

### 8.3.8    TQT trials in patients

TQT trials in healthy volunteers are now routinely performed in drug development, and the issues summarized above are regularly considered in the design of TQT trials that are tailored to the relevant drug's properties. The situation becomes more challenging if a TQT trial cannot be performed in healthy subjects, for example because of the toxicity of the drug. Some trials in oncology have been performed recently using less stringent designs in patients [38–40]. In those cases, supra-therapeutic doses often cannot be applied, the number of ECGs that can be taken may be restricted, and the use of controls has been questioned. However, the interpretation of the results of such trials occasionally has been difficult if QT liability could not be ruled out [41, 42]. In these cases, a comprehensive evaluation of the risk–benefit balance must be performed, which might lead to drug approval with restrictions [43].

## 8.4    Statistical analysis: thorough QT/QTc study

### 8.4.1    Data

#### 8.4.1.1    Hierarchical data structure

ECG data obtained from a TQT trial with a cross-over design have a hierarchical, cross-classified structure [44]. Each subject undergoes several treatment periods. In each treatment period, triple 10-second ECGs are obtained at various time points. For each ECG, the intervals (such as QT and RR intervals) are typically measured in three to five wave forms (Figure 8.4).

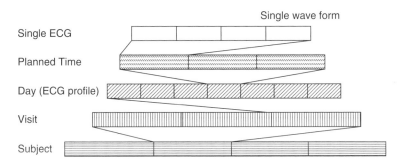

**Figure 8.4**    Hierarchical data structure of ECG interval data from 10-second ECGs. Adapted from [44].

As mentioned earlier, in some TQT studies each treatment period is preceded by a baseline day to account for circadian variation, creating a rich pool of baseline data. When full 24-hour baseline profiles are available, correction slopes for calculation of heart rate corrected QTc interval data can be estimated from the baseline profiles (see Section 8.4.2). Otherwise, heart rate correction may be performed using the data from the placebo arm of the trial. Since many recent studies no longer include full baseline profiles for each treatment arm, we assume in the following that heart correction is done using the data from the placebo arm of the trial.

### 8.4.1.2   Typical trial design

A schematic outline of a typical trial design might look as follows. Each subject undergoes at least three treatment periods with the following treatments in randomized sequence:

1. Active drug whose potential for QT prolongation is to be assessed.

2. Placebo control treatment.

3. Active control treatment with a drug known to cause QT prolongation (usually moxifloxacin), in order to validate the sensitivity of trial to detect QT prolongation when present.

In each treatment period, ECGs are obtained at various time points before (at baseline) and after drug administration.

As mentioned in Section 8.3, usually at least two doses of the active drug are investigated in a TQT study, namely both a therapeutic and one or more supra-therapeutic doses, so that a TQT study includes at least four treatments. TQT studies are high-order cross-over trials with repeated measures data over several time points within each treatment period.

### 8.4.1.3   Data averaging

When ECG intervals are measured in several (three to five) wave forms for each ECG, it is recommended to average the data on wave-form level to obtain one value (for QT and RR) on the ECG level. When data are analyse on the original scale (QT and RR interval as measured), the arithmetic mean would be calculated on the wave-form level; when data are analyse on the logarithmic scale, the arithmetic mean on the logarithmic scale, corresponding to the geometric mean on the original scale, would be calculated on the wave-form level.

### 8.4.1.4   Notation

Let $QT_{ijk}(m)$ be the QT interval measured for subject $i(i = 1, \ldots, N)$ on treatment $j$ $(j = 1, \ldots, J)$ at repeated measures time point $k(k = 1, \ldots, K)$, where, when needed, $m$ indicates that subject $i$ received randomized treatment $j$ in the $m$th treatment period. We define $Y_{ijk}(m) = f(QT_{ijk}(m))$, where $f(\cdot)$ is a suitable monotonic transformation, usually either the identity function or the natural logarithm [44, 45]. Similarly, let $RR_{ijk}$ be the RR interval measured simultaneously with $QT_{ijk}$, and $X_{ijk} = f(RR_{ijk})$. If QT and RR interval data have been measured for several wave forms per ECG, then $QT_{ijk}(m)$ and $RR_{ijk}$ are assumed to represent the averages over the replicate wave forms, as described in Section 8.4.1.3 above.

## 8.4.2    Heart rate correction

### 8.4.2.1    Association of QT interval with heart rate and RR interval

It is well known that the QT interval is associated with the heart rate. When a subject's heart rate changes, because of natural variability, circadian rhythm, physical exercise, drug treatment, or for any other reason, the QT interval changes in an inverse fashion: the higher the heart rate, the shorter the QT interval. The RR interval (that is, the inverse of the heart rate) therefore has a positive correlation with the QT interval: the longer the RR interval, the longer the QT interval. The positive correlation between RR and QT interval is plausible or suggested by the fact that the QT interval is "nested" in the RR interval.

### 8.4.2.2    Confounding effect of changes in heart rate; Need for heart rate correction

The association between the RR interval and the QT interval can complicate or confound the assessment of drug-induced QT prolongation when the drug in question has an effect on the heart rate or, equivalently, on the RR interval. The potential of a drug to prolong the QT interval could be "masked" if that drug decreases the RR interval (increases heart rate). Conversely, a drug that does not prolong the QT interval may appear to do so if the drug increases the RR interval (decreases heart rate). Therefore, when a drug affects the RR interval, the drug's effect on the QT interval must be distinguished from changes in the QT interval that are due merely to changes in the RR interval [46]. For this reason, QT interval data are routinely "corrected" for the RR length interval using various correction formulas or procedures, to obtain a value known as the QTc interval (the heart rate corrected QT interval) which is hoped to be independent of the RR interval length, or at least less dependent on the RR interval than the QT interval itself [6].

### 8.4.2.3    Principle of heart rate correction

Heart rate correction "normalizes" the measured QT interval to a specific "reference" heart rate, usually 60 bpm, which is equivalent to a reference RR interval of $RR_R = 1$ s. Let QT and RR be simultaneous measurements of the QT and RR intervals. Furthermore, let $y = f(QT)$ and $x = f(RR)$ where $f(\cdot)$ is the transformation referred to in Section 8.4.1 (usually either the identity function or the natural logarithm). Then the QTc interval is obtained through the equation

$$y^c = y = E(y|x) + E(y|x_R) .\tag{8.1}$$

That is, after suitable transformation of the QT and RR interval, the transformed corrected QT interval, $y^c$, is obtained by subtracting the expectation of $y$ conditional on $x = f(RR)$ (i.e., conditional on the RR interval), and adding the expectation of $y$ conditional on $x = x_R = f(RR_R)$, namely conditional on the reference RR interval $RR_R$. The QTc interval is obtained by back-transforming to the original scale,

$$QTc = f^{-1}(y^c) .\tag{8.2}$$

In order to perform heart rate correction, therefore, it is necessary to model and estimate the conditional expectation $E(y|x)$. Different models and estimation methods for $E(y|x)$ lead to different heart rate correction methods. In practice, most heart rate correction methods employ a linear model of the form

$$E(y|x) = \alpha + \beta(x - x_R)\tag{8.3}$$

for the conditional expectation $E(y|x)$ [46–48]. Using equation (8.1), the QTc interval is then obtained as

$$
\begin{aligned}
y^c &= y - E(y \mid x) + E(y \mid x_R) \\
&= y - [\alpha + \beta(x - x)] + [\alpha + \beta(x - x_R)] \\
&= y + \beta(x - x_R)
\end{aligned}
$$

and back-transformed to the original scale,

$$ \text{QTc} = f^{-1}\{f(\text{QT}) + \beta[f(\text{RR}_R) - f(\text{RR})]\} \ . \tag{8.4} $$

When $f(\cdot)$ is the log transformation, the RR interval is expressed in seconds, $\text{RR}_R = 1$ s, and equation (8.4) simplifies to

$$ \text{QTc} = \text{QT RR}^{-\beta} \ . \tag{8.5} $$

Similarly, when $f(\cdot)$ is the identity function, both the QT and RR interval are expressed in seconds and, when $\text{RR}_R = 1$ s,

$$ \text{QTc} = \text{QT} + \beta \ (1 = \text{RR}) \ . \tag{8.6} $$

In practice, the slope parameter $\beta$ in equations (8.3)–(8.6) must be estimated, and the QTc interval is obtained by replacing $\beta$ in those equations by a suitable estimate. When the conditional expectation $E(y|x)$ is modeled through a linear model such as in (8.3), different heart rate correction methods are distinguished by how the linear model is fitted to the data, and to which data the model is fitted. In the remainder of this section, various explicit heart rate correction methods are discussed, namely, methods for calculating QTc.

### 8.4.2.4   "Off-drug data driven" correction

In an "off-drug data driven" correction the linear model (8.3) is fitted to "off-drug" data, that is, placebo or baseline data from a TQT study. In the following, we assume that for each subject included in the TQT study to be analysed a single "off drug" series of observations (repeated measures) of QT and RR interval data is available. This series of observations will usually be collected during the placebo treatment period of the trial. Richer pools of "off drug" data (i.e., multiple "off drug" profiles per subject) might be available when full 24-hour baseline profiles are taken for each study period. However, recently fewer studies have included time-matched baselines as this might not be cost-effective.

We assume in what follows that the linear regression model (8.3) is fitted to the placebo data from a TQT study, that is, a single "off drug" data profile per subject. Where appropriate, we will indicate how to accommodate multiple "off-drug" profiles in the respective regression models for the estimation of heart rate correction slopes.

### 8.4.2.5   Individual correction; Fixed-effects model

The basic model (8.3) can be fitted to data in various ways. One option is to fit the model individually to the data of the subjects in a TQT study, that is, one simple linear regression fit (intercept and slope parameter) per subject. The regression model for a given subject's placebo data is of the form

$$y_{Pk} = \alpha_P + \beta_P x_{Pk} + e_{Pk} ,$$ (8.7)

where $y_{Pk} = f(QT_{Pk})$ is the observation, under placebo (P) treatment, at the $k$th repeated measures time point $(k = 1, \ldots, K)$, $x_{Pk} = f(RR_{Pk})$ is the RR interval measurement corresponding to $QT_{Pk}$, and $e_{Pk}$ is the corresponding residual. Fitting model (8.7) to the placebo data of each subject separately is equivalent to fitting the following model to the placebo data of all subjects jointly:

$$y_{iPk} = \alpha_{iP} + \beta_{iP} x_{iPk} + e_{iPk} .$$ (8.8)

SAS PROC MIXED code for model (8.8) is as follows:

```
/* Model (8.8): Individual heart rate correction (Fixed effects
model) */
PROC MIXED;
  CLASS subject;
  MODEL y = subject subject*x;
RUN;
```

Model (8.8) yields individual slope estimates $\hat{\beta}_P$ $(i = 1, \ldots, N)$ for the subjects in the study. Using those parameter estimates, and referring back to equation (8.2), the heart rate corrected QT interval data are obtained as

$$QTc_{ijk} = f^{-1}[y_{ijk} + \hat{\beta}_P (x_R - x_{ijk}) .$$ (8.9)

### 8.4.2.6 Individual correction; random-effects model

Alternatively to the fixed-effects model (8.3), a particular type of mixed model, namely a random-coefficients model, can be fitted to the placebo data of all study subjects jointly:

$$y_{iPk} = (\alpha_{iP} + s_i) + (\beta_{iP} + v_i) x_{iPk} + e_{iPk} .$$ (8.10)

Model (8.10) includes random subject effects $s_i$ representing individual random deviations from the "population" intercept $\alpha_P$ and random coefficients $v_i$ representing individual random deviations from the "population" slope $\beta_P$; the $2 \times 2$ covariance matrix of the random coefficients $[s_i, v_i]'$ is assumed to be unstructured [40, 44]. SAS PROC MIXED code for model (8.10) is as follows:

```
/* Model (8.10): Individual heart rate correction (Random
coefficients model)*/
PROC MIXED;
  CLASS subject; MODEL y = x;
  RANDOM INT subject / SUBJECT=subject TYPE=UN;
RUN;
```

Similarly to model (8.8), model (8.10) yields individual slope estimates $\hat{\beta}_{iP} = \hat{\beta}_P + \hat{v}_i$, $i = 1, \ldots, N$. Using those random-effects estimates, the QTc interval data can again be obtained as in equation (8.9).

### 8.4.2.7    Population correction; random-coefficients model

The fixed-effects parameter $\beta_P$ in the random-coefficients model (8.10) can be interpreted as the "population" slope for the study population, since $E(v_i) = 0$ so that $\beta_P$ represents the mean of the individual slopes $\beta_P + v_i$ [44, 48]. Thus, using the estimate $\hat{\beta}_P$ for $\beta_P$ from model (8.10), "population" corrected QT interval data can be obtained from equation (8.9).

### 8.4.2.8    Population correction; simple linear regression

Many traditional population correction methods amount to fitting a simple linear regression model of the form

$$y_{iPk} = \alpha_P + \beta_P x_{iPk} + e_{iPk} . \tag{8.11}$$

In model (8.11) we note the absence of subject-specific intercepts such as in models (8.8) and (8.9). As Ring [44] points out, "population heart rate corrections have often been derived based on a pool of data points originating from a large number of subjects, each of whom usually contributed only very few data points. Population correction parameters were then derived based on [simple] linear regression ... In these investigations, the subject level was often neglected."

Quite apart from the fact that a model such as equation (8.11) usually does not take account of the correlation of QT interval data within subject, the absence of individual subject intercepts, whether fixed as in model (8.8) or random as in model (8.10), can cause severe bias in the slope estimate $\beta$ [49]; see also the estimates in the last column of Table III of [44]. Thus population heart rate correction using a simple linear regression model as in equation (8.11) cannot be recommended.

### 8.4.2.9    "Fixed" correction

So-called "fixed" correction formulas, such as those of Fridericia [50], Bazett [51], and the Framingham correction [52], are obtained when the slope parameter $\beta$ in model (8.3) is not estimated from the data of the TQT trial at hand, but "fixed" at values obtained from historical data.

The correction methods of Fridericia and Bazett essentially use log-linear correction equation (8.5) with slopes of $\hat{\beta}_P = \frac{1}{3}$ (Fridericia) and $\hat{\beta}_P = \frac{1}{2}$ (Bazett), respectively. Thus we have Fridericia's well-known cube root formula,

$$QTcF = QT/\sqrt[3]{RR},$$

and the equally well-known square root formula of Bazett,

$$QTcB = QT/\sqrt[2]{RR}.$$

It should be noted that Fridericia's and Bazett's estimates of $1/3$ and $1/2$ for $\beta_P$ were obtained from relatively small "convenience samples" (39 and 50 subjects, respectively), and no statistical methods were employed in their derivation [47]. Furthermore, since Fridericia's and Bazett's slope estimates were obtained using simple linear regression models that did not fit individual subject intercepts, it is not surprising that their estimates tend to be somewhat higher than slope estimates obtained using models such as (8.8) and (8.10).

The Framingham correction formula is obtained using the linear correction equation (8.6), with $\hat{\beta} = 0.154$; thus

$$QTcFr = QT - 0.154\,(RR - 1),$$

where both QT and RR interval lengths are given in seconds.

### 8.4.2.10   One-step versus two-step analysis of heart rate corrected QT prolongation

Once the QTc interval has been calculated, QT prolongation is assessed by comparing the QTc interval data for active drug with the QTc interval data for placebo. Thus an assessment of heart rate corrected QT prolongation conventionally proceeds in two steps [46]: In the first step, the QT interval data (as measured) are corrected for the effect of heart rate, using one of the two classes of correction procedures discussed above: either (i) "off-drug data driven" correction where the slope estimate from a regression of placebo (off-drug) QT data against heart rate is used to calculate QTc data; or (ii) "fixed" correction where one of a number of published correction formulas is used to calculate QTc data as a function of QT and HR. Thereafter, in the second step, the QTc data of active and placebo treatment are compared statistically (see Section 8.4.5 for relevant analysis models). In principle, then, after the correction step, QTc data are analysed statistically in the same manner as the measured QT and RR interval data are analysed.

More recently, Li *et al.* [46] and other authors have pointed out that, from a statistician's perspective, a so-called "one-step" statistical analysis of both active treatment and placebo QT data, using mixed model analysis of covariance (where RR is fitted as a covariate) would be preferable to the two-step approach. Mixed model analysis of covariance models for one-step analysis of QT interval data will be discussed in detail in Section 8.4.5.

### 8.4.2.11   Analysis variables

The association of the QT and RR interval and potential confounding effect of drug-induced changes in heart rate might suggest that QT prolongation should be assessed (only) after heart rate correction. However, as the ICH E14 (2005) guidance document states, it is not yet clear whether cardiac arrhythmia is more closely related to an increase in the absolute (i.e., uncorrected) QT interval or to an increase in QTc. As long is this clinical question is open, both QT and QTc data have to be studied. Furthermore, since it is not yet clear what is the best heart rate correction approach, the ICH E14 guidance document [6] suggests that all drug applications submit QT interval data corrected using Bazett's and Fridericia's correction formulas, in addition to QT interval data using any other formula or method that the applicant might choose to use.

In summary, therefore, under current regulatory requirements statistical analysis of the data of a TQT study will routinely involve, as a minimum, analysis of the following sets of data:

1. Data "as measured":

   a. QT interval data (as measured): investigate drug effect on "uncorrected" QT interval

   b. RR interval data (as measured): investigate drug effect on RR interval (or heart rate).

2. Heart rate corrected QT interval:

   a. QTcF: QT interval data corrected using Fridericia's correction

   b. QTcB: QT interval data corrected using Bazett's correction.

3. Additional analyses@

   a. QTc data calculated using other correction formulas

   b. "one-step" analysis of (heart rate corrected) QT prolongation (Section 8.4.5).

The data "as measured" (QT and RR interval data) are compared statistically as outlined in Section 8.4.4, using mixed analysis of variance (ANOVA) models such as those described in Section 8.4.5. QTc interval data are routinely analysed in the same manner (e.g., [49]). However, depending on the type of heart rate correction method, interval estimates of the treatment contrast from the two-step procedure might not have the correct coverage [43].

## 8.4.3    A general framework for the assessment of QT prolongation

The appropriate assessment of QT prolongation remains an open question, and a potentially confusing array of heart rate correction methods, and associated statistical methods, is available. As pointed out above, it is not yet known whether an increase in the uncorrected or in the heart rate corrected QT interval is the best predictor of cardiac arrhythmia. Thus it is necessary to analyse both "absolute" (uncorrected) and heart rate corrected QT prolongation. More seriously, it is not clear which of the many heart correction methods is the most appropriate, so that the current regulatory guidelines require the application of various heart rate correction methods and statistical analysis of the resulting data (Section 8.4.2).

### 8.4.3.1    Marginal versus conditional QT prolongation

In an attempt to provide a basis for the discussion and comparison of various methods, Schall and Ring [54] proposed a general framework for the assessment of QT prolongation. Within this framework, the relationship between uncorrected and heart rate corrected QT prolongation, as well the relationships between different heart rate correction methods were outlined.

Specifically, as in Section 8.4.2 above, let $y = f(QT)$ and $y = f(QT)$ be the (possibly transformed) QT and RR interval measurements. Schall and Ring [54] defined the assessment of "uncorrected" or "absolute" QT prolongation as a between-treatment (active versus placebo) comparison of the marginal distributions of the QT data $y_A$ of active treatment, and $y_P$ of placebo treatment, referring to such a comparison as an assessment of marginal QT prolongation. Similarly, they defined the assessment of "heart rate corrected" QT prolongation as a between-treatment comparison of the conditional distributions of $y_A$ and $y_P$ given a particular RR interval measurement $x = f(RR)$ (see also [55, Section 2.3]), referring to such a comparison as an assessment of *conditional* QT prolongation.

In practice, the comparison of marginal and conditional distributions of QT interval data focuses on the marginal means $E(y_A) = \mu_A$ and $E(y_P) = \mu_P$ and on the conditional means $E(y_A|x)$ and $E(y_P|x)$ of $y_A$ and $y_P$. In the terminology of the relevant ICH guidance [6, Section 3.2.1] a comparison of means constitutes an analysis of the "central tendency" of QT interval data. In particular, the extent of QT prolongation is characterized by the between-treatment (active–placebo) contrasts of marginal and of conditional means, respectively. Thus

$$\gamma_m = \mu_A - \mu_P$$

is the treatment contrast characterizing marginal QT prolongation, and

$$\gamma_c(x) = E(y_A|x) - E(y_P|x) \tag{8.12}$$

is a treatment contrast characterizing conditional QT prolongation. Note that $\gamma_c(x)$ in general is a function of $x$.

### 8.4.3.2   Linear/log-linear model for conditional expectation of QT interval

Equation (8.12) does not necessarily require a linear model for the conditional means, and in principle $E(y_A|x)$ and $E(y_P|x)$ and, consequently, $\gamma(x)$ can be estimated using nonlinear or nonparametric regression techniques. However, the usual assumption is that $E(y_A|x)$ and $E(y_P|x)$ can be written as linear functions of $x$, as in equation (8.3) above, namely

$$E(y_i|x) = \alpha_i + \beta_i(x - x_R), \quad i = A, P. \tag{8.13}$$

In model (8.13) one can allow, in general, for different (non-parallel) slopes $\beta_A$ and $\beta_P$ for active and placebo treatment, respectively. The slopes would be different if drug treatment "changes the correction factor" (here denoted by $\beta$) [9].

In terms of the parameters of model (8.13), the treatment contrast for conditional QT prolongation, namely $\gamma_c(x)$ in equation (8.12), can be written as

$$\gamma_c(x) = E(y_A|x) - E(y_P|x) = \alpha_A - \alpha_P + (\beta_A - \beta_P)(x - x_R). \tag{8.14}$$

### 8.4.3.3   Relative merits of heart rate correction procedures within the general framework

When, in model (8.14), the slopes are equal $(\beta_A = \beta_P)$, $\gamma_c(x)$ simplifies to

$$\gamma_c(x) = \alpha_A - \alpha_P,$$

so that conditional QT prolongation is characterized globally (independent of $x$ or of the RR interval) by the difference in intercepts $\alpha_A - \alpha_P$. The contrast of intercepts $\alpha_A - \alpha_P$ is often viewed almost as the "definition" of conditional (i.e., heart-rate corrected) QT prolongation. However, in general, when the slopes are not equal, the extent of conditional QT prolongation, $\gamma_c(x)$, depends on $x = f(RR)$, and $\gamma_c(x)$ is equal to $\alpha_A - \alpha_P$ *only* if we condition on $x = x_R$, that is, we are interested in the conditional QT prolongation at the reference RR interval $x_R$.

Schall and Ring [54] showed that the two-step procedure with data-driven correction provides an unbiased estimate for the expected conditional QT prolongation, $\gamma_c(v_A)$, where $v_A$ is the mean RR interval in the active treatment group. Thus the expectation is taken with respect to the distribution of the RR interval data under active treatment. This treatment contrast in principle is clinically meaningful, and might well be more meaningful than the conditional QT prolongation at some poorly chosen reference RR interval. However, a TQT study in healthy volunteers may not be suitable for estimating the average heart rate under active treatment *in the target population*. Furthermore, interval estimates of the treatment contrast from the two-step procedure might not have the correct coverage [47]: when data-driven correction methods are used, multiple QT values are corrected using the same slope estimate. The resulting correlation between QTc data (and reduction of error degrees of freedom) is not taken into account when the data are analysed. Consequently, CIs for between-treatment differences from the two-step procedure may have coverage smaller than their nominal coverage so that the two-step procedure might not be valid statistically.

Schall and Ring [54] also argued that fixed correction methods are not appropriate for assessment of conditional QT prolongation in TQT studies. Depending on the effect of active treatment on the average RR interval, fixed correction can falsely suggest conditional QT prolongation, or mask its presence. The Bazett correction is particularly notorious in this regard because Bazett's regression slope tends to be considerably larger than regression slopes estimated from modern databases using appropriate analysis models (see, for example, [44, 47, 48]). Bazett's procedure will falsely suggest QT prolongation for drugs that increase heart rate, and will mask QT prolongation for drugs that decrease heart rate. (No harm is done only when active treatment does not shift the average heart rate, but only because in this case correction has no effect and is redundant.) A case in point is the analysis published by Shah and Hajian [48]: active treatment increased the average heart rate by about 10 bpm, and therefore decreased the average RR interval (their Table II); furthermore, the slope estimate from the one-step procedure assuming equal slopes (an assumption supported by the data) was 0.292, which is only slightly smaller than the Fridericia slope of $1/3$ but considerably smaller than Bazett's slope of $1/2$. Data analysis using the one-step method suggested QT shortening, while the two-step method using Bazett's fixed correction suggested QT prolongation; the two-step method using Fridericia's fixed correction suggested QT shortening, but less extensive than the QT shortening estimated by the one-step method. Thus the results of the one-step procedure and of the two-step procedure using Bazett's correction are completely contradictory, but are as predicted by the discussion in Schall and Ring [54, Section 4.3]. Thus, all fixed correction methods are potentially biased, and the bias of Bazett's method is the most severe. There may be no alternative to the use of a fixed correction when single or very sparse ECG data are evaluated, such as in routine clinical practice; in this case the Fridericia correction is probably preferable to the Bazett correction because Fridericia's regression slope of $1/3$ is likely to be associated with less bias than Bazett's slope of $1/2$. In the statistical analysis of TQT studies fixed correction methods should not be used.

The so-called one-step procedure, by fitting model (8.13) simultaneously to both active and placebo data, has at least two advantages: the procedure can provide unbiased estimates of the parameters of the model, and therefore the procedure can provide a "complete" characterization of conditional QT prolongation since $\gamma_c(x)$ can be estimated over any range of RR interval values of interest. Furthermore, and this point has been made by many authors, if an appropriate error model for the one-step procedure is specified, usually a linear or log-linear mixed model, then point estimates for $\gamma_c(x)$ are efficient, and the interval estimates have correct coverage. Another advantage of the one-step procedure is that QT prolongation is assessed directly through analysis of QT data (under a model that contains the RR interval as a covariate): it is not necessary to calculate explicitly any QTc values. The choice of a QT correction method (e.g., data driven with "population" slopes, data driven with "individual" slopes, or data driven with shrinkage of individual slopes) is replaced by the equivalent choice of an appropriate mixed model for the QT data, fixed and random effects. Lastly, within the "one-step" approach, it is possible in principle to model the QT–RR relationship using nonlinear or nonparametric regression models. Thus, if one is not convinced that the linear or log-linear modeling of the QT–RR relationship is adequate, nonparametric regression methods can be used.

In summary, we recommend assessing conditional QT prolongation using a one-step procedure, in practice by fitting a linear or log-linear mixed model. This might in generally require allowing for non-parallel regression slopes for the different treatments, although in our experience the assumption of parallel slopes is usually consistent with the data. Mixed analysis of covariance models for this purpose will be discussed in Section 8.4.5.

## 8.4.4    Statistical inference: Proof of "Lack of QT prolongation"

The ICH E14 guidance document distinguishes between "analyses of central tendency" [6, Section 3.2.1] and "categorical analyses" [6, Section 3.2.2]. An analysis of central tendency, which we consider now, focuses on "the largest time-matched mean difference between [active] drug and placebo over the collection period" [6, Section 3.2.1]. An analysis of central tendency of QT data therefore involves statistical inference about the active–placebo contrasts of treatment means, $\tau_{Ak} - \tau_{Pk}$ (i.e., the time-matched mean differences), for all repeated measures time points $k = 1, \ldots, K$.

As we have seen in Section 8.4.2, the treatment contrasts $\tau_{Ak} - \tau_{Pk}(k = 1, \ldots, K)$, in the first instance, refer to differences in mean QT interval between treatments. If a "two-step" procedure for assessment of heart rate corrected QT prolongation is used, the treatment contrasts $\tau_{Ak} - \tau_{Pk}$ also may refer to differences in mean QTc interval. If a one-step procedure is used, $\tau_{Ak} - \tau_{Pk}$ may refer to treatment contrasts in the context of a (mixed) analysis of covariance model.

Whatever the analysis variable or heart rate correction method employed, the aim of a TQT study is to show "lack of QT prolongation". Specifically, the largest of time-matched mean differences $\tau_{Ak} - \tau_{Pk}(k = 1, \ldots, K)$ must be shown to be sufficiently small; equivalently, all treatment contrasts $\tau_{Ak} - \tau_{Pk}(k = 1, \ldots, K)$ must be shown to be small. Therefore, as in a non-inferiority study, the largest treatment contrast (over all time points) must be shown not to exceed a certain upper limit $\Delta$. Here $\Delta$, which fulfils the role of the "non-inferiority delta" of a non-inferiority study, is a regulatory constant.

Thus statistical inference for TQT studies can be outlined as follows (e.g., [49]). Let $\tau_{Ak} - \tau_{Pk}$ denote the active–placebo treatment contrast at repeated measures time point $k, k = 1, \ldots, K$. Then the null hypothesis

$$H_0 : \tau_{Ak} - \tau_{Pk} \geq \Delta \text{ for at least one } k$$

is tested against the alternative

$$H_1 : \tau_{Ak} - \tau_{Pk} < \Delta \text{ for all } k = 1, \ldots, K.$$

The regulatory constant $\Delta$ represents a clinically insignificant change in mean QT prolongation. The ICH E14 guidance document specifies $\Delta = 10$ ms (when the QT interval data are analysed on the original scale).

In practice, the test of $H_0$ is carried out by calculating two-sided 90% CIs for the $K$ treatment contrasts $\tau_{Ak} - \tau_{Pk}, k = 1, \ldots, K$; then $H_0$ is rejected, and "lack of QT prolongation" for the active dose in question is declared, if the upper bounds of the CIs for all $K$ treatment contrasts are below $\Delta$. Statistical inference for TQT studies, therefore, requires point and interval estimation of the contrasts $\tau_{Ak} - \tau_{Pk}$ for repeated measures time points $k = 1, \ldots, K$.

If QT interval data are analysed on the logarithmic scale, so that $\tau_{Ak} - \tau_{Pk}$ represents a treatment contrast of means of logarithmically transformed QT interval data under active and placebo treatment, respectively, an equivalence delta of $\Delta = \log(1.025)$ can be motivated on the log scale [54]. If $\Delta = 10$ ms is the maximum permissible mean QT prolongation on the difference scale, and if 400 ms is the average QT interval in an untreated healthy volunteer, then $\delta = 410/400 = 1.025$ is the maximum permissible QT prolongation on the ratio scale, and therefore $\Delta = \log(1.025)$ is the maximum permissible mean QT prolongation on the logarithmic scale.

## 8.4.5    Mixed models for data from TQT studies

### 8.4.5.1    Marginal QT prolongation and heart rate data

Schall and Ring [56] proposed the following mixed model for the analysis of QT interval data:

$$ y_{ijk(m)} = \mu + b_{ijk}\gamma + \pi_m + \tau_j + \zeta_k + b_{ijk}\gamma_k + \pi_{mk} + \tau_{jk} + s_{ik} + e_{ijk} . \tag{8.15} $$

Here $y_{ijk(m)}$ is the observation for the $i$th subject and the $j$th treatment at the $k$th repeated measures time point ($k = 1, \ldots, K$); $\mu$ is the intercept; $b_{ijk}$ is the baseline value for subject $i$, treatment $j$, and time $k$ (the index $k$ allows for time-matched baseline values); $\gamma$ is the associated covariate effect; $\pi_m$ is the $m$th period effect; $\tau_j$ is the $j$th treatment effect; $\zeta_k$ is the $k$th time effect; $\gamma_k$ is the interaction effect of baseline and time; $\pi_{mk}$ is the interaction effect of period and time; $\tau_{jk}$ is the interaction effect of treatment and time; $s_{ik}$ is the random effect of subject $i$ at time $k$; and $e_{ijk}$ is the random error for subject $i$, treatment $j$, and time $k$. The $s_{ik}$ are assumed independent of the $e_{ijk}$ and mutually independent across index $i$ (subject), while the $e_{ijk}$ are assumed independent across indices $i$ and $j$ (subject and treatment).

To accommodate the covariance between the subject effects $s_{ik}$ over the $K$ time points and, similarly, to accommodate the covariance between the error terms $e_{ijk}$ over time, the covariance structure of the $K$-variate random vectors $\mathbf{s}_i = (s_{i1}, \ldots, s_{iK})'$ and $\mathbf{e}_{ijk} = (e_{ij_1}, \ldots, e_{ijK})'$ is modeled as follows. Consistent with the notation of Jones and Kenward [57, pp. 234–235] and of [58], we write $\mathrm{cov}(\mathbf{s}_i) = \mathbf{G}_{K \times K}$ and $\mathrm{cov}(\mathbf{e}_{ij}) = \mathbf{R}_{K \times K}$. In the terminology of [57, pp. 246–248] the matrices $\mathbf{G}$ and $\mathbf{R}$ model the covariance structure of the repeated measurements respectively between and within treatment periods.

The following SAS PROC MIXED code can be used to carry out the calculations for equation (8.15) with unstructured covariance patterns specified for both $\mathbf{G}$ and $\mathbf{R}$:

```
/* Model (8.15): RMC Model for Assessment of Marginal QT
   Prolongation */
PROC MIXED;
  CLASS subject treat period time;
  MODEL y = b period treat time b*time period*time treat*time
          / DDFM=KR;
  RANDOM time / SUBJECT=subject TYPE=UN;
  REPEATED time / SUBJECT=subject*treat TYPE=UN;
RUN;
```

Schall and Ring [56] called model (8.15) the repeated measures cross-over (RMC) model. Depending on the study design and study population, the basic model (8.15) might be extended, for example, by including a gender effect (e.g., [44]).

The RMC model (8.15) models the covariance structure of the RMC data in a particular way. Schall and Ring also considered a covariance pattern model with saturated covariance structure,

$$ y_{ijk(m)} = \mu + b_{ijk}\gamma + \pi_m + \tau_j + \zeta_k + b_{ijk}\gamma_k + \pi_{mk} + \tau_{jk} + e_{ijk} , \tag{8.16} $$

which is expression (8.15) without the $s_{ik}$ term. The covariance structure of the residuals $e_{ijk}$ and, therefore, of the observations $y_{ijk(m)}$ is specified as $cov(\mathbf{e}_i) = cov(e_{iA1}, \ldots, e_{iPK}) = \mathbf{V}$, an unstructured covariance matrix of dimension $2K \times 2K$. The SAS PROC MIXED code for carrying out the calculations using model (8.16) is as follows:

```
/* Model (8.16): Saturated Model for Assessment of Marginal QT
   Prolongation */
PROC MIXED;
  CLASS subject treat period time;
  MODEL y = b period treat time b*time period*time treat*time
  REPEATED treat*time / SUBJECT=subject TYPE=UN;
RUN;
```

Schall and Ring showed by simulation that point estimates for treatment contrasts under the RMC and the saturated models are similar, and have similar precision. Furthermore, the coverage properties of CIs for treatment contrasts under both models were shown to be adequate. In contrast, they showed that CIs under a mixed model proposed earlier [53] did not have adequate coverage properties and the model thus cannot be recommended for the statistical analysis of QT data.

### 8.4.5.2   One-step assessment of conditional QT prolongation

To assess QT prolongation corrected for the RR interval, Schall [59] introduced a covariate $x_{ijk}$ into model (8.15), in the manner of [48] and [46]:

$$y_{ijk(m)} = \mu + b_{ijk}\gamma + x_{ijk}\beta + \pi_m + \tau_j + \zeta_k + b_{ijk}\gamma_k + x_{ijk}\beta_j + \pi_{mk} + \tau_{jk} + s_{ik} + e_{ijk} . \quad (8.17)$$

Here the $\beta + \beta_j$ are the fixed regression slopes of $y_{ijk}$ against $x_{ijk}$ (the "population" slopes of $f(QT)$ against $f(RR)$) that allow for possibly treatment-dependent slopes. All of the other terms, including the specifications of the covariance models $cov(\mathbf{s}_i) = \mathbf{G}$ and $cov(\mathbf{e}_{ij}) = \mathbf{R}$, remain the same as in model (8.15). The model originally proposed by Schall [59] included only a single slope parameter $\beta$. The SAS PROC MIXED code for carrying out the calculations using model (8.17) with unstructured covariance matrices is as follows:

```
/* Model (8.17): RMC Model for Assessment of Conditional QT
   Prolongation */
PROC MIXED;
  CLASS subject treat period time;
  MODEL y = b x period treat treat*x time b*time period*time
           treat*time / DDFM=KR;
  RANDOM time / SUBJECT=subject TYPE=UN;
  REPEATED time / SUBJECT=subject*treat TYPE=UN;
RUN;
```

Between-treatment covariance is modeled in equation (8.17) through the random subject by time effects $s_{ik}$ (allowing unstructured covariance patterns for the $s_{ik}$ over time). Within-treatment covariance is modeled by using an unstructured covariance pattern for the residuals. In the terminology of [60], model (8.17) combines the elements of a random-effects and of a covariance pattern model.

Alternatively, the random effects $s_{ik}$ in model (8.17) can be replaced by subject-specific random intercepts and slopes [46, 48, 59], to express the individual nature of the relationship between QT and RR interval [45] by adding random intercept ($u_i$) and slope ($v_i$) terms for subject $i$:

$$y_{ijk(m)} = \mu + b_{ijk}\gamma + x_{ijk}\beta + \pi_m + \tau_j + x_{ijk}\beta_j + \zeta_k + b_{ijk}\gamma_k + \pi_{mk} + \tau_{jk} + u_i + x_{ijk}v_i + e_{ijk}.$$
(8.18)

The $u_i$ and $v_i$ are assumed independent across subjects (index $i$), and independent of the $e_{ijk}$. Furthermore, $E[(u_i, v_i)'] = \mathbf{0}$ and $cov[(u_i, v_i)'] = \mathbf{G}_1$, the $2 \times 2$ covariance matrix of the random coefficients. Model (8.18) combines the elements of a random-coefficients and of a covariance pattern model because between-treatment correlation is modeled by the random coefficients $u_i$ and $v_i$, while within-treatment correlation is modeled through an unstructured covariance pattern for the residuals as in model (8.15).

The SAS PROC MIXED code for carrying out the calculations using model (8.18) with unstructured covariance matrices is as follows:

```
/* Model (8.18): Random Coefficients Model for Assessment of
   Conditional QT Prolongation */
PROC MIXED;
  CLASS subject treat period time;
  MODEL y = b x period treat treat*x time b*time period*time
            treat*time / DDFM=KR;
  RANDOM INT x / SUBJECT=subject TYPE=UN;
  REPEATED time / SUBJECT=subject*treat TYPE=UN;
RUN;
```

Finally, model (8.16) can be extended by using a saturated covariance structure, and we can also fit a mixed model with saturated covariance structure, namely

$$y_{ijk(m)} = \mu + b_{ijk}\gamma + x_{ijk}\beta + \pi_m + \tau_j + x_{ijk}\beta_j + \zeta_k + b_{ijk}\gamma_k + \pi_{mk} + \tau_{jk} + e_{ijk}.$$
(8.19)

All of the effects in this model are interpreted as in equation (8.17), but the covariance structure of the residuals $e_{ijk}$ and, therefore, of the observations $y_{ijk(m)}$ is specified as $cov(\mathbf{e}_i) = cov(e_{iJ1}, \ldots, e_{iJK}) = \mathbf{V}$, an arbitrary non-singular covariance matrix of dimension $2K \times 2K$ (if the data for two treatments is analysed). The SAS PROC MIXED code for carrying out the calculations using model (8.19) is as follows:

```
/* Model (8.19): Saturated Covariance Model for Assessment of
   Conditional QT Prolongation */
PROC MIXED;
  CLASS subject treat period time;
  MODEL y = b x period treat time b*time period*time treat*time
         / DDFM=KR;
  REPEATED treat*time / SUBJECT=subject TYPE=UN;
RUN;
```

Schall [59] found that point estimates of treatment contrasts from all the three models (8.17)–(8.19) are similar. Treatment contrasts from all three models have similar precision and all three models are suitable for the one-step assessment of conditional QT prolongation.

The particular mixed model considered by Li *et al.* [46] and Shah and Hajian [48], a random-coefficients model with independent and identically distributed residuals, is not robust; the model potentially leads to both under- and overestimation of standard errors of treatment contrasts, and therefore the model cannot be recommended for one-step analysis of conditional QT prolongation.

### 8.4.5.3  Relationship between baseline and covariance structure

Section 8.3.3 considers the choice of baseline in the design of TQT trials. The mixed models in section 8.4.5 above focus on identifying the covariates for the analysis of QT prolongation, but do not adapt the covariance structure to the various baseline options.

Li *et al.* [61] closed that gap by providing the structures of covariance matrices the QTc change from baseline for the main definitions of time-matched baselines (time-matched baseline in each period or at first period only, averaged time-matched baseline etc.) for TQT trials with crossover design. A particular advantage is that the risk of inflating the statistical type I error (because of potential misspecification of the covariance structure) is reduced, as the variance of the treatment contrast is being analytically derived.

Furthermore this approach allows one to compare the statistical efficiency of the baseline definitions analytically by using additional assumptions on the covariance structure of the residuals (eijk). These assumptions can be motivated using data from previous TQT studies. The main result is that the variance of the estimator of $\Delta\Delta QT$ is lower for the time-matched baseline from the first period only than for time-matched baselines of each period, hence the former method is recommended by Li *et al.* [61] from a cost and efficiency perspective.

## 8.5  Examples of ECG trial designs and analyses from the literature

In this section we discuss a number of trial designs and analyses that have been performed. These examples provide insight into typical options and considerations when planning new TQT trials. Although TQT trials are nowadays a standard requirement, they should be planned carefully with the aim of demonstrating the absence of QT prolongation and to avoid unnecessary costs and effort.

### 8.5.1  Parallel trial: Nalmefene

Nalmefene is a competitive opioid receptor antagonist, marketed for reducing alcohol consumption in alcohol-dependent patients [62]. The TQT trial was performed with a parallel, multiple-dose design and four treatment arms. Nalmefene was given as 20 and 80 mg oral tablets and matching placebo once daily for 7 days, blinded. Moxifloxacin 400 mg as the active control was given open label on day 7 only, following 6 days of placebo. The 20 mg dose is the therapeutic dose level of nalmefene, while the 80 mg dose provides 4.4-fold pharmacokinetic exposure as a safety margin according to ICH E14.

EGGs were obtained on the baseline day and on day 7, so that the primary endpoint was the individually heart rate corrected (QTcI) time-matched change from baseline, evaluated using a repeated measurements ANCOVA. Two hundred and seventy subjects were randomized into the study (no details of a power calculation were provided), of whom 245 were evaluated for the primary endpoint.

QTcI was slightly increased at day 7 between 1 and 12 hours after treatment for both doses of nalmefene; the average placebo-adjusted QTcI change from baseline was 3–6 ms. Although at some time points these differences represent a statistically significant difference between placebo and nalmefene, the upper limits of all 90% confidence intervals were below 10 ms, and no dose–response relationship was apparent. Moxifloxacin showed the expected effect of 6–10 ms increase of QTcI against placebo, and the 90% CI was twice above the margin of 5 ms.

This trial is an example of a straightforward parallel design. The baseline day ensures that within-subject comparisons of QTcI can be performed for a potential exposure–response analysis. The sample size of more than 60 subjects per group might indicate that the study was powered under the assumption of a slight (but not clinically relevant) QT effect of the new drug.

## 8.5.2   Cross-over trial: Linagliptin

Linagliptin is an antidiabetic drug. Since type II diabetes is very prevalent, drugs for this indication should have large safety margins (see also the next section) [18]. Therefore, the linagliptin TQT trial used a 20-fold supra-therapeutic dose (100 mg), the therapeutic dose of 5 mg, as well as matching placebo. Because of this large overdose, and in the absence of cumulating metabolites, the trial was performed using a single dose of moxifloxacin 400 mg given open-label.

Despite the long wash-out period of 6 weeks between two treatments (based on the long pharmacokinetic terminal half-life of the drug), a cross-over design was chosen for the trial. Baseline measurements consisted of three triple ECGs recorded pre-dose in the morning prior to each drug administration, followed by 10 time points with triple ECG recordings up to 24 hours post baseline.

Change from baseline of QTcI was selected as the primary analysis variable, and a repeated measures mixed model was used for the primary analysis. As there was no indication of a QTc effect during early clinical development, a power of 90% was specified for achievement of the trial objectives, which led to a sample size of 40 subjects (44 subjects were randomized in order to accommodate potential drop-outs).

The trial data suggested that the heart rate was slightly increased (by up to 4 bpm) by the supra-therapeutic dose; this was deemed to be clinically not relevant because of the large overdose. Because of the shift in heart rate it was, however, important that the heart rate correction of the QT interval was performed adequately. Individual heart rate correction was applied based on a mixed model as described in [44]. The upper limit of the 90% CI of the placebo-corrected change from baseline of QTcI was below 5 ms for all repeated measures time points, hence lack of QT prolongation could be demonstrated. Both results (dose-dependent change of heart rate and no change of QTcI) were confirmed in an exposure–response analysis. In addition, moxifloxacin showed the expected QT prolongation effect of about 10 ms, with the lower limit of the 90% CI exceeding 5 ms at 3 and 4 hours post dose.

Overall, the cross-over design was considered efficient for this trial, as there was no need to record a baseline day. The use of three triple ECGs at baseline reduced the standard error of the change from baseline adequately, and yielded a sufficient number of ECGs for determination of the individual heart rate corrections. Despite the long duration of the trial (about 4 months for each subject), only one subject discontinued prematurely from the trial.

### 8.5.3   Cross-over with minor QTc effect: Sitagliptin

Sitagliptin belongs to the same class of drugs as linagliptin [17]. Therefore, this TQT trial also used a substantial multiple of the therapeutic dose to demonstrate the safety of the drug. The design was a four-treatment, single-dose cross-over trial with pre-dose baseline ECG measurements and seven post-baseline ECG recordings (with five replicates) up to 12 hours post dose. Sitagliptin 100 and 800 mg, placebo and moxifloxacin were administered in blinded fashion. The Fridericia corrected QT interval QTcF was used as the primary analysis variable.

Eighty-six subjects were randomized in this trial but only 79 subjects completed at least two trial periods, and apparently less than 73 subjects completed the trial. The heart rate was not altered by any of the treatments, but the supra-therapeutic dose showed a slight prolongation of mean QTcF effect compared to placebo at 3 hours post dose, which is also the time to maximum drug concentration ($T_{max}$). At this time, the mean prolongation of QTcF was 8 ms with an upper limit of the 90% CI of 11 ms, thus slightly above the regulatory margin. Furthermore, the exposure–response analysis indicated a positive relationship.

The fact that the QTcF effect was seen only with a large supra-therapeutic of dose eight times the therapeutic dose, the fact that the drug is mostly excreted unchanged (hence little impact of CYP interactions is expected), and the absence of a relevant QT effect at the therapeutic dose led to a favourable outcome for the labeling for this drug. Regulatory authorities indicated that the characterization of the drug's potential to alter ventricular polarization was considered to be satisfactory. Hence the label indicated the finding of marginal QT prolongation at supra-therapeutic doses, without, however, containing any precautions and warnings. This evaluation and finding by the regulatory authorities is positive for the planning of future TQT trials in that sponsors are not discouraged from choosing large multiples of the therapeutic dose for a TQT study because the overall picture in relation to the dose–response curve is considered when evaluating the safety and risk–benefit profile of a drug. This was the case even though the trial formally did not demonstrate lack of QT prolongation at the supra-therapeutic dose.

This trial also illustrates the rationale for not excluding the therapeutic dose from a TQT trial. When a supra-therapeutic dose is investigated in a TQT trial, excluding the therapeutic dose sometimes is suggested in order to reduce costs. Although one can extrapolate the potential QTc effect of the lower therapeutic dose from an exposure–response analysis of the supra-therapeutic dose, one might not be able to address fully some concerns (e.g., a nonlinear exposure response). Furthermore, direct statistical proof of the absence of QTc effect at the therapeutic dose will always be a convincing argument.

Finally, it should be noted that the width of the 90% CI of the change from baseline was 6 ms in this sitagliptin trial, which was very similar to the linagliptin trial which used half the number of the subjects and three ECGs per time point (compared with five ECGs for sitagliptin). Hence, the variability of the QT measurements in the sitagliptin trial appears to have been at least 50% larger than that of the linagliptin trial, which emphasizes the importance of the quality of the QT interval determination on the statistical efficiency of the trial. The sitagliptin trial used fully automated measurement of the QT intervals from a Holter ECG, while the linagliptin trial used a semi-automatic approach with manual over-read from dedicated 10-second ECGs.

### 8.5.4    TQT study with heart rate changes but without QTc effect: Darifenacin

Darifenacin is indicated for the treatment of overactive bladder [63]. The TQT study was performed before the release of ICH E14, although most requirements of the guideline were fulfilled. The study was designed with four treatments in parallel, multiple-dose fashion over 6 days. It appears that the treatments were given open-label, but the ECG evaluations were performed blinded with regard to treatment and time point. The four treatments were placebo, moxifloxacin 400 mg, the therapeutic dose of 15 mg and a supra-therapeutic dose of 75 mg. Triplicate ECGs were recorded at 14 time points at baseline day −1 and at day 6, and the primary endpoint was derived using change from mean baseline. The final publication included detailed outcomes (change from baseline and placebo-corrected change from baseline) of the uncorrected QT interval as well as of QTcF and QTcB, where QTcF had been specified prospectively as primary analysis variable.

One hundred and eighty eight subjects were randomized into the trial (about 48 subjects per arm) and 179 subjects were included in the analysis. The trial included a (blinded) stratification of the genotypes with regard to poor and extended metabolizers. Because of the intended patient population, about half of the patients were in the age range 45–65 years, which meant that the mean heart rate at baseline was about 80 bpm.

Regarding the trial results the authors wrote: "There were no clinically relevant mean changes in heart rate (mean changes versus placebo at Tmax were +4, +6, and 6 beats per minute in the darifenacin 15 mg, darifenacin 75 mg, and moxifloxacin groups, respectively)." However, these changes were indeed statistically relevant for the outcome of the trial. From the figures presented it can be determined that following moxifloxacin treatment very little change in heart was seen, while the heart rate was increased in the other treatment groups.

As a consequence of the drug effect on heart rate the drug effect on QT, QTcF, and QTcB varied greatly: For QTcF, both dose levels of darifenacin showed very little effect on the placebo-corrected change from baseline; moxifloxacin had a QTcF effect of about 12 ms. The effect of darifenacin on the uncorrected QT interval was clearly negative (−5 to − 8 ms) and for QTcB somewhat positive (about 2 ms for both dose levels). Because of the heart rate change in the placebo group, the placebo-corrected change from baseline of QT and QTcB of moxifloxacin was also different, although the heart rate in the moxifloxacin group was not changed.

Overall, this trial demonstrates the importance of the choice of adequate heart rate correction methods in TQT trials. Many drugs change the heart rate, but the heart rate corrected QT interval might well be unchanged, if determined correctly. Fortunately, the Fridericia correction is often quite adequate, but newer methods as outlined in the previous section would have improved the estimation and could have led to higher power in this trial.

Lastly, for TQT trials it is advisable always to report in detail changes in heart rate, even if those changes are deemed clinically not to be relevant.

### 8.5.5    Trial with both changes in HR and QT(c): Tolterodine

Tolterodine is another drug for the treatment of overactive bladder [64]. This is an example of a TQT study where unchanged QT intervals on treatment in combination with an increase in heart rate imply that treatment prolongs the heart rate corrected QT interval. Furthermore, the trial results suggest that the magnitude of the apparent QTc effect can depend on the method used for measuring the QT interval – fully automatic or manual.

This was a double-blind (with respect to tolterodine and placebo) four-way multiple dose (4 days) cross-over trial. Tolterodine was administered in a therapeutic dose (2 mg twice daily) and in a supra-therapeutic dose (4 mg twice daily), while the other two treatments were placebo and moxifloxacin. Forty-eight subjects were randomized and the primary analysis variable was QTcF.

With manually measured ECG intervals, the uncorrected QT interval was almost unchanged in steady state after 4 days of treatment. The mean heart rate was slightly increased by 2 bpm (2 mg) and 6 bpm (4 mg), respectively, while it was stable for moxi-floxacin, compared with placebo. The increase in heart rate implied that mean QTcF increased by 5 and 12 ms, respectively, for the two doses of tolterodine. Hence, the therapeutic dose level just passed the non-inferiority test against placebo, while for the supra-therapeutic dose lack of QTcF prolongation could not be shown.

For the automatically read QT intervals, the magnitude of QT prolongation was slightly lower, with mean QT effects of −3 and −6 ms, and mean QTcF effects of 1 and 6 ms. With this method, both doses would have passed the non-inferiority test. Interestingly, the magnitude of the QT effect of moxifloxacin also depended on the method of measurement: the manual method suggested a QTcF effect of about 19 ms, much larger than for most other TQT trials.

The label information for tolterodine contains the full results of this TQT study, including the different methods of measurement. The "precautions" section states that the QT effect should be considered, specifically for patients with a history of QT prolongation. However, it is also stated that for this drug there is no association between the QT prolongation and TdP in the post-marketing surveillance.

## 8.5.6    Boosting the exposure with pharmacokinetic interactions: Domperidone

For some drugs it is not possible to administer supra-therapeutic doses in TQT trials due to expected side effects. In this case, one might be able to increase concentrations of the investigational drug by co-administration of another drug that limits the metabolism of the investigational drug. Ritonavir and ketaconazole are CYP3A4 inhibitors which are most frequently considered for this purpose [24]. While ritonavir does not to prolong the QT interval [20], ketaconazole appears to have some QT liability.

In this QT study of domperidone (a dopamine antagonist), ketaconazole was chosen both as interacting drug and as active control. The study used double-blind, double-dummy medication, with multiple doses for 7 days (four doses of domperidone 10 mg at intervals of 4 hours daily, and two doses of ketoconazole 200 mg twice daily). QTcF was the primary analysis variable. The study was performed on only 24 subjects (14 of them male), which meant that the study was not fully powered for a TQT trial.

Boosting by ketoconazole led to a threefold increase in plasma concentrations of domperidone. The heart rate was virtually not altered by any of the treatments, compared to placebo. Both drugs alone caused some QT prolongation in men, namely 5 ms for domperidone and 9 ms for ketoconazole. For the combination therapy, the QTcF effect was around 16 ms, which is slightly less than expected when assuming a linear exposure– response relationship for the increased exposure of domperidone. However, all 90% CIs were very wide as there were only 14 subjects in the male subgroup.

In women the QTc effects of the single drugs were slightly negative, if at all different from placebo, and slightly positive for the combination. This result was unexpected and might be a false negative, as typically women are more prone to QT prolongation than men. Further studies would be needed to confirm the apparent lack of QT effect of domperidone in women. The inclusion of a moxifloxacin arm would have been advantageous in this study to check the susceptibility of the study population to QT prolongation.

In summary, boosting using pharmacokinetic interactions might be an option for increasing plasma exposure of a drug. However, the use of an agent that prolongs QT cannot be recommended, as the interpretation of the study results might be difficult.

### 8.5.7    Double placebo TQT cross-over design

An investigation of QT prolongation of empagliflozin, a new antidiabetic drug (SGLT-2 inhibitor) was recently carried out using a new, efficient cross-over design [32]. During early clinical development, there was no indication of changes of the heart rate or QT(c) interval by this drug.

The design is based on the fact that all comparisons in TQT trials are comparisons of an active drug versus placebo. There is no comparison between two active treatments. Administrating the (blinded) placebo treatment in two periods reduced the variance of the endpoint differences between active and placebo; overall a reduction of about 14% of the standard error is expected. Details provided in [35] and [37] show that this implies that the same power can be achieved with 30 instead of 40 subjects. Hence in total, 30 subjects × 5 periods =150 treatment periods were needed, compared to 160 treatment periods in the conventional four-period cross-over design.

## 8.6    Other issues in cardiovascular safety

The investigation of potential QTc prolongation to assess the risk of TdP is the focus of cardiac safety analysis, and is relevant to almost all new investigational drugs. However, the field of cardiovascular safety is wider than the mere investigation of QT prolongation. Examples of other areas in need of study are drug-induced changes of ECG intervals different from QT (PR interval prolongation, increase of QRS interval) as well as changes in the morphology or conduction of ECGs. The thorough investigation of markers such as blood pressure or safety laboratory measurements has also been discussed [10].

Hard cardiovascular outcomes such as myocardial infarction, stroke, or congestive heart failure can be observed with sufficient frequency only in large patient populations. Thus large outcome studies would be required in order to either detect or rule out significant risk of these events due to a drug. In the therapeutic area of diabetes, this approach is now formalized, since all new antidiabetic therapies need to demonstrate cardiovascular safety.

In 2008, the Food and Drug Administration (FDA) released the guidance "Diabetes Mellitus Evaluating Cardiovascular Risk in New Antidiabetic Therapies to Treat Type 2 Diabetes" [65] which changed the clinical development of glucose- lowering drugs. Before this time, it was sufficient to demonstrate antidiabetic activity in terms of lowering blood glucose levels and subsequently a reduction of the biomarker HbA1c hemoglobin after at least 3 months of therapy [66]. A lowering of HbA1c was assumed to decrease the risk of cardiovascular and other diabetic side effects because several studies had indicated that increased levels are associated with both microvascular and macrovascular complications (e.g., [67]).

## 8.6.1   Rosiglitazone

Rosiglitazone was approved in the USA in 1999 based on its glucose-lowering effects. A meta-analysis of adverse cardiovascular events associated with this drug was published in 2007 [68] suggesting a borderline, but statistically significant, increased risk of myocardial infarction when compared to other antidiabetic medications (odds ratio (OR) 1.43, 95% CI (1.03, 1.98)). Furthermore, an increased risk of cardiovascular death was observed, though not statistically significant (OR 1.64, 95% CI (0.98, 2.74)). Both effects appeared to contradict the intended treatment effect of rosiglitazone.

The meta-analysis was based on a number of rather small trials. At that time, a large open-label, randomized cardiac outcome trial with rosiglitazone (RECORD trial, started in 2006) was being conducted. Because of the publicity due to the publication of the meta-analysis, it was decided to perform an interim analysis to assess the safety profile of the drug. In this interim analysis, no increased risk of cardiovascular death or hospitalizations was found (OR 0.99, 95% CI 0.85–1.16) [69]. Instead an increased risk for heart failure (which was known) and an increased risk for bone fracture (which was a new finding) were identified. These results were confirmed in the final analysis [70].

With these different findings regarding the cardiovascular safety of rosiglitazone the over-all assessment of the risk–benefit profile of the drug became complex, and led to various regulatory actions in different parts of the world. The drug prescription was limited, but the approval was withdrawn only in the EU.

## 8.6.2   Requirements of the FDA guidance

The FDA guidance [65] recommends studying the major adverse cardiovascular events (MACE). MACE is a composite endpoint, typically defined as experiencing one of the events "cardiovascular mortality, myocardial infarction, or stroke". MACE may also include "hospitalization for acute coronary syndrome or urgent revascularization procedures". The aim is to compare the risk of MACE endpoints when patients take the new drug with the risk of treatment with placebo or standard care.

The guideline recommends a two-stage approach to establish cardiovascular safety for new investigational drugs. The first stage comprises a meta-analysis of all *pre-marketing* (Phase 2 + 3) clinical trials performed for submission for approval. As indicated, the typical objective of these trials is to confirm the glucose-lowering effects of the new drug in medium-length periods (3–12 months), so that they often study a few hundred patients each.

The meta-analysis across these trials should be performed based on a previously estab-lished analysis plan to evaluate the risk ratio for the MACE endpoints. Both the point estimate and the 95% CI of relevant risk ratios are assessed as a basis for approval and post-marketing commitments. The potential outcomes are listed in Table 8.1.

The sample size and the duration of the treatment periods within the drug development program should be planned accordingly, to rule out a risk ratio that is larger than 1.8, as the total investment of the program depends on the outcome of this meta-analysis. For a relative risk of 1.0 and balanced number of patients per treatment, in total 91 events should occur in order to have 80% power and 122 events for 90% power [71].

If the pre-marketing data lead to a 95% CI for the risk ratio that excludes the value 1.8, but not 1.3, then a dedicated cardiovascular outcome trial should be performed as a post-marketing commitment. This trial is typically a long-term outcome trial with the primary objective of investigating MACE endpoints in a population having a higher risk of cardiovascular events. The decision on whether this trial is analysed as stand-alone trial, or whether the trial should extend the meta-analysis, is left to the sponsor (but the decision needs to be made before carrying out the first meta-analysis).

If the estimated upper limit of the 95% CI is lower than 1.3 based on pre-marketing data alone, the post-marketing cardiovascular outcome trial may be waived. However, the waiver is not always granted, for example when the study population in the clinical trials differs from the intended patient population (when the general risk for cardiovascular events in the trial population is significantly lower than in an average population). To ensure the quality of the reporting of CV events, all events should be centrally adjudicated by an independent committee, in phase 2-3 trials as well as in dedicated outcome trials.

An example of a sponsor initiated meta-analysis is [72], which assessed MACE endpoints during the Phase 3 program of linagliptin. In total 5239 patients were included in the analysis, with a median follow up of 6 months. The analysis found a benefit of linagliptin, with a hazard ratio of 0.34 (95% CI: 0.16–0.70), based on 11 events for patients on linagliptin and 23 events for patients on placebo. This result was, however, not accepted by the FDA as evidence for a waiver of the cardiovascular outcome trial, primarily because the overall number of events was deemed too low. The reason for the low number of observed events was, firstly, the rather short follow up period. Secondly, the Phase 3 program had been performed in a "normal" diabetic patient population, while the FDA guideline recommends to "include patients at higher risk of cardiovascular events, such as patients with relatively advanced disease, elderly patients, and patients with some degree of renal impairment."

Following the FDA decision, two cardiovascular outcome trials of linagliptin have been initiated and are expected to report results in 2017. The first trial (CAROLINE) compares the cardiovascular outcome of treatment with linagliptin and glimepiride, respectively. As the cardiovascular safety of glimepiride has not been established yet, it was deemed necessary to perform also a direct comparison of linagliptin with placebo, which is currently conducted as the CARMELINA trial.

The first major trial of an antidiabetic treatment which has reported cardiovascular outcomes according to the new guidance is SAVOR-TIMI 53 [73]. This trial compared saxagliptin 5 mg and placebo with a median follow up time of 2.1 years in a total of 16,492 patients. The primary endpoint (MACE) occurred with a very similar frequency in both treatment arms

**Table 8.1** Inference on risk ratio for new drug against placebo and associated conclusions recommended in the guideline.

| Upper limit of 95% CI for risk ratio | Conclusion | |
|---|---|---|
| | Approval | Post-marketing commitment |
| ≥ 1.8 | Not adequate to support approval | – |
| [1.3, 1.8)[a] | Based on overall risk–benefit profile | Post-marketing trial required to demonstrate RR < 1.3 |
| < 1.3 | Based on overall risk–benefit profile | Post-marketing trial may not be required |

[a] With reassuring point estimate.

so that the hazard ratio estimate of 1.00 (95% CI: 0.89–1.12) fulfilled the criterion of the FDA guideline for non-inferiority. However, one of the secondary endpoints, hospitalization for heart failure, showed inferiority of the active drug to placebo, with a hazard ratio estimate of 1.27 (95% CI: 1.07–1.51). This secondary endpoint was considered only in an exploratory fashion, but it could indicate a potential risk of saxagliptin different from MACE. The conclusion of the authors was that "although saxagliptin improves glycemic control, other approaches are necessary to reduce cardiovascular risk in patients with diabetes."

In summary, the general objective of the FDA guidance is to establish the (cardiovascular) safety in a large patient population. The number of patients studied will be larger than in most other therapeutic areas, but in the light of the large number of patients who need glucose-lowering therapies this approach appears to be justified.

## 8.6.3    Impact on the development of antidiabetic drugs

The impact of the FDA guidance on the development of antidiabetic drugs has been discussed by several authors [71, 74, 75], focusing on whether the objectives and the sample sizes of trials changed compared to the time before the release of the guidance, based on the published information (e.g., in clinicaltrials.gov). Bethel [74] compared the time periods 2005–2008 and 2008–2011 and found that the proportion of open-label trials decreased over time (38% vs 42%) while the proportion of double-blind trials increased (58% vs 52%). A similar change was observed regarding the number of trials which investigated a moderate number of 100–1000 patients (63% vs 56%), although this change was primarily caused by a reduction of those trials which did not state their sample size adequately (from 6% to 1%).

Another significant change was the larger number of Phase 2 trials between 2008 and 2011 compared to the earlier time frame (29% vs 23%), while the number of Phase 3 trials decreased (40% vs 46%). This finding might, however, be confounded by the drug development cycles: the class of upcoming DPP-4 inhibitors and other incretinine therapies had mostly completed their Phase 2 program in 2005 and started their Phase 3 trials in that period. Current new classes of antidiabetic drugs had, on the other hand, started most of their Phase 2 trials after 2008.

The major changes, however, were the initiation of a large number of cardiovascular outcome trials. Only eight cardiovascular outcome studies were conducted between 2005 and 2008 (and only three of them were started during this period), with a total of about 22 000 patients. After 2008, 16 new trials with cardiovascular outcome objectives were initiated, with a total of 112 000 patients. Since February 2011, at least three additional trials have been initiated.

These trials were planned and started for all new compounds, with sample sizes of more than 5000 patients. The number of patients must be balanced against the duration of the trials, as 611 events are required to in order to have 90% power to demonstrate that the risk ratio in the trial is below 1.3, if the true risk ratio is 1.0.

The costs of these trials are substantial, even if they are often handled pragmatically to mimic the real-world situation. To recruit and maintain about 10 000 patients in a trial requires intensive support for the trial center and excellent logistics. New monitoring methods need to be established which review the (blinded) data centrally at the sponsor for medical or data quality monitoring, to identify those centers for which local monitoring would lead to the highest improvements in quality [76]. Thorough planning of outcome trials is crucial for their success, and intense involvement of regulatory agencies is required to clarify the suitability of their design components.

### 8.6.4    General impact on biomarker validation

When the relationship between the biomarker HbA1c and cardiovascular risk was established, it was generally believed that this biomarker could serve as a surrogate endpoint in the evaluation of antidiabetic therapies. Today, although HbA1c still has a major role in assessing the glucose-lowering potential of a drug during its development, it no longer is considered to be the primary criterion for risk–benefit assessment since drugs can present cardiovascular (or other) side effects independently of their main molecular pathways.

Furthermore, the ACCORD trial found that antidiabetic therapies should not lower HbA1c to values which are close to normal in healthy people [77]. The ACCORD trial compared intensive glucose monitoring (aiming for an HbA1c $\leq$ 6.0%) with standard therapies (7.0% $\leq$ HbA1c $\leq$ 7.9%). Patients in the intensive monitoring group had no reduction of cardiovascular events, more hypoglycaemias, and overall higher mortality.

This phenomenon is one example of a biomarker for which an observational relationship to hard clinical endpoints has been established (prognostic biomarker), but which might need to be assessed differently when used for evaluating the potential of a drug to affect the medical condition (predictive biomarker). The recent ICH E16 guideline [78] outlines general recommendations for validating biomarkers and their use during drug approval. In this light, the FDA guidance on cardiovascular risk assessment can be seen as a specific implementation of the ICH E16 guideline in the field of diabetes, as the FDA guidance clarifies that the drug-specific investigation of cardiovascular risks can be supported but not replaced by biomarker assessment.

## References

[1]  Yap, Y.G. and Camm, A.J. (2003) Drug induced QT prolongation and torsades de pointes. *Heart*, **89**, 1363–1372.

[2]  Lipicky, R.J. (1993) A viewpoint on drugs that prolong the QTc interval. *American Journal of Cardiology*, **76**, 53B–54B.

[3]  Committee for Proprietary Medicinal Products "The assessment of the potential for QT interval prolongation by non–cardiovascular medicinal products", CPMP/986/96, 1–6 (1997).

[4]  Health Canada. "Assessment of the QT prolongation potential of non–antiarrhythmic drugs", http://www.fda.gov/ohrms/dockets/ac/03/briefing/pubs/canada.pdf. Health Canada Therapeutic Products Directorate. (2001).

[5]  ICH Expert Working Group. "The non–clinical evaluation of the potential for delayed ventricular repolarization (QT interval prolongation) by human pharmaceuticals S7B", http://www.ich.org /fileadmin/Public_Web_Site/ICH_Products/Guidelines/Safety/S7B/Step4/S7B_Guideline.pdf. International Conference on Harmonization. (2005). Accessed 8–5–2013.

[6]  ICH Expert Working Group. "The clinical evaluation of QT/QTc interval prolongation and proarrhythmic potential for non–antiarrhythmic drugs E14", http://www.ich.org/fileadmin/Public_ Web_Site/ICH_Products/Guidelines/Efficacy/E14/E14_Guideline.pdf. International Conference on Harmonization. (2005).

[7]  Dmitrienko, A., Sides, G., Winters, K. *et al.* (2005) Electrocardiogram reference ranges derived from a standardized clinical trial population. *Drug Information Journal*, **39**, 395–406.

[8] Shah, R.R. (2002) Drug–induced prolongation of the QT interval: regulatory dilemmas and implications for approval and labelling of a new chemical entity. *Fundamental & Clinical Pharmacology*, **16**, 147–156.

[9] Garnett, C., Zhu, H., Malik, M. *et al.* (2012) Methodologies to characterize the QT/corrected QT interval in the presences of drug–induced heart rate changes or other autonomic effects. *American Heart Journal*, **163**, 912–930.

[10] Piccini, J.P., Whellan, D.J., Berridge, B.R. *et al.* (2009) Current challenges in the evaluation of cardiac safety during drug development: Translational medicine meets the Critical Path Initiative. *American Heart Journal*, **158**, 317–326.

[11] Park, E., Willard, J., Bi, D. *et al.* (2013) The impact of drug–related QT prolongation on FDA regulatory decisions. *International Journal of Cardiology*, **168**, 4975–4976.

[12] Darpo, B., Garnett, C., Benson, C.T. *et al.* (2014) Cardiac Safety Research Consortium: Can the thorough QT/QTc study be replaced by early QT assessment in routine clinical pharmacology studies? Scientific update and a research proposal for a path forward. *American Heart Journal*, **168**, 262–272.

[13] Kleiman, R.B., Shah, R.R. and Morganroth, J.A. (2014) Replacing the thorough QT study: reflections of a baby in the bath water. *British Journal of Clinical Pharmacology*, **78**, 195–201.

[14] Fossa, A.A., Zhou, M., Brennan, N. *et al.* (2014) Use of continuous ECG for improvements in assessing the standing response as a positive control for QT prolongation. *Annals of Noninvasive Electrocardiology*, **19**, 82–89.

[15] Garnett, C.E., Beasley, N., Bhattaram, V.A. *et al.* (2008) Concentration–QT relationships play a key role in the evaluation of proarrhythmic risk during regulatory review. *Journal of Clinical Pharmacology*, **48**, 13–18.

[16] Morganroth, J.A. (2004) A definitive or thorough phase 1 QT ECG trial as a requirement fo drug safety assessment. *Journal of Electrocardiology*, **37**, 25–29.

[17] Bloomfield, D.M., Krishna, R., Hreniuk, D. *et al.* (2009) A thorough QTc study to assess the effect of sitagliptin, a DPP4 inhibitor, on ventricular repolarization in health subjects. *Journal of Clinical Pharmacology*, **49**, 937–946.

[18] Ring, A., Port, A., Graefe–Mody, E.U. *et al.* (2011) The DPP–4 inhibitor linagliptin does not prolong the QT interval at therapeutic and supratherapeutic doses. *Journal of Clinical Pharmacology*, **72**, 39–50.

[19] Koenen–Bergmann, M., Revollo, I., Ring, A. and Haertter, S. (2009) Pramipexole does not prolong the QTc interval. *European Journal of Neurology*, **16**, 538.

[20] Sarapa, N., Nickens, D.J., Raber, S.R. *et al.* (2008) Ritonavir 100mg does not cause QTc prolongation in healthy subjects: A possible role as CYP3A inhibitor in thorough QTc studies. *Clinical Pharmacology & Therapeutics*, **83**, 153.

[21] Huettner, S., Ring, A., Sabo, J. P., Hoesl, C. E., Ballow, C., Roszko, P., Macgregor, T. R., and Robinson, P. "no significant ECG effects are observed with therapeutic and supra–therapeutic doses of tipranavir coadministered with ritonavir (TPV/r)", *47th Interscience Conference on Antimicrobial Agents and Chemotherapy, Chicago.*, A1422–(2007).

[22] Zhang, X., Jordan, P., Cristea, L. *et al.* (2012) Thorough QT/QTc study of ritonavir–boosted saquinavir following multiple–dose administration of therapeutic and supratherapeutic doses in healthy participants. *Journal of Clinical Pharmacology*, **52**, 520–529.

[23] Mok, N.S., Lo, Y.K., Tsui, P.T. and Lam, C.W. (2005) Ketoconazole induced torsades de pointes without concomitant use of QT interval–prolonging drug. *Journal of Cardiovascular Electrophysiology*, **16**, 1375–1377.

[24] Boyce, M.J., Baisley, K.J. and Warrington, S.J. (2012) Phamacokinetic interaction between domperidone and ketoconazole leads to QT prolongation in healthy volunteers: a randomized,

placebo–controlled double–blind, crossover study. *British Journal of Clinical Pharmacology*, **73**, 411–421.

[25] South African Medicines Control Council (2006) Interaction between ketoconazole and domperidone and the risk of QT prolongation – important safety information. *South African Medical Journal*, **96**, 596.

[26] Glomb, P. and Ring, A. "Use of baseline ECGs in the evaluation of thorough QT studies with crossover design.", http://www.biopharmnet.com/doc/2008_04_15_poster.pdf. Biopharmnet. (2008).

[27] Zhang, X., Silkey, M., Schumacher, M. *et al.* (2009) Period correction of the QTc of moxifloxacin with multiple predose baseline ECGs is the least variable of 4 methods tested. *Journal of Clinical Pharmacology*, **49**, 534–539.

[28] Tian, H., Qiao, W. and Natarajan, J. (2010) A comparison of several methods for analyzing data from thorough QT studies. *Journal of Biopharmaceutical Statistics*, **20**, 632–640.

[29] Tsong, Y. and Zhang, J.N. (2010) Further Discussion on the Design and Analysis of Thorough QTc Clinical Trials: Guest Editors' Notes. *Journal of Biopharmaceutical Statistics*, **20**, 493–496.

[30] Eaton, M.L., Muirhead, R.J., Mancuso, J.Y. and Lolluri, S. (2005) A confidence interval for the maximal mean QT interval change due to drug effect. *Drug Information Journal*, **40**, 267–271.

[31] Anand, S.P., Murray, S.C. and Koch, G.G. (2010) Sample size calculations for crossover thorough QT studies: satisfaction of regulatory threshold and assay sensitivity. *Journal of Biopharmaceutical Statistics*, **20**, 587–603.

[32] Hosmane, B., Locke, C. and Chiu, Y.L. (2010) Sample size and power estimation in "thorough" QT/QTc studies with parallel group design. *J Biopharm Stat*, **20**, 578–586.

[33] Meng, Z., Kringle, R., Chen, X. and Zhao, P.L. (2010) Sample size calculation for thorough QT/QTc study considering various factors related to multiple time points. *Journal of Biopharmaceutical Statistics*, **20**, 563–577.

[34] Natekar, M., Hingorani, P., Gupta, P. *et al.* (2011) Effect of number of replicate electrocardiograms recorded at each time point in a thorough QT study on sample size and study cost. *Journal of Clinical Pharmacology*, **51**, 908–914.

[35] Julious, S.A. (2012) Seven useful designs. *Pharmaceutical Statistics*, **11**, 24–31.

[36] Ring, A., Brand, T., Macha, S., Breithaupt–Groegler, K., Simons, G., Walter, B., Woerle, H. J., and Broedl, U. C. "The sodium glucose cotransporter 2 inhibitor empagliflozin does not prolong QT interval in a thorough QT study (Submitted for publication)", (2013).

[37] Ring, A., Walter, B., Larbalestier, A., and Chanter, D. "An efficient crossover design for thorough QT studies", *GMS Med.Inf.Biom.Epidemiol.*, **6**(*1*): Doc 06, 1–12 (2010).

[38] Bello, C.L., Mulay, M., Huang, X. *et al.* (2009) Electrocardiographic characterization of the QTc interval in patients with advanced solid tumors: pharmacokinetic–pharmacodynamic evaluation of sunitinib. *Clinical Cancer Research*, **15**, 7045–7052.

[39] Kitagawa, K., Kawada, K., Morita, S. *et al.* (2012) Prospective evaluation of corrected QT intervals and arrhythmias after exposure to epirubicin, cyclophasphamide, and 5–fluorouracil in women with breast cancer. *Annals of Oncology*, **23**, 743–747.

[40] Yavas, O., Yazici, M., Eren, O. *et al.* (2008) The acute effect of tropisetron on ECG parameters in cancer patients. *Support Care Cancer*, **16**, 1011–1015.

[41] Morganroth, J.A., Shah, R.R. and Scott, J.W. (2010) Evaluation and management of cardiac safety using the electrocardiogram in oncology clinical trials: focus on cardiac repolarization (QTc interval). *Clinical Pharmacology & Therapeutics*, **87**, 166–174.

[42] Smith, L.H. (2012) Toursade de pointes, prolonged QT intervals, and patients with cancer. *Clinical Journal of Oncologic Nursing*, **16**, 125–128.

[43] Thornton, K., Kim, G., Maher, V.E. *et al.* (2012) Vandetanib for the Treatment of Symptomatic or Progressive Medullary Thyroid Cancer in Patients with Unresectable Locally Advanced or Metastatic Disease: U.S. Food and Drug Administration Drug Approval Summary. *Clinical Cancer Research*, **18**, 3722–3730.

[44] Ring, A. (2010) Statistical models for the heart rate correction of the QT interval. *Statistics in Medicine*, **29**, 786–796.

[45] Malik, M., Frbom, P., Batchvarov, V. *et al.* (2002) Relation between QT and RR intervals is highly individual among healthy subjects: implications for heart rate correction of the QT interval. *Heart*, **87**, 220–228.

[46] Li, L., Desai, M., Desta, Z. and Flockhart, D. (2004) QT analysis: a complex answer to a "simple" problem. *Statistics in Medicine*, **23**, 2625–2643.

[47] Dmitrienko, A. and Smith, B. (2003) Repeated–measures models in the analysis of QT intervals. *Pharmaceutical Statistics*, **2**, 175–190.

[48] Shah, A. and Hajian, G. (2003) A maximum likelihood approach for estimating the QT correction factor using mixed effects model. *Statistics in Medicine*, **22**, 1901–1909.

[49] Malik, M., Hnatkova, K. and Batchvarov, V. (2004) Differences between study–specific and subject–specific heart rate corrections of the QT interval in investigations of drug induced QTc prolongation. *Pacing and Clinical Electrophysiology*, **27**, 791–800.

[50] Fridericia, L.S. (1920) Die systelendauer im elektrokardiogramm bei normalen menschen und bei herzkranken. Teil I: Beziehung swischen der pulsfrequenz und der dauer des ventrikelektrokardiogramms bei nermalen menschen in der ruhe. *Acta Medica Scandinavica*, **53**, 469–486.

[51] Bazett, J.C. (1920) An analysis of time relations of electrocardiograms. *Heart*, **7**, 353–367.

[52] Sagie, A., Larson, M.G., Goldberg, R.J. *et al.* (1992) An improved method for adjusting the QT interval for heart rate (the Framingham Heart Study). *American Journal of Cardiology*, **70**, 797–801.

[53] Patterson, S., Agin, M.A., Anziano, R. *et al.* (2005) Investigating drug–induced QT and QTc prolongation in the clinic: A review of statistical design and analysis considerations. *Drug Information Journal*, **39**, 243–266.

[54] Schall, R. and Ring, A. (2010) Statistical characterization of QT prolongation. *Journal of Biopharmaceutical Statistics*, **20**, 543–562.

[55] Senn, S. and Julious, S. (2009) Measurement in clinical trials: a neglected issue for statisticians? *Statistics in Medicine*, **28**, 3189–3225.

[56] Schall, R. and Ring, A. (2011) Mixed models for data from thorough QT studies: Part 1. Assessment of marginal QT prolongation. *Pharmaceutical Statistics*, **10**, 265–276.

[57] Jones, B. and Kenward, M.G. (2003) *Design and Analysis of Cross–Over Trials*, 2th *edition* edn, Chapman and Hall/CRC Press, London.

[58] SAS Institute (2010) *SAS/STAT 9.22 User's Guide*, SAS Institute, Cary, NC.

[59] Schall, R. (2011) Mixed models for data from thorough QT trials: Part 2. One–step assessment of conditional QT prolongation. *Pharmaceutical Statistics*, **10**, 301.

[60] Brown, H. and Prescott, R. (2006) *Applied Mixed Models in Medicine*, 2th *edition* edn, Wiley, Hoboken.

[61] Li, W., Maes, A., Quinlan, M. and Anand, S. (2013) Interdependence of baseline correction method and covariance structure for crossover TQT studies. *Journal of Biopharmaceutical Statistics*, **23**, 82–87.

[62] Matz, J., Graff, C., Vainio, P.J. *et al.* (2011) Effect of nalmefene 20 and 80 mg on the corrected QT interval and T–wave morphology. *Clinical Drug Investigation*, **31**, 799–811.

[63] Serra, D.B., Affrime, M.B., Bedigian, M.P. *et al.* (2005) QT and QTc interval with standard and

supratherapeutic doses of darifenacin, a muscarinic M3 selective receptor antagonist for the treatment of overactive bladder. *Journal of Clinical Pharmacology*, **45**, 1038–1047.

[64] Malhotra, B.K., Glue, P., Seeney, K. *et al.* (2007) Thorough QT study with recommended and supratherapeutic doses of tolterodine. *Clinical Pharmacology & Therapeutics*, **81**, 377–385.

[65] FDA. "Diabetes mellitus evaluating cardiovascular risk in new antidiabetic therapies to treat Type 2 diabetes: Guidance for industry", http://www.fda.gov/downloads/Drugs/Guidance ComplianceRegulatoryInformation/Guidances/ucm071627.pdf. Food and Drug Administration. (2008).

[66] Fleming, A. (1999) FDA approach to the reguation of drugs for diabetes. *American Heart Journal*, **138**, S338–S345.

[67] Stratton, I.M., Adler, A.I., Neil, H.A. *et al.* (2000) Association of glycaemia with macrovascular and microvascular complications of type 2 diabetes (UKPDS 35): prospective observational study. *British Medical Journal*, **321**, 405–412.

[68] Nissen, S.E. and Wolski, K. (2007) Effect of rosiglitazone on the risk of myocardial infarction and death from cardiovascular causes. *New England Journal of Medicine*, **356**, 2457–2471.

[69] Home, P.D., Pocock, S.J., Beck–Nielsen, H. *et al.* (2007) Rosiglitazone evaluated for cardiovascular outcomes – an interim analysis. *New England Journal of Medicine*, **357**, 28–38.

[70] Home, P.D., Pocock, S.J., Beck–Nielsen, H. *et al.* (2009) Rosiglitazone evaluated for cardiovascular outcomes in oral agent combinathion therapy for Type 2 diabetes (RECORD). *Lancet*, **373**, 2125–2135.

[71] Zannad, F., Stough, W.G., Pocock, S.J. *et al.* (2012) Diabetes clinical trials: helped or hindered by the current shift in regulatory requirements? *European Heart Journal*, **33**, 1049–1057.

[72] Johansen, O.E., Neubacher, D., von Eynatten, M. *et al.* (2012) Cardiovascular safety with linagliptin in patients with type 2 diabetes: a pre–specified, prospective, and adjudicated meta–analysis from a aloarge phase III program. *Cardiovascular Diabetology*, **11**, 3.

[73] Scirica, B.M., Bhatt, D.L., Braunwald, E. *et al.* (2013) Saxagliptin and cardiovascular outcomes in patients with Type 2 diabetes mellitus. *New England Journal of Medicine*, **369**, 1317–1326.

[74] Bethel, M.A. and Sourij, H. (2012) Impact of FDA guidance for developing diabetes drugs on trial design: from policy to practice. *Current Cardiology Reports*, **14**, 59–69.

[75] Viereck, C. and Boundes, P. (2011) An analysis of the impact of FDA's guidelines for addressing cardiovascular risk of drugs for type 2 diabetes. *Contemporary Clinical Trials*, **32**, 324–332.

[76] Venet, D., Doffange, E., Burzykowski, T. *et al.* (2012) A statistical approach to central monitoring of data quality in clinical trials. *Clinical Trials*, **9**, 205–213.

[77] ACCORD Study Group (2010) Effects of intensive blood–pressure control in Type 2 diabetes mellitus. *New England Journal of Medicine*, **362**, 1575–1585.

[78] ICH Expert Working Group. "Biomarkers related to drug or biotechnology product development: Context, structure and format of qualification submissions E16", http://www.ich.org/fileadmin /Public_Web_Site/ICH_Products/Guidelines/Efficacy/E16/Step4/E16_Step_4.pdf. International Conference on Harmonization. (2010).

# 9

# Hepatotoxicity

## Donald C. Trost

*Director, Intelligent Systems, Ativa Medical, 1000 Westgate Drive, Suite 100, St Paul, MN, 55114 USA*

## 9.1  Introduction

The liver plays a central role in metabolism. Knowing how the liver works and which observable effects are normal, which are pathological, which are pharmacological, and which signal potential liver toxicity is essential for understanding the effects of pharmacologically active compounds on the liver and for providing effective, informative, and useful statistical analyses. This chapter focuses on the harmful pharmacological effects, referred to collectively as drug-induced liver injury (DILI). Most of the observable effects are not specific to a particular lesion, at least individually, necessitating both multivariate and longitudinal approaches.

Section 9.2 discusses the liver from both the organ level and the cellular level. There is a brief review of the major diseases of the liver and how they impact the primary liver tests. These diseases may mimic DILI and need to be understood in the pharmaceutical context. Some of the key features for each blood analyte are included.

Section 9.3 focuses on DILI. It reviews the literature and describes the toxicological effects that drugs have on the liver. This is followed by a review of the US Food and Drug Administration (FDA) guidance on the pre-marketing clinical evaluation of DILI and other clinical trial issues.

Classical statistical approaches to the detection of DILI in clinical trial data are presented in Section 9.4. These cover some probability distribution issues along with several methods for constructing reference limits, which are needed for detecting the DILI signal. Statisticians

*Statistical Methods for Evaluating Safety in Medical Product Development*, First Edition.
Edited by A. Lawrence Gould.
© 2015 John Wiley & Sons, Ltd. Published 2015 by John Wiley & Sons, Ltd.

reading this chapter are expected to have a solid background in descriptive statistics and graphical displays of laboratory data. Therefore, these topics are not covered.

Some relatively new ideas are presented in Section 9.5. These are based on the use of stochastic process models to describe the dynamic (longitudinal) changes that occur when DILI exists in the study subject. These models are not fully developed and good software is not commonly available. Mixed-effect models are used for illustration.

Efficacy may be population-based, but safety should be patient-based. This chapter tries to illuminate some of the statistical problems related to the evaluation of DILI in drug clinical trials and points the reader in several directions where good solutions may exist. The idea of individualized reference limits or models of disease is relatively foreign to both the medical and statistical establishments. It is hoped this chapter will stimulate some new thinking in this direction.

## 9.2    Liver biology and chemistry

### 9.2.1    Liver function

#### 9.2.1.1    Organ level

The liver is the primary detoxifying organ and thus a major location of drug metabolism. It weighs about 1500 g, or about 2.5% of body weight. It is the primary organ of waste excretion along with the kidney. Blood flows through the liver from the portal vein ($\sim$70%) and the hepatic artery ($\sim$30%). The portal vein, hepatic artery, and intrahepatic bile duct run in parallel throughout the liver, branching about 20 times [1]. The portal vein is a direct connection between the intestine and the liver. All oral compounds enter the liver through this "first pass" route. Any compound that is not metabolized in the first pass circulates through the body and re-enters the liver via the hepatic artery as well.

The liver also is an engine for converting digested nutrients into usable molecules:

- Carbohydrates are converted to energy, the excess carbohydrates are converted to glycogen for storage and converted back when energy is needed, and excess glycogen is converted to fat.

- Amino acids are converted to proteins, and excess amino acids are converted to carbohydrates.

- Triglycerides are converted to carbohydrates, and excess triglycerides are converted to fat.

- Amino acids and nucleic acids are converted to urea and excreted in the bile.

The commonly measured liver enzymes are significant facilitators of nutrient metabolism. Drugs can interfere with many of these metabolic steps.

At the organ level, the liver can be viewed as three connected systems: the hepatocyte (liver cell), the biliary tract, and the reticuloendothelial system [2]. The hepatocyte is where the fundamental biochemical processes occur. The liver synthesizes over 90% of all proteins in the body and 100% of some proteins such as albumin and coagulation factors. The primary function of the biliary tract is the excretion of bilirubin, a metabolic product of hemoglobin. The reticuloendothelial system conjugates bilirubin which is not water soluble with a molecule that makes it water soluble. The conjugated bilirubin is then excreted in the bile.

The liver has a strong regenerative capability. Some 80% of the liver has to be destroyed before the liver cannot regenerate itself. This is why most patients recover from DILI. When the liver function is severely diminished, the levels of all liver-related analytes will generally be normal or low.

### 9.2.1.2 Cellular level

The primary liver cell is the hepatocyte [2]. It contains some important enzymes such as aspartate aminotransferase (AST), alanine aminotransferase (ALT), lactate dehydrogenase (LD), alkaline phosphatase (ALP), and γ-glutamyl transferase (GGT) that are used to assess DILI. AST and ALT are involved in the conversion reactions of amino acids and require the cofactor pyridoxal phosphate (vitamin $B_6$). ALT has two known isoenzymes, ALT1 and ALT2 [3]. ALT1 is found in the liver, while ALT2 is not. LD catalyzes the interconversion of lactate and pyruvate, an important step in the glycolysis (carbohydrate) pathway. It has five known isoenzymes, $LD_1$–$LD_5$. Only $LD_5$ is found in the liver. Typically, in drug studies only the total LD is measured, if at all. ALP is found in several tissues. Its function is somewhat ubiquitous and ill defined. It has at least four distinct isoenzymes found in bone, the biliary tract, the intestine, and the placenta. Usually total ALP is measured to assess biliary function. Only if bone and liver ALP origins need to be distinguished are the isoenzymes measured. GGT regulates the transport of amino acids across cell membranes, and is sometimes used to determine if ALP elevations are due to liver or bone since they tend to rise together. However, GGT is very sensitive to various liver insults such as alcohol consumption and considered by many to be uninformative because of its lack of specificity. Preliminary results in the analysis of DILI suggest that GGT may contain more information, and possibly more specificity, when analyzed multivariately [4]. Several other enzymes may be useful in DILI but are not generally available for clinical trial use.

As stated above, most of the proteins in the body are made in the liver. Typically total protein (the sum of albumin and globulin) and albumin are measured in the serum for drug safety monitoring. Globulin is hard to measure and is generally obtained by subtraction. The coagulation proteins are assessed by measuring how fast the blood clots via the international normalized ratio (INR), formerly prothrombin time (PT).

Hemoglobin is mostly metabolized to bilirubin outside the liver and transported in the blood to the liver attached to albumin. The unconjugated bilirubin enters the hepatocyte via passive diffusion and active transport. It then attaches to the smooth endoplasmic reticulum where it is conjugated (made water soluble). From there it is transported to the cell membrane on edge of the hepatocyte that is connected to the bile canaliculus where it enters the bile. The bile passes into the intestine where bacteria break it down further to urobilinogen and urobilin, which can be reabsorbed into the blood or excreted in the feces. Total bilirubin in the serum is the sum of the unconjugated and conjugated bilirubin. The total and conjugated forms can be measured directly. The conjugated bilirubin is sometimes called direct bilirubin. The unconjugated bilirubin value is obtained by subtraction, or indirectly. The unconjugated bilirubin is sometimes called indirect bilirubin.

Secondary liver cells include Kupffer cells and hepatic stellate cells, which are part of the reticuloendothelial system. Kupffer cells are specialized macrophages. These cells are important in homeostasis and the modulation of acute liver injury and chronic liver responses to injury [5]. Hepatic stellate cells are located between the hepatocyte and sinusoidal epithelial cells. In normal conditions, they are inactive and store vitamin A [6]. When the liver is injured, they become an engine of fibrosis.

## 9.2.2    Liver pathology

### 9.2.2.1    Pathology terminology

Medical literature and clinical discussions are full of technical pathology terms that are seldom defined or explained to those not clinically trained. Some key terms that are relevant to drug safety are the following:

- Apoptosis – a normal process of biologically programmed single-cell death.

- Cholestasis – a stoppage of the flow of bile.

- Fibrosis – the formation of collagen fibers in the tissue.

- Hepatitis – inflammation of the liver.

- Idiosyncratic – an abnormality that is peculiar to an individual person. In common usage, it really means "unpredictable."

- Inflammation – a complicated local reaction of tissue to injury involving the vasodilation, vascular congestion, movement of plasma and white blood cells into the tissue, and the release of signaling proteins. An inflammatory process is usually labeled with the "-itis" suffix.

- Lesion – any pathological or traumatic loss of form or function.

- Necrosis – the abnormal death of groups of cells.

- Steatosis – the fatty degeneration of tissue.

Occasionally these terms are misused and can be confusing to those trying to understand the biology. For example, and especially in drug safety, the term "idiosyncratic" tends to be used by clinicians whenever the cause is unknown. The implication is that no pattern is discoverable; therefore, no attempt to find a pattern should be pursued. A statistician should assume that a pattern exists but has not been discovered, rather than it being a one-of-a-kind reaction (implied by the term) that is not amenable to statistical analysis. True idiosyncratic drug reactions may exist, but should not be assumed without some analytical proof.

### 9.2.2.2    Infectious and inflammatory diseases

Acute viral hepatitis [7] is a viral infection that causes acute liver necrosis and inflammation. Its incubation period is days to weeks, potentially confounding a DILI reaction. AST and ALT are elevated as high as $10 \times$ ULN (upper limit of normal). ALP, INR, total and direct bilirubin may be elevated as well. Viral antibodies, antigens, RNA, and DNA are measured to confirm or rule out the diagnosis. There are at least five known viral diseases (A, B, etc.) in this category.

Chronic hepatitis [8] is defined by chronic liver necrosis and inflammation from various causes including viral hepatitis, autoimmunity, alcohol abuse, and metabolic disorders. AST and ALT are elevated 2–5 × ULN in the inactive form and elevated 10–25 × ULN in the active form. ALP and GGT are usually elevated. Total and direct bilirubin and INR are usually normal. Serum immunoglobulins may be slightly elevated. Viral antibodies, antigens, RNA, and DNA are measured to confirm or rule out the diagnosis. A liver biopsy is usually required to confirm or rule out the diagnosis and to assess the severity of the disease.

Autoimmune hepatitis [8] is caused by the immune system attacking the liver. The liver test findings are similar to those of chronic hepatitis except that the serum immunoglobulins may be very elevated. Investigation of this disorder requires the use of various antibody tests such as antinuclear antibody (ANA). A liver biopsy may be required.

### 9.2.2.3   Neoplastic and other space occupying lesions (liver masses)

Many space-occupying lesions can be found in the liver. These include malignant lesions such as metastatic cancer, lymphoma, hepatocellular carcinoma, cholangiocarcinoma, and angiosarcoma. Other lesions include hemangiomas, adenomas, cysts, abscesses, granulomas, and focal nodular hyperplasia. Isolated elevations in ALP and LD are associated with mass lesions [9, 10].

### 9.2.2.4   Inherited and metabolic disorders

Hereditary hemochromatosis is an inherited disorder of iron metabolism where iron accumulates in the body, especially in the liver and pancreas [1]. It is the most common inherited liver disorder [11]. Liver enzymes are elevated in about 25% of cases [12]. Serum iron, transferrin saturation, and ferritin are typically increased. A liver biopsy is required to evaluate the extent of liver damage.

The disease $\alpha_1$-antitripsin deficiency is present in about 1 in 2000 live births [11, 13]. It can cause organ damage at any age, primarily the liver and the lungs. Liver signs show up as early as about 1 month of age as persistent jaundice and mild to moderate conjugated bilirubin and aminotransferase elevations. All stages of liver disease can be found at this age, including fulminant liver failure (very rapid liver failure following symptom emergence). In adults, the disease can show up as chronic hepatitis, cryptogenic cirrhosis, and hepatocellular carcinoma. The diagnosis is established by a low serum $\alpha_1$-antitrypsin level and phenotyping by isoelectric focusing or electrophoresis. Liver biopsy is used to determine the degree of fibrosis.

Wilson disease (also called Wilson's disease and hepatolenticular degeneration) is an inherited disorder where copper accumulates in the liver [11]. This disease may show up as elevated aminotransferases in asymptomatic patients, but many other clinical signs are usually present as well. Diagnosis is confirmed by a low serum ceruloplasmin level and a high 24-hour urine copper excretion. Without treatment the patient's liver disease progresses to liver failure. A biopsy is usually not required.

Non-alcoholic fatty liver disease (NAFLD) is commonly seen in obese, diabetic, and hyperlipidemic non-alcoholic patients [11]. It can progress to non-alcoholic steatohepatitis (NASH) and cirrhosis. Liver enzymes levels are generally elevated, which is usually an incidental finding. The diagnosis is made by history and exclusion of other liver diseases. A biopsy is required for a definitive diagnosis.

Porphyria is a group of diseases caused by defects in heme synthesis some of which involve the liver [11]. Liver involvement usually shows up as asymptomatic liver enzyme elevations. The clinical presentation and various tests are required to establish the diagnosis of a specific porphyria.

Lipid storage disease is a variety of diseases where lipid accumulates in the tissues [11]. These diseases include Gaucher's disease, Niemann–Pick disease, abetalipoproteinemia, Fabry's disease, Tangier disease, and types 1 and 5 hyperlipoproteinemia. Liver enzymes may be elevated when there is liver involvement. A biopsy is required to make the diagnosis.

Amyloidosis is a systemic disease of amyloid accumulation in various organs and commonly involves the liver [11, 14]. Mildly elevated liver enzyme levels may be seen, ALP and INR in particular. Serum albumin may be decreased with kidney involvement. Elevated bilirubin is an ominous sign. A biopsy is required to identify the presence of tissue amyloid.

### 9.2.2.5  Systemic disorders

Many other systemic diseases can affect the liver [15]. Inflammatory bowel disease (IBD) may extend to the biliary tree, causing sclerosing cholangitis. Elevated ALP or GGT may be the first sign. IBD can also lead to autoimmune hepatitis, drug toxicity, malnutrition and metabolic disturbances, systemic infections, hypercoagulability, and sequelae involving the liver. Liver injury can be caused by heart disease such as congestive heart failure, congenital heart disease, and acute ischemic shock. Any of the liver tests can be affected due to passive congestion in the liver or reduced cardiac output. Sickle cell disease involves the liver in about 10% of cases. Sickle cell crisis can mimic viral hepatitis, acute cholecystitis, or choledocholithiasis and can have markedly elevated bilirubin and ALP. Infrequently, sickle cell disease manifests intrahepatic cholestasis that can progress to liver failure.

### 9.2.2.6  Biliary tract disease

The primary pathology of the biliary tract related to DILI is cholestasis. Cholestasis can be either intrahepatic (inside the liver) or extrahepatic (outside the liver). DILI includes only intrahepatic cholestasis [16]. Bile acts as a detergent to solubilize dietary lipids. Cholestasis can lead to the fecal excretion of excess non-absorbed fat. In the longer term, this can lead a deficiency of fat-soluble vitamins. Cholestasis leads to significantly elevated ALP and GGT but normal or slightly elevated aminotransferases. Bilirubin may not be elevated until late stages of cholestasis. Other causes of cholestasis include gallstones, cancer, pancreatic disease, intrinsic biliary tract disease, cysts, parasites, AIDS, lymph node enlargement, viral and alcoholic hepatitis, and congenital anomalies.

### 9.2.2.7  Fibrosis, cirrhosis, and end-stage liver disease

Liver fibrosis occurs when the hepatic stellate cells are activated [6]. In the process, they lose their vitamin A, convert into contractile myofibroblasts, and secrete collagen, proteoglycans, and glycoproteins to form a wall between the hepatocyte and the plasma. Laboratory tests may show a low platelet count, AST/ALT > 1, elevated serum bilirubin, decreased serum albumin, increased INR, elevated α-fetoprotein, and the presence of rheumatoid factor or high-serum globulins. Ultrasound should be used to rule out liver masses [8].

Cirrhosis is the end stage of any chronic liver disease characterized by diffuse fibrosis and a nodular architecture [6]. The most common causes are chronic hepatitis C, alcoholic liver disease, NAFLD, and chronic hepatitis B. Cholestatic, autoimmune, and metabolic diseases also contribute to the list. Cirrhosis can be compensated or decompensated. Compensated cirrhosis can be mostly asymptomatic and diagnosed inadvertently in up to one third of cases. The laboratory blood tests may include any combination of high bilirubin, high AST, high GGT, low albumin, low platelets (most sensitive), and high INR. A liver biopsy may be required to confirm the diagnosis. A patient with decompensated cirrhosis manifests ascites, variceal bleeding, hepatic encephalopathy, or jaundice.

#### 9.2.2.8    Acute liver failure

Acute liver failure (ALF) is defined as a coagulation abnormality (e.g., INR > 1.5) and any mental alteration in an illness with less than 26 weeks' duration [17]. The American Association for the Study of Liver Diseases (AASLD) recommends that any patient with moderate to severe acute hepatitis have an immediate INR and mental evaluation. Once ALF is established, immediate hospitalization is mandatory, and intensive care is preferred along with planning for a liver transplantation.

The criteria for liver transplantation can shed some light on which factors are important for identifying potentially fatal DILI. The King's College Criteria for Liver Transplantation [18, 19] for patients with ALF are as follows: with acetaminophen, either blood pH < 7.30 or (INR > 6.5 and serum creatinine > 3.4 mf/dL); without acetaminophen, either INR > 6.5 or any three of the following:

- Age under 10 years or over 40 years

- A probable cause of non-A, non-B hepatitis, halothane hepatitis, or idiosyncratic drug reaction

- Onset of jaundice more than 7 days prior to the onset of encephalopathy

- INR > 3.5

- Serum bilirubin > 17.6 mg/dL.

## 9.2.3    Clinical laboratory tests for liver status

### 9.2.3.1    Sampling sources

The most common hepatic source for analytical samples is the venous blood using a needle [10, 20]. This obviously requires the liver substances to flow into or out of the bloodstream via normal physiological processes or the liver cell membranes have to be damaged enough to leak the substances into the blood space. The blood provides three primary types of samples:

Whole blood = plasma + red cells + white cells + platelets + other cells
Plasma = serum + coagulation proteins
Serum = water + organic compounds + inorganic compounds.

Serum is the most common biological sample for chemistry analysis. It is obtained by letting the blood clot, which takes several minutes, and separating the fluid from the solid material. For plasma, the sample tube contains an anticoagulant that prevents the clotting process, and the fluid is separated from the cells using a centrifuge. Whole blood is the most common sample for hematology analysis. It is mixed with an anticoagulant and used as is or stained for microscopic or automated examination of the cells. Some chemistry analytes are equivalent among serum, plasma, and whole blood, some are approximately equivalent, and some are definitely not equivalent. Any statistical analysis must consider the exchangeability of these tests and the analytical laboratory methods should be clearly defined in the study protocol if they are not exchangeable.

Urine is sometimes used to detect liver abnormalities. It is the easiest sample to obtain and least invasive, but also the least useful. For DILI, urine should not be used in clinical studies where blood is being drawn anyway.

A biopsy of the liver can be very specific if the lesion is microscopically visible and not just biochemical in nature. A biopsy is the hardest sample to obtain. It is highly invasive, expensive, and potentially life-threatening. It could be useful to have the biopsy sample in DILI cases but this is generally impractical and can be unethical. Also if the lesion is localized, a biopsy may miss it completely.

### 9.2.3.2 Serum enzymes

Liver enzymes are sometimes referred to as "liver function tests," but they do not measure liver function [21, 22]. An enzyme is a protein that catalyzes a biochemical reaction. Unlike other clinical chemistry measurements, enzyme analysis results are based on kinetic tests. This means that the measurement is the speed of the chemical reaction, not the enzyme concentration. In most normal cases, the rate of change in the concentration of some reaction product is proportional to the concentration of the enzyme:

$$\frac{d[\text{product}]}{dt} = k[\text{enzyme}]$$

where [A] usually, but not always, means "concentration of A." The reaction product can be several coupled reactions away from the enzyme-catalyzed reaction, introducing potentially magnifying error effects. Enzyme kinetics (activity) can be affected by several extraneous variables. These include temperature, pH, conformation, mixture of isoenzymes, and the presence of interfering substances. One example is that vitamin $B_6$ is required as a cofactor for aminotransferase catalyzed reactions. If the laboratory procedure does not add vitamin $B_6$ to the assay, a subject with a low vitamin $B_6$ level will have a aminotransferase activity that is lower than it should be, causing enzyme elevations to be missed. Another common example relevant to international drug trials is that many laboratories, especially those outside the United States, use a reaction temperature of 30°C rather than 37°C. This can make data pooling among laboratories quite challenging, but this source of variability can be controlled by specifying the enzymatic methods to be used or choosing laboratories that use the same analytical procedures.

For the evaluation of liver damage in drug safety, it is the concentration of enzyme in the blood that is important, not its activity. Therefore the assumption of proportionality between activity and concentration is critical. Liver enzymes get into the blood primarily by leakage from the liver cells. Elevations of these enzymes over normal, or homeostatic, levels in the blood occur when the liver cell membranes become leakier because of cell damage or death or when the enzyme is induced to higher concentrations in the liver cells by metabolic processes.

Selected liver-related enzyme properties and stability requirements are as follows [21, 23]:

- AST (aspartate aminotransferase, aspartate transaminase, glutamate oxaloacetate transaminase, GOT)

  — Tissue sources (in decreasing order of concentration, relative to serum) – heart (8000), liver, skeletal muscles, kidneys, pancreas, spleen, lungs, erythrocytes (15), all other cells.

  — Approximate serum half-life – 12 hours, depends on isoenzyme mixture.

— Stability – 24 hours at room temperature/ 7 days with vitamin B6 added to sample, 28 days at 4°C, over 1 year at −20°C.

— Sources of systematic measurement error – hemolysis, high-dose vitamin C, deficiency of vitamin $B_6$, extreme exercise, intramuscular injections, and obesity.

- ALT (alanine aminotransferase, alanine transaminase, glutamate pyruvate transaminase, GPT)

— Tissue sources – liver (3000), kidneys, heart, skeletal muscles, pancreas, spleen, lungs, erythrocytes (7) – in cytosol and mitochrondria.

— Approximate serum half-life – 48 hours, depends on isoenzyme mixture.

— Stability – not stable at any temperature, activity decreases with time.

— Sources of systematic measurement error – hemolysis, deficiency of vitamin B6, obesity, alcohol use.

- GGT (γ-glutamyl transferase, gamma-glutamyl transferase, glutamyl transpeptidase)

— Tissue sources – kidney, liver, pancreas, prostate – in cell membranes and microsomes.

— Approximate serum half-life – 2–4 weeks.

— Stability – 1 month at 4 °C, 1 year at −20°C.

— Sources of systematic measurement error – high-dose vitamin C, alcohol use.

- LD (lactate dehydrogenase, LDH)

— Tissue sources – liver (150 000), heart, kidney, skeletal muscle, erythrocytes (500), all other cells including tumors – in cytosol only.

— Approximate serum half-life – 48 hours, depends on isoenzyme mixture.

— Stability – store at room temperature only, do not refrigerate, or freeze.

— Sources of systematic measurement error – hemolysis, alcohol use.

- ALP (alkaline phosphatase)

— Tissue sources – intestine, kidney, bone, liver, placenta, all other cells – at or in the cell membrane.

— Approximate serum half-life – 48 hours, depends on isoenzyme mixture.

— Stability – not stable at room temperature (increases activity), 0–4°C for 2–3 days, 1 month at −25°C.

— Sources of systematic measurement error – high dose vitamin C, alcohol use.

As is evident from the properties above, elevated "liver" enzymes do not always come from the liver and normal enzymes levels in the laboratory are not always normal in the subject. It is very important to know how much time has elapsed between the sample collection and the sample analysis. This often is ignored in practice but, if drug safety is important, then knowing both the sampling time and the analysis time is very important. Much depends on how the sample is handled and what procedure is used to obtain the result. Almost all sample-related errors cause the result to be lower than it should be, thus potentially masking a safety problem.

Hemolysis is a special issue in the assessment of liver changes, especially enzymes. It means the breakage (or leakage) of erythrocytes (red blood cells), causing spurious elevations in the test results. Hemolysis can occur *in vivo* due to disease or drugs. Although not the topic of this chapter, these causes should be ruled out in any drug trial before attributing the hemolysis to something else. Obviously, the sample handling has no primary impact on these causes but may secondarily make the hemolysis worse after phlebotomy. The primary *in vitro* cause is the improper handling of a blood sample, and occasionally improper acquisition technique. The longer the erythrocytes are left in the blood fluid, the more likely they are to leak or break. For various reasons, sometimes clinical sites are not as prompt as they should be in separating the cells from the fluid. Hemolysis causes major increases in serum potassium, AST, and LD. It causes smaller increases in ALT, ALP, total protein, and albumin. It may also cause a decrease in bilirubin. Since free serum hemoglobin, which should be a good measure of cell leakage, is usually not measured, potassium is a reasonable flag for hemolysis, especially if it is outside the reference limits along with AST or LD. At present no data-driven rule is available for identifying errant laboratory results due to hemolysis, efforts at solution notwithstanding. It should be straightforward to construct a decision rule if the right training data are collected. A lot of money can be wasted chasing falsely elevated liver tests.

### 9.2.3.3   Hematologic components

The blood cells have little relevance to DILI other than the cell lysis or leakage that causes spurious results. However, the erythrocytes are the primary tissue storing hemoglobin, which is metabolized to bilirubin and eliminated by the liver [24]. About 70% of bilirubin comes from the degradation of erythrocytes, another 15% comes from the liver, and smaller amounts come from the kidneys and bone marrow [2]. Total bilirubin consists of conjugated and unconjugated fractions. Typically, the total and conjugated forms are measured directly while the unconjugated form is determined by subtraction. Elevations of total bilirubin due to DILI are from conjugated bilirubin leaking into the blood compartment.

The primary cause of sample instability for bilirubin is light exposure, which converts it into a different compound. For blood samples used for bilirubin determinations, the clinical protocol should state explicitly that the exposure to light should be minimized as much as possible. Hemolysis and lipemia can interfere with bilirubin measurement.

### 9.2.3.4   Serum proteins

The liver is the site of synthesis of most plasma proteins except immunoglobulins and protein hormones, for example, insulin [25]. Albumin is the most abundant plasma protein, approximately half of the protein mass. Its primary function is the maintenance of body fluid distribution between the intravascular space and the extravascular space via osmosis. Its second main function is the transport of compounds in the blood that are not water soluble or that have a high ionic charge. Other functions include amino acid source for peripheral tissues, antioxidant, buffering agent, regulation of capillary permeability, and mitigation of the inflammatory response.

In liver disease, albumin synthesis is not affected until over 95% of the liver function is lost. However, immune response, leakage into extravascular spaces, and inhibition of synthesis by drugs and toxins can reduce blood levels without severe loss of liver function. Other causes of low albumin levels are genetic, inflammatory, urinary, gastrointestinal, and dietary. Albumin samples are stable for 72 hours at 4°C, 6 months at −20°C, and indefinitely at −70°C. Systematic measurement error can be caused by lipemia, hemolysis, and upright posture.

Posture influences the concentration of all proteins including the enzymes. When a person lies in a horizontal position for an extended period such as sleep time, the fluid equilibrates osmotically between the intravascular space and the extravascular space. This establishes the baseline concentrations of proteins in the blood. When a person assumes an upright posture (standing or sitting), the effect of gravity comes into play and counters osmotic forces. During the waking hours, enough fluid moves from the intravascular space to the extravascular space to increase the concentration of non-permeable substances in blood by as much as 10%, that is, the denominator decreases in the concentration calculation while the numerator is constant. Thus, any blood proteins measured to assess liver status should be measured at the same time of day or analyzed with an adjustment for circadian variation.

Serum total protein is an approximation of the sum of all the proteins in the blood. It is usually proportional to the number of peptide bonds exposed on the surface of the "average" protein. If the drug or patient's conditions cause the proteins to unfold or fold more tightly, then an apparent increase or decrease in protein concentration might occur without any change in the underlying protein concentration. The frequency or significance of these protein changes is not known but should be considered when abnormal protein values are observed. The stability and systematic measurement errors for total protein are the same as those for albumin.

Globulins are usually not measured directly unless protein electrophoresis is performed. They usually are obtained by subtracting the albumin measurement from the total protein measurement. Electrophoresis and specific globulin measurements generally are not done in drug clinical trials unless needed to answer a specific question. Globulins, or the albumin–globulin ratio, if specified in the clinical protocol, should not be ordered from the lab, but calculated by the statistician, unless it can be verified that the there is no charge for providing the number. Reference values can be derived from those for total protein and albumin using the cross-correlations provided herein or elsewhere [26].

### 9.2.3.5  Coagulation

Most clotting proteins are synthesized in the liver. PT has been used traditionally to access the integrity of the extrinsic pathway of the coagulation cascade: factor VII, factor VIIa, factor X, factor Xa, factor V, factor Va, prothrombin, thrombin, fibrinogen, fibrin, polymerized fibrin. If any one of these factors is deficient, malformed, or inhibited, the PT will be prolonged [2]. The measurement of PT requires a plasma sample with citrate to block the coagulation and therefore necessitates a specific sample specimen. Historically, PT has been a highly variable measurement because the thromboplastin used in the assay had large variation in its activity, which varied from lot to lot for the same reagent manufacturer. In the 1970s, the World Health Organization created a method of standardization so that each batch of thromboplastin has a number called the international sensitivity index (ISI) associated with it that is used to adjust the PT results [27]. The adjusted value is called the international normalization ratio which has the formula

$$\mathrm{INR} = \left( \frac{\text{patient PT}}{\text{normal geometric mean PT}} \right)^{\mathrm{ISI}}.$$

PT still is the underlying fundamental measurement. It is the waiting time between the start of the coagulation reaction, trigged by laboratory procedures, and the end of clot formation.

It is stable in a sample stored for up to 2 hours at room temperature and for 4 hours at 4°C. This implies that shipping to a central laboratory may lead to an erroneous result.

Systematic measurement error can occur when hemolysis, prolonged storage, or vitamin K deficiency is present.

Although the INR has been around for about 25 years, it is not universally used. A protocol design should never specify PT when a screening test for coagulation or liver disorders is desired, but should specify INR instead. Otherwise PT cannot be statistically analyzed, even within a single laboratory, unless the INR can be calculated with ancillary information provided by the laboratory.

### 9.2.4   Other clinical manifestations of liver abnormalities

Many symptoms of liver disease are non-specific [7, 9]. These include fatigue, nausea, weakness, anorexia, and flu-like symptoms. Jaundice, dark urine, light stools, pruritus (itching), and vague right upper quadrant abdominal pain are more specific for liver disease.

Physical findings are not usually diagnostic alone but complement other diagnostic tests. Jaundice, hepatomegaly, splenomegaly, spider angiomata (small dilated arteries in the skin of the face, neck, upper arms, and upper trunk radiating from a central point like a spider web), palmar erythema, and excoriations are typical liver disease findings. Findings associated with liver failure include muscle wasting, ascites, edema, dilated abdominal veins, hepatic fetor (sweet smelling breath), asterixis (a flapping of the hand when extended), mental confusion, stupor, and coma. In males, gynecomastia (enlarged breasts), testicular atrophy, and loss of male-pattern baldness hair distribution are common, especially in alcoholics.

The end stage of liver disease is cirrhosis [6]. At first, the body compensates for the dysfunction of the liver. In the end, compensation is not possible and the patient dies. In compensated cirrhosis, decreased libido, sleep disturbances, muscle atrophy, spider angiomata, palmar erythema, and splenomegaly, and male-specific findings mentioned above may be present. A liver biopsy may be needed to confirm this diagnosis. In decompensated cirrhosis, ascites (80% of cases), gastroesophageal variceal hemorrhage, and hepatic encephalopathy (asterixis, fetor, inverted sleep pattern, forgetfulness, confusion, bizarre behavior, disorientation, lethargy, coma) may be present. A liver biopsy is generally not needed to make this diagnosis.

Some of the key risk factors for liver disease include alcohol use, medication history including over-the-counter products, herbal remedies, and birth control pills, personal habits, sexual activity, travel, exposure to high-risk persons, abuse of injectable drugs, transfusion history and other exposure to blood or blood products, occupation, and family history of liver disease [9].

## 9.3   Drug-induced liver injury

### 9.3.1   Literature review

DILI has been around since the first drugs were given to patients, but did not become a focused topic of drug safety until relatively recently [28]. Although the hepatic toxicity of various compounds has been known for many years and significant efforts have been put into pre-clinical toxicology studies routinely, there had been little effort to quantify hepatic toxicity in patients until it became a noticeable reason for regulatory withdrawal of drugs from the market. There is a long list of drugs associated with hepatic toxicity which can be found in the LiverTox database at the National Institute of Diabetes and Digestive and Kidney Diseases (NIDDK) website of the National Institutes of Health (NIH): http://www.livertox.nih.gov.

In 1997, the Acute Liver Failure Study Group was formed to collect and analyze data prospectively to help understand the etiology of ALF. In 1998, the United Kingdom limited the availability of acetaminophen (paracetamol), which was suspected to be a major contributor to the number of ALF cases in the UK, and saw a concomitant drop in hospital admissions and deaths due to ALF [29]. In 2000, at an NIH symposium on DILI, Lee described the impact of drugs, especially acetaminophen, as a cause of ALF [30]. Early results of the Study Group suggested that 36% of ALF cases were due to acetaminophen alone and another 16% were due to idiosyncratic drug reactions. This seemed to catch everyone in attendance by surprise (including this author and FDA regulators). In a formal analysis performed later, it was found that more than 50% of ALF cases could be attributed to DILI, with over 40% due to acetaminophen alone [31]. For various reasons, in spite of all this evidence, no regulatory action of significance regarding acetaminophen was taken in the US until 2011 [32].

Lee published one of the first major reviews of DILI [33]. This paper gave one of the first in-depth descriptions of the clinical aspects of DILI. Additional reviews have subsequently been published [34–38]. None have identified or significantly contributed to the quantitative methods for detecting and assessing DILI.

The Drug-Induced Liver Injury Network (DILIN), sponsored by the NIDDK, was formed in 2004 [39]. This is a prospective epidemiological study to collect data and biological samples to improve the body of knowledge related to DILI. Patients are identified by either self-referral or provider referral at the study site or surrounding area. This study includes two categories of patients: "standard DILI" (no prior known liver disease) or "liver DILI" (prior known liver disease). Liver injury at DILI onset is classified into one of three groups depending on the $R$ ratio at onset: hepatocellular ($R > 5$), cholestatic ($R < 2$), or mixed ($2 < R < 5$). The $R$ ratio is defined as the ratio of measured ALT divided by its ULN and measured ALP divided by its ULN. Other testing and inclusion–exclusion criteria are applied.

## 9.3.2    Liver toxicology

Drugs cause many types of hepatic injury [28, 40]. Both acute and chronic types of morphological injury occur. Acute conditions have a sudden onset and can last for a few months. Chronic conditions have a slow insidious onset or are an extension of an acute condition and can last for the life of the patient. Sometimes the term "subacute" is used as a condition in-between the two, but it is generally ill defined.

Acute lesions are cytotoxic (hepatocellular), cholestatic, combined cytotoxic and cholestatic, or vascular. The microanatomy of the liver can be conceptualized as a lattice of hexagonal groupings of cells with the termini of the portal vein at the edges and the beginning of the central hepatic vein in the center of each group [24, 41]. These are called liver acini or lobules. At the vertices are the portal triads – the portal vein (nutrients and drugs), the hepatic artery (oxygen and drugs), and the bile duct plus lymphatics and nerves. Blood flows from the outside inward and bile flows from the inside outward. A metabolic zone can be thought of as the triangle formed by the central vein and two portal triads. Although concentrations have a continuous gradient from outside to inside the lobule, toxicologists have discretized it into three zones, with Zone 1 (outside) having the highest drug concentration and Zone 3 (inside) the lowest due to metabolism. The chemical components used as liver tests have different distributions in the three zones. Zone 1 tends to be specialized for carbohydrate, amino acid, and fatty acid metabolism, the urea cycle, cholesterol synthesis, and bile acid secretion, while Zone 3 tends to be specialized for energy management and detoxifying reactions. The distributions of some zonal functions or components are relatively stable over time, while others vary according to exposure to blood components.

The necrosis of hepatocytes due to DILI can be either zonal or non-zonal [28]. Some drugs effect mostly Zone 1 and others mostly Zone 3, while Zone 2 tends not to have specific responses other than extensions from Zones 1 and 3. Zonal necrosis tends to cause relatively limited injury and preserves regenerative function if the offending drug is discontinued early enough. Idiosyncratic drug reactions tend to cause non-zonal necrosis, which can destroy large segments of the liver and may lead to fibrosis and cirrhosis.

In subnecrotic states, the liver shows degenerative changes. One of these changes is steatosis [28, 42]. There are two types of steatosis: microvesicular and macrovesicular. Both are seen in DILI. In macrosteatosis, a single large fat droplet fills the cytoplasmic space and displaces the nucleus. In microsteatosis, tiny fat droplets are formed that spread throughout the cytoplasm. Macrosteatosis, in the absence of other lesions, has a good long-term prognosis and rarely leads to fibrosis or cirrhosis. Microsteatosis, on the other hand, appears to have a grave prognosis and is believed to be caused by disruption of mitochondrial β-oxidation (a step in the conversion of fatty acids to energy) [43]. Without a liver biopsy, it is not possible to distinguish these lesions using liver tests.

There are two main types of acute cholestatic injury – canalicular and hepatocanalicular [28]. These types are difficult to distinguish with laboratory tests. Besides an elevated serum bilirubin, canalicular cholestasis has normal to mildly elevated aminotransferases and ALP; hepatocanalicular has moderately elevated aminotransferases and elevated ALP due to focal necrosis and portal inflammation. Many diseases besides DILI cause intrahepatic cholestasis. These include alcoholic liver disease, viral hepatitis, and metabolic diseases. In addition, some drugs cause a mixture of necrosis and cholestasis.

Some drugs can cause acute vascular injury [28]. One type of injury is hepatic vein thrombosis. It causes congestion (blood stasis) and Zone 3 necrosis along with some fibrosis. Another is veno-occlusive disease of hepatic venules. It starts with Zone 3 necrosis and progresses to fibrosis that reduces hepatic venule flow. In drug studies, this would probably mimic mild, zonal necrosis. Diagnosis would require a liver biopsy.

Chronic DILI is usually an extension of the acute forms [28] and is not likely to be observed in drug trials because of their relatively brief duration. However, it may appear in the post-marketing phase but would probably only be associated with a drug the patient was on at the time of diagnosis unless there was a specific need to gather past medication history. In addition, longer-term exposure may lead to granuloma formation, neoplasms, and pigment deposition. Whenever a sufficient number of DILI cases occur during a drug development program, it may be informative to conduct a long-term follow-up of these cases along with appropriately selected matched controls.

Clinically, drug reactions are described as either intrinsic or idiosyncratic [44, 45]. Intrinsic reactions are relatively frequent, dose-dependent, and predictable. Idiosyncratic reactions are infrequent, have a variable time of onset from initial exposure, and have a varying presentation in different individuals. This type of idiosyncrasy generally does not match the standard pathology definition. Idiosyncratic drug reactions are classified as allergic and non-allergic reactions [44].

Hepatocellular reactions are the most common, comprise about 90% of cases, and rarely progress to ALF. They are diagnosed by a characteristic pattern of liver tests [45].

Pathologically, these reactions cause liver necrosis and inflammation. The necrosis can be zonal, diffuse, or massive. The inflammation in the liver usually is dominated by lymphocytes and esosinophils.

Cholestatic reactions are the next most common [45]. Pure cholestasis is almost exclusively limited to oral contraceptives, anabolic steroids, and sex hormone antagonists. It leads to significantly elevated ALP and GGT, and normal or slightly increased amino-transferases. Bilirubin may or may not be elevated. More frequently the reaction is a mixture of cholestasis and hepatocellular damage. Acute cholestatic hepatitis manifests intrahepatic cholestasis, some necrosis, bile duct injury, and inflammation, mostly neutrophils. It generally takes longer to recover, up to 6 months or more.

Immunoallergic reactions are usually accompanied by hypersensitivity findings such as fever, rash, and elevated serum eosinophils [45]. These reactions usually present within the first week of exposure. Subsequent exposures tend to have shorter onset times and are more severe. Although liver damage might not be clinically apparent, the liver tests might be expected to resemble those of autoimmune or chronic hepatitis. Antibody and cytokine tests may be useful here.

Amacher recently described the state of pre-clinical liver biomarker use and discovery [46]. He discussed a number of liver tests that are not currently used in clinical practice. Some of these may not be commercially available to use in a clinical trial. If pre-clinical liver findings are specific and are strongly linked to the compound under study, then clinical trials should incorporate them. Just because the central laboratory does not have these on the menu, it should not be used as an excuse for not using it. If a drug is slated to earn hundreds of millions of dollars, it is possibly unethical not to spend a few million dollars to develop a commercially or experimentally usable test to help define the safety of a drug proposed for marketing. New biomarkers should improve safety in general, may help define reactions currently deemed to be idiosyncratic, and may allow drugs to be marketed to those patients not at risk, when the drug would otherwise not be approved for use or be withdrawn from marketing due to liver safety reasons.

### 9.3.3  Clinical trial design

In 2009, the FDA issued a drug safety guidance for industry to create a better quantitative structure for the regulatory evaluation of DILI in pre-marketing clinical trials [37]. The recommendations are paraphrased as follows:

- Signals of severe DILI
  - Excess number of aminotransferase elevations over $3 \times$ ULN compared to control group
  - Marked aminotransferase elevations (over $5 \times$ ULN) in modest numbers significantly greater than control group
  - One or more "Hy's law" cases
- Issues for consideration
  - Patients with pre-existing liver abnormalities or disease (generally no reason to exclude)

— Detection of DILI (liver tests every 2–4 weeks, then every 2–3 months if no sign of DILI after 3 or more months)

— Confirmation of DILI (ALT, AST, ALP, and total bilirubin in 48–72 hours following aminotransferase over 3 × ULN repeated until return to baseline)

— Close observation, if DILI threshold crossed, defined as

  • repeat liver tests two to three times weekly

  • more detailed history of prior or concurrent diseases

  • concomitant drug (including over-the-counter and dietary/herbal supplements), alcohol use, recreational drug use, and special diets

  • rule out acute viral hepatitis, autoimmune or alcoholic hepatitis, NASH, hypoxic/ischemic liver events, and biliary tract disease

  • additional laboratory testing as appropriate

— The decision to discontinue study drug should be considered if

  • ALT or AST over 8 × ULN

  • ALT or AST over 5 × ULN for more than 2 weeks

  • (ALT or AST over 3 × ULN) and (total bilirubin over 2 × ULN or INR over 1.5)

  • ALT or AST over 3 × ULN and new fatigue, nausea, vomiting, right upper quadrant pain or tenderness, fever, rash, and/or eosinophilia (over 5%)

— Follow-up of patient to resolution (until return to normal or to baseline)

— Rule for rechallenge.

It is important that every statistician and clinician involved in the clinical trial read and understand the content of this guidance and know its limitations. All Phase 3 protocols should include these recommendations unless better rules apply or unless the regulatory medical reviewer suggests (for good reason) otherwise. Unfortunately, this is only a quasi-quantitative approach typical of clinical thinking.

The guidance above suggests liver tests generally should not be used to exclude subjects from clinical trials. When outliers are excluded from the study, the measurements at subsequent visits will "regress from the mean" because they were inside the cutoff boundary by chance. This is the opposite of regression to the mean [47]. This phenomenon may lead to unnecessary follow-up on new elevated values and probably increases the noise level, masking real signals.

Given the ubiquitous presence of acetaminophen in over-the-counter medications [48] and its major contribution to the incidence of ALF [31], it may be wise to attempt to collect acetaminophen use data during a clinical trial. It may even be important enough to obtain blood levels at baseline, during the trial, or after a liver signal is detected, whichever is feasible and relevant.

The statistician needs to be aware of protocol design issues and the relevance of clinical components that can aid in or confound the analysis of liver test data. As suggested in the FDA guidance, additional testing may be used to follow liver reactions during a clinical trial.

However, this tends to happen only to those patients who passed some test threshold. This can introduce several biases [49]. Although they are certainly relevant to individual subject inferences, it is probably not appropriate to use these follow-up data points when comparing treatment groups.

## 9.4 Classical statistical approaches to the detection of hepatic toxicity

The data used in this chapter are a subset of the data that can be found in the supplemental files published elsewhere [50] and consist of the eight liver analytes, age, relative visit day, and blinded identifiers for study, subject, and clinical laboratory from untreated or placebo subjects that were seen over several years. There were a total of 5483 records/visits for 1755 male subjects between the ages of 20 and 40 years that were tested at 52 laboratories. Neither the subjects nor the laboratories are necessarily unique because of the coding and blinding, but it is likely that the vast majority of subjects is unique and mostly came from Phase 1 trials. The median time interval between observations was 4 days. The calculations were carried out using R [51] and the lattice graphics package [52].

### 9.4.1 Statistical distributions of analytes

Some graphical displays and statistics from the data set are presented. The baseline distributions are shown in Figure 9.1. Most of the subjects were under 30 years old. The analyte distributions as transformed were approximately normal at baseline. The laboratory variability is demonstrated in Figure 9.2. Figure 9.3 shows the stability of the distributions over the time of observation. Descriptive statistics for the means, samples sizes, and number of visits are given in Table 9.1 and the covariances and cross-correlations are given in Table 9.2. The small number of visits per subject makes the estimation of dynamic parameters difficult.

### 9.4.2 Reference limits

Reference limits are known by many names: normal ranges, normal limits, reference intervals, and multivariately as reference regions [53]. Sometimes the term "tolerance limits" is used, but this really is something different. Also, reference regions are not confidence intervals. Technically, reference limits are parameters that define the boundaries (level sets) of a probability density function – point pairs in the degenerate univariate case and surfaces in the multivariate case – that include an observed laboratory test value with probability $p$. In other words, if a vector $\mathbf{X}$ has a distribution with density $f_{\mathbf{X}}(\mathbf{x})$, then the reference limits corresponding to a level $p$ consist of the boundary of values of $X$ such that for an appropriately chosen constant $h(p)$, (a) $f_{\mathbf{X}}(\mathbf{x}) \geq h(p)$ and (b) the probability content of this set of $\mathbf{X}$ values is $p$. In the following text, the sample mean and variance have the usual definitions:

$$\bar{x} = \frac{1}{n}\sum_{i=1}^{n} x_i \quad \text{and} \quad s^2 = \frac{1}{n-1}\sum_{i=1}^{n}(x_i - \bar{x})^2,$$

where $n$ denotes the sample size. In multivariate expressions, $r$ denotes the dimension of the random vector under consideration.

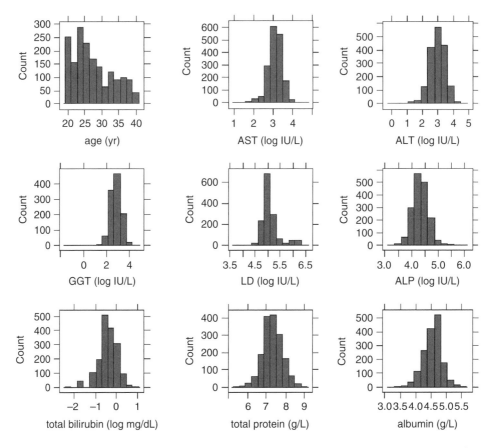

**Figure 9.1**    Frequency distributions of subject age and laboratory analyte values at baseline.

The data are assumed to have been transformed if necessary in what follows, so that the assumption of multivariate normality is tenable (see also [54, 55]). The fundamental equation for a reference region of a multivariate normal distribution is the implicit function of an ellipsoidal surface $g(\mathbf{Z}_p)$ with $\mathbf{Z}_p$ being the parameter of interest such that

$$g(\mathbf{Z}_p) = (\mathbf{Z}_p - \boldsymbol{\mu})'\, \boldsymbol{\Sigma}^{-1}(\mathbf{Z}_p - \boldsymbol{\mu}) - \chi_r^2(p) = 0, \tag{9.1}$$

where $\boldsymbol{\mu}$ is the $r \times 1$ mean vector, $\boldsymbol{\Sigma}$ is the $r \times r$ covariance matrix, $\mathbf{Z}_p$ is the $r \times 1$ non-random solution vector defining the boundary of the surface that contains the central $100p\%$ of the distribution, and $\chi_r^2(p)$ is the $100p^{\text{th}}$ percentile of a central chi-squared distribution with $r$ degrees of freedom.

When $r = 1$ (univariate case), equation (9.1) reduces to the familiar form

$$\zeta_p = \mu \pm \sigma\sqrt{\chi_1^2(p)}.$$

The chi-squared term is used here instead of the classical $z$-score to show the analogy with the non-degenerate multivariate case rather than the analogy with a confidence interval.

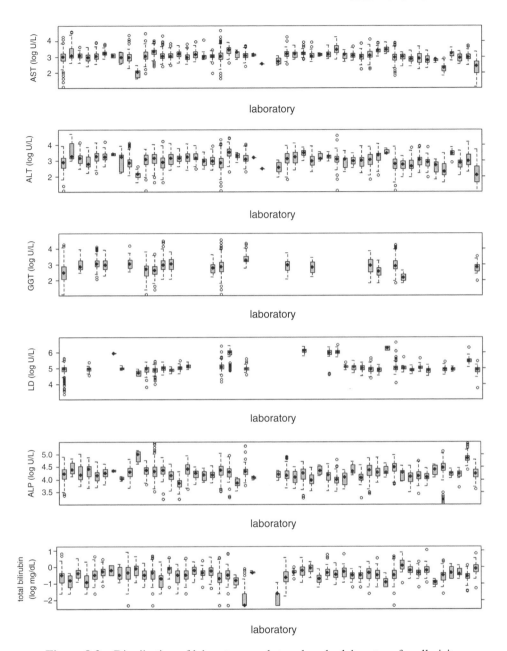

**Figure 9.2**    Distribution of laboratory analyte values by laboratory for all visits.

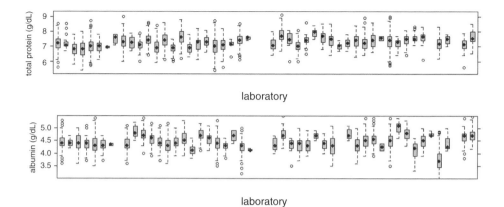

**Figure 9.2**  (*continued*)

The maximum likelihood (ML) estimator for $\zeta_p$ is

$$\widehat{\zeta}_p = \bar{x} \pm s\sqrt{\chi_1^2(p)}, \tag{9.2}$$

obtained by plugging in the ML estimates for the normal distribution. The population mean and variance of $\widehat{\zeta}_p$ are

$$\mathrm{E}[\widehat{\zeta}_p] = \mu \pm \sigma\sqrt{\chi_1^2(p)}\frac{2}{n-1}\frac{\Gamma(n/2)}{\Gamma((n-1)/2)} = \mu \pm \sigma\xi\sqrt{\chi_1^2(p)},$$

$$\mathrm{V}[\widehat{\zeta}_p] = \sigma^2\left\{\frac{1}{n} + \chi_1^2(p)(1-\xi^2)\right\}, \tag{9.3}$$

respectively, where $\Gamma$ denotes the usual gamma function. Routines for computing this function are readily available in statistical software packages. It is well known that ML estimators can be biased and inefficient for small samples. Sample sizes are almost never asymptotic when reference limits are estimated.

A better estimator might be one that is unbiased minimum variance (UMV). Since $\mathrm{E}(s) = \xi\sigma$, replacing $s$ with $\widehat{s} = s/\xi$ in equation (9.2) gives an unbiased estimator of $\widehat{\zeta}_p$,

$$\widehat{\zeta}_p = \bar{x} \pm \widehat{s}\sqrt{\chi_1^2(p)},$$

which has a population mean and variance of

$$\mathrm{E}[\widehat{\zeta}_p] = \mu \pm \sigma\sqrt{\chi_1^2(p)},$$

$$\mathrm{V}[\widehat{\zeta}_p] = \sigma^2\left(\frac{1}{n} + \chi_1^2(p)(\xi^{-2}-1)\right). \tag{9.4}$$

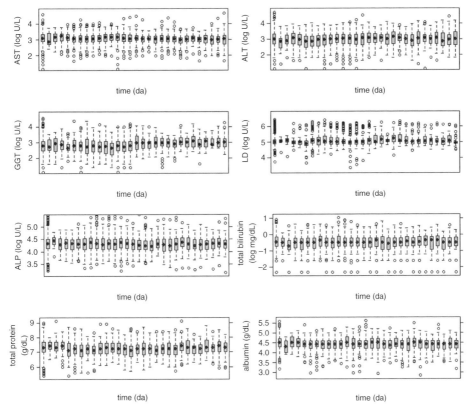

**Figure 9.3** Distribution of laboratory analyte values by time.

This estimator does not have an obvious multivariate analog. Correcting for bias in fact makes little difference in the properties of the estimators, at least for likely reference sample sizes:

| $n$ | 5 | 10 | 15 | 20 | 25 | 30 | 35 | 40 | 45 | 50 | 60 | 80 | 100 |
|---|---|---|---|---|---|---|---|---|---|---|---|---|---|
| $\xi$ | 0.940 | 0.973 | 0.982 | 0.987 | 0.990 | 0.991 | 0.993 | 0.994 | 0.994 | 0.995 | 0.996 | 0.997 | 0.997 |
| $1 - \xi^2$ | 0.116 | 0.054 | 0.035 | 0.026 | 0.021 | 0.017 | 0.015 | 0.013 | 0.011 | 0.010 | 0.008 | 0.006 | 0.005 |
| $\xi^{-2} - 1$ | 0.132 | 0.057 | 0.036 | 0.027 | 0.021 | 0.017 | 0.015 | 0.013 | 0.011 | 0.010 | 0.009 | 0.006 | 0.005 |

For reference sample sizes of 25 observations or more, the bias correction factor $\xi$ is about equal to 1, which means that the ML estimator is essentially unbiased, and the variances in equations (9.3) and (9.4) are indistinguishable. Directly estimating the quadratic form in equation (9.1), the Mahalanobis distance, provides another possibility for improving the ML estimator under multivariate normality; further details are provided in [56].

**Table 9.1**  Crude estimates of analyte means and standard errors (se) for baseline values and all values.

|  | AST | ALT | GGT | LD | ALP | Bilirubin | Protein | Albumin |
|---|---|---|---|---|---|---|---|---|
| Baseline mean | 3.09 | 2.98 | 2.80 | 5.09 | 4.33 | −0.46 | 7.33 | 4.53 |
| Overall mean | 3.06 | 2.98 | 2.82 | 5.08 | 4.32 | −0.51 | 7.27 | 4.45 |
| Baseline se | 0.0088 | 0.012 | 0.015 | 0.0092 | 0.0073 | 0.0108 | 0.0125 | 0.0076 |
| Overall se | 0.0050 | 0.0066 | 0.010 | 0.0065 | 0.0043 | 0.0068 | 0.0077 | 0.0050 |
| Baseline $n$ | 1746 | 1745 | 1127 | 1443 | 1742 | 1693 | 1671 | 1610 |
| Overall $n$ | 5439 | 5429 | 2912 | 3325 | 5411 | 5377 | 4442 | 4339 |
| Mean visits | 3.1 | 3.1 | 2.6 | 2.3 | 3.1 | 3.2 | 2.7 | 2.7 |

**Table 9.2**  Crude estimates of analyte covariances and cross-correlations (shaded) for baseline values (top) and all values (bottom).

|  | AST | ALT | GGT | LD | ALP | Bilirubin | Protein | Albumin |
|---|---|---|---|---|---|---|---|---|
| AST | 0.135 | 0.129 | 0.019 | 0.041 | 0.001 | −0.004 | −0.001 | −0.004 |
|  | 0.134 | 0.112 | 0.020 | 0.053 | −0.006 | 0.006 | 0.016 | 0.015 |
| ALT | 0.684 | 0.262 | 0.072 | 0.053 | −0.006 | −0.006 | −0.007 | −0.009 |
|  | 0.632 | 0.240 | 0.073 | 0.047 | −0.006 | −0.003 | 0.009 | 0.006 |
| GGT | 0.102 | 0.275 | 0.267 | 0.008 | 0.006 | −0.022 | 0.019 | −0.011 |
|  | 0.106 | 0.271 | 0.314 | 0.005 | 0.010 | −0.052 | 0.029 | −0.012 |
| LD | 0.303 | 0.291 | 0.068 | 0.122 | 0.012 | 0.008 | −0.006 | 0.003 |
|  | 0.352 | 0.249 | 0.035 | 0.141 | 0.002 | 0.015 | 0.001 | 0.000 |
| ALP | 0.012 | −0.035 | 0.039 | 0.112 | 0.094 | −0.013 | 0.012 | 0.013 |
|  | −0.054 | −0.037 | 0.059 | 0.014 | 0.099 | −0.014 | 0.015 | 0.017 |
| Bilirubin | −0.025 | −0.025 | −0.096 | 0.048 | −0.096 | 0.199 | 0.043 | 0.025 |
|  | 0.036 | −0.013 | −0.176 | 0.076 | −0.087 | 0.247 | 0.037 | 0.027 |
| Protein | −0.005 | −0.028 | 0.075 | −0.034 | 0.076 | 0.191 | 0.259 | 0.083 |
|  | 0.083 | 0.037 | 0.102 | 0.006 | 0.092 | 0.152 | 0.260 | 0.090 |
| Albumin | −0.033 | −0.056 | −0.075 | 0.032 | 0.139 | 0.184 | 0.531 | 0.094 |
|  | 0.122 | 0.035 | −0.069 | 0.001 | 0.165 | 0.171 | 0.530 | 0.110 |

It may be just semantics, but since there is no implied hypothesis test about the value of $\mathbf{Z}_p$, a confidence interval is not really appropriate. This is a good place to use the term tolerance interval, which is the interval that contains the true parameter with probability $1 - \alpha$ [57]. The $100(1 - \alpha)\%$ tolerance intervals for either the ML or the UMV estimate are defined by

$$P\left(AF_{r \cdot n-r}\left(\frac{\alpha}{2}, n\chi_r^2\,(\text{p})\right) - B < g(\mathbf{Z}_\text{p}) < AF_{r \cdot n-r}\left(1 - \frac{\alpha}{2}, n\chi_r^2\,(\text{p})\right) - B\right) = 1 - \alpha,$$

where $A = r(n-1)/n(n-r)$ and $B = \chi_r^2(p)$ for the ML estimate $(\hat{\mathbf{Z}}_p)$, and $A = r(n-1)(n-r-2)/n^2(n-r)$ and $B = r/n + \chi_r^2(p)$ for the UMV estimate $(\tilde{\mathbf{Z}}_p)$. These tolerance intervals can be used to determine the sample size needed to achieve a specified surface thickness for a $100p\%$ reference region with probability $1 - \alpha$. Results for $10 < n < 10\,000$ and selected dimensions in the interval $1 < r < 100$ are published in [56], Figure 3.

Wellek presents some approaches to constructing multivariate references regions [58]. These are generally analogs of Bonferroni-type rectangular regions, with many of the same inadequacies. If rectangular regions are required for some historical reason, then his approach is a reasonable one to consider. However, his rationale for using rectangular regions and against using ellipsoidal regions includes the premises that (i) at least one analyte has to be outside its marginal reference limit, (ii) rectangular regions are easier to interpret, and (iii) his methods are less dependent on strong distributional assumptions.

The first premise is archaic. This is a historical remnant of the pre-computer era. In the past, there was not a quick method for constructing a multivariate rule or for evaluating a vector of analyte results. All that physicians could do was to compare each result with some corresponding normal interval supplied by the laboratory. If a vector result was outside the ellipsoidal boundary, there was no way to know, and therefore, such a result has never been considered to be relevant clinically. Until we do the research, this view is naïve. There is no reason why an organization evaluating drug safety should adhere to archaic clinical thinking.

The second premise has some merit, but only because medical practice is still in the "dark ages" with respect to quantitative methods, partially related to the reasons in the previous paragraph. Biological systems are very complex and not fully comprehensible by practicing physicians, or anyone else. What they believe to be their deep understanding of human biology is really just a gross oversimplification of what the underlying processes really are. Systems biology is just currently scratching the surface. Clinical interpretations are based on these oversimplifications that can be taught in a medical curriculum and memorized in some systematic way and that help rationalize treatment decisions, but may or may not approximate the true biology. Biology is not linear and there is no reason why decision rules should be linear either. A biologically significant result should be one that exceeds the boundaries of analytical precision, not boundaries of convenience.

The third premise is one used commonly by statisticians, who believe it is better to make no assumptions about the probability model and have no worries about committing a Type I error than to make strong assumptions about the probability model and have to explain the findings, which may be surprising to the clinical establishment. Due to the abundance of data, the distributions of most common analytes can be known to a high level of accuracy. Even those with some approximation error generally are more efficient from a sample size viewpoint than distribution-free, assumption-free, or assumption-weak approaches. These strong models are likely to reduce the Type II error, perhaps at the expense of the Type I error, but this should be preferable when analyzing data to find drug safety signals. For liver tests, normal or lognormal distributions should be used for analysis and signal detection. There is really no need for distribution-free methods. These methods tend to be superior for heavy-tailed distributions that are found in economics and physics but are essentially non-existent in biology. Sometimes heavy tails are seen in normal laboratory test data, but these are generally due to a contamination, not the natural distribution. Occasionally construction of ratios by clinicians can lead to Cauchy-like distributions.

If a multivariate definition of abnormal is unacceptable or "uninterpretable," then perhaps conditional reference limits [59] for each analyte would give a middle ground. They could be evaluated in the same coordinates as the original data and would contain information about the other test results along with some of the cross-correlation information:

$$\zeta_p(x_1|\mathbf{x}_2) = \mu_1 + \mathbf{\Sigma}_{12}\mathbf{\Sigma}_{22}^{-1}(\mathbf{x}_2 - \mathbf{\mu}_2) \pm \sqrt{\chi_1^2(p)(\sigma_{11}^2 - \mathbf{\Sigma}_{12}\mathbf{\Sigma}_{22}^{-1}\mathbf{\Sigma}_{21})},$$

where the normal distribution parameters are partitioned as $\mathbf{\mu} = \begin{bmatrix} \mu_1 & \mathbf{\mu}_2 \end{bmatrix}'$ and

$$\mathbf{\Sigma} = \begin{bmatrix} \sigma_{11}^2 & \mathbf{\Sigma}_{12} \\ \mathbf{\Sigma}_{21} & \mathbf{\Sigma}_{22} \end{bmatrix}.$$

Different estimation approaches could be applied here, but the ML estimation procedure is obviously easiest to implement. This is effectively a regression model approach with a "Type III sum-of-squares" interpretation. Rather than using marginal or conditional limits only, a multivariate region could be used to determine the overall abnormality to control the Type I error and the conditional limits would then provide interpretability as to which analytes are in play. It seems that the conditional approach may have both increased sensitivity and specificity as compared to the marginal approach, although clinicians find it somewhat "disorienting" to have values declared abnormal inside the marginal limits.

A generalized approach to some of the interval estimation methods above has recently been published [60]. It discusses some of the background of interval standards and the terminology of different types of intervals.

### 9.4.3   Hy's rule and other empirical methods

Since the 1980s when cholesterol-lowering clinical trials became popular, elevated liver enzyme activities have been a frequent concern, starting with the Lipid Research Clinics Coronary Primary Prevention Trial [61, 62], which used a non-systemically active compound, cholestyramine. This drug binds bile acid, a cholesterol product, in the intestine and prevents the bile from being reabsorbed, thus removing cholesterol from the body via fecal excretion. It was found that some of the trial patients had elevated AST and LD. These enzymes had been measured primarily for coronary event evaluation. This was a surprise to clinicians since cholestyramine was not expected to have systemic effects [61, 62]. Not too long afterward, clinical trials with lovastatin and pravastatin also revealed similar elevations of liver transaminase activities. A noted hepatologist, Hyman Zimmerman, an expert in hepatotoxicity [28, 63], was consulted on some or all of these liver findings. It is said that he had a rule-of-thumb that AST and ALT levels of about 100 were clinically significant for detecting hepatotoxicity, which is about three times the ULN for these tests. In the late 1980s, this became the *de facto* regulatory standard for identifying hepatotoxicity in drug trials and is still in use today, with little scientific basis.

There are several problems with this standard. The method to establish the ULN, the upper reference limit, is not standardized among clinical laboratories – some use normal distribution assumptions, some use lognormal assumptions, some use distribution-free methods, and others do something else including looking them up in a textbook. Most use sample sizes that are too small. Not only are the statistical methods not standardized in spite of standards being issued [53], but the chemical analysis methods are not standardized. From a local clinical viewpoint, this variation does not matter much because it is internally consistent and this is the primary reason there is no movement to standardize across laboratories. However, the variations in methods make this number externally inconsistent and subject to manipulation. For instance, a company conducting clinical trials for drug approval can choose laboratories that have overestimated the ULN, making the incidence of liver test elevations lower than that of the competitors.

The methods described in Section 9.4.2 should be used to calculate reference limits from clinical trial data that have a suitable control group rather than using those limits supplied by the laboratory. Pooling data across laboratories is described in Section 9.5.2. This allows the limits to be calculated properly and consistently and allows a better interpretation of what the limits mean.

An example of a purely empirical approach to evaluating DILI is described by Lee [45], Table 152-4. It is a scoring system incorporating drug exposure, the time course of liver tests, risk factors, concomitant drugs, and rechallenge results. It is called the Roussel-Uclaf causality assessment method (RUCAM). It was designed to be used by experienced clinicians. The utility of the instrument in detecting or quantifying DILI in drug development is unclear.

Senior gave a good review of the regulatory viewpoint for evaluating DILI using ULN criteria and the history of "Hy's law," or "Hy's rule," named after Hyman Zimmerman [35]. Unfortunately, these rules still have the flaws of the ULN determination and rectangular (Euclidean) regions in a non-Euclidean world, are only quasi-quantitative, and are clinically derived without a good quantitative scientific basis. Hy's rule is generally defined as a rectangular region specified by $ALT > 3 \times ULN$ and total bilirubin greater than $2 \times ULN$. ALT has a poor predictive value for serious DILI. Hy's rule probably improves this considerably [64]. In fairness, some of these flaws are caused by the rarity of serious DILI in data sets suitable for rigorous statistical analysis and the ethical problems of allowing subjects to continue on a drug until a definite diagnosis can be made.

A graphical software tool called "eDISH" (evaluation of Drug-Induced Serious Hepatotoxicity) has been developed to aid in the review of liver data submitted for regulatory approval [64]. It is an enhanced version of Hy's rule-based drug review, especially by clinical reviewers. It is unclear whether or not this tool offers better analysis of DILI than something a statistician could develop with minimal effort using standard statistical software. It still has the properties of Hy's rule.

# 9.5   Stochastic process models for liver homeostasis

## 9.5.1   The Ornstein–Uhlenbeck process model

It has been demonstrated that, in a subset of treated subjects for some compounds, the vector of liver test values defines a trajectory over time that is not parallel with the coordinate axes [4]. This seems to suggest that the real disease/reaction patterns are nonlinear and multivariate in the laboratory test space. Appropriate models need to be developed to capture this dynamic information and to assess its clinical significance. The methods in this section have been applied to healthy normal subjects to build dynamic models to create a more accurate definition of what it means to be healthy normal [50]. However, they have not yet been extended to model the dynamic reactions of treated patients to their treatments.

Laboratory measurement values in healthy individuals are not constant over time, but instead vary randomly from time to time in a predictable way, at least in principle. In the presence of, say, liver damage, one would expect to see values oscillating outside the predictable region corresponding to the healthy state, and this could signal the presence of toxicity, possibly more sensitively, and sooner than conventional methods based on laboratory normal ranges. The physical analog of this situation is that of an object attached to a spring and driven by a force over time about an equilibrium point. In physics, the equation of motion of an object of mass $m$ fixed at the equilibrium point $\mu$ by a spring with Hook's constant $\rho$ in a uniform friction medium with friction coefficient $\phi$, driven by a force over time $F(t)$, is

$$m\frac{d^2y}{dt^2} + \phi\frac{dy}{dt} + \rho(y - \mu) = F(t). \tag{9.5}$$

With a few modifications, this seems like a reasonable starting point for modeling the dynamics of a blood analyte. In the healthy state, this model should be somewhat simpler. For instance, if the acceleration $d^2y/dt^2$ is assumed to be zero at dynamic equilibrium, the equation simplifies to

$$\frac{dy}{dt} = -\frac{\rho}{\phi}(y - \mu) + \frac{1}{\phi}F(t). \tag{9.6}$$

This equation does not depend on the mass. A natural forcing function for a continuous biological dynamic system is Brownian motion, that is, independent, random Gaussian excursions. Simplistically, a stochastic process is a random variable that is a function of time. A mathematical model of Brownian motion, the standard Brownian motion (Wiener) process $B(t)$, can be defined by three characteristics [65–68]:

1. $B(t)$ is a continuous stochastic process with $B(0) = 0$,

2. $E[B(t)] = 0$ and $E[B(s)B(t)] = \min(s, t)$ for all $s, t > 0$, and

3. $B(t) \sim N(0, t)$.

An $r$-dimensional standard Brownian motion process is defined similarly. A standard Brownian motion process can be rescaled to another Brownian motion process, that is, $B(t)/\sigma^2 = B(\sigma^2 t)$, in distribution. Since a Brownian motion process is not differentiable, when inserting it as a forcing function into the equation above, it is more proper to use a differential form called a stochastic differential equation (SDE) such that

$$dY = -\alpha(Y - \mu)dt + \theta dB, \tag{9.7}$$

where the coefficients of (9.6) have been reparameterized and the variables $Y$ and $B$ are stochastic processes. This SDE is a special case of a diffusion process where $\alpha$ is called the diffusion coefficient and $\theta$ is called the drift coefficient.

In the context of liver homeostasis (biological dynamic equilibrium), the diffusion coefficient can be thought of as the strength of the "homeostatic" force and the drift coefficient as the strength of the opposing "thermal" force. The latter drives the system, keeps it in motion, and increases entropy, while the former keeps the system in a dynamic equilibrium or steady state and decreases the entropy. These coefficients could be key biological parameters (biomarkers) that are constant in a healthy individual and time-varying or space-varying in a pathological or pharmacological state. If the variational patterns of these coefficients are regular and specific, they may have important diagnostic and clinical significance, even for an individual whose analyte values are within the reference region. In other words, any non-random change in the system is a potential signal of an abnormal condition. This concept might be called "pathodynamics," an analog to thermodynamics. A pathodynamics (disease-related) SDE may require an acceleration term or something more complicated.

The homeostatic SDE in equation (9.7) can be solved using Itô calculus without the use of derivatives and is a representation of a mean-reverting Ornstein–Uhlenbeck (OU) process. The general aspects of Itô calculus and martingale theory are beyond the scope of this book and can be found elsewhere [65–67]. The solution to this equation is a Gaussian stochastic process induced by the Brownian motion process such that

$$Y(t) = \mu + e^{-\alpha(t-s)}(Y(s) - \mu) + e^{-\alpha(t-s)} \int_s^t e^{\alpha(u-s)}\theta dB(u)$$

for $0 \le s < t$. This OU process is normal with conditional mean

$$E[Y(t)|Y(s)] = \mu + e^{-\alpha(t-s)}(Y(s) - \mu) + \theta e^{-\alpha t} \int_s^t e^{\alpha u} dE[B(u)|Y(s)]$$

$$= \mu + e^{-\alpha(t-s)}(Y(s) - \mu) \tag{9.8}$$

and conditional variance

$$V[Y(t)|Y(s)] = \theta^2 e^{-2\alpha t} \int_s^t e^{2\alpha u} dV[B(u)|Y(s)] = \theta^2 e^{-2\alpha t} \int_s^t e^{2\alpha u} du$$

$$= \frac{\theta^2}{2\alpha}(1 - e^{-2\alpha(t-s)}).$$

It should be noted that the variance depends only on the measurement times and not on the values of the process. It is straightforward to show that $Y(t) \sim N(\mu, \theta^2/2\alpha)$. The derivation of the multivariate OU process is analogous using the $r \times r$ matrix exponential function $e^{At}$. It should also be noted that

$$E[(Y(s) - \mu)(Y(t) - \mu)] = E[E[(Y(s) - \mu)(Y(t) - \mu)|Y(s)]]$$

$$= E[(Y(s) - \mu)E[Y(t) - \mu|Y(s)]]$$

$$= E[(Y(s) - \mu)((-e^{-\alpha(t-s)})\mu + e^{-\alpha(t-s)}Y(s))]$$

$$= E[(Y(s) - \mu)(e^{-\alpha(t-s)}Y(s))] = \frac{\theta^2}{2\alpha}e^{-\alpha(t-s)}$$

for $0 \le s < t$. This indicates that the autocorrelation of the process is $e^{-\alpha(t-s)}$ and that the joint distribution of two consecutive measurements is multivariate normal with mean $\begin{bmatrix} \mu & \mu \end{bmatrix}'$ and covariance

$$\frac{\theta^2}{2\alpha} \begin{bmatrix} 1 & e^{-\alpha(t-s)} \\ e^{-\alpha(t-s)} & 1 \end{bmatrix}.$$

It can be shown that this OU process is Markovian and is equivalent to an AR(1) process as described in the time series literature [69] and has been suggested for constructing subject-based reference limits [70]. However, time series estimation algorithms essentially all require frequent, equally spaced observation times, which do not exist in liver test results. Therefore, time series approaches will not be discussed here.

Under the assumption that the healthy liver analytes follow an OU process, the conditional reference limits for an individual subject at time $t$ given a previous observation $Y(s)$ are

$$\zeta_p(s,t|Y(s)) = \mu + e^{-\alpha(t-s)}(Y(s) - \mu) \pm \sqrt{\chi_1^2(p)}\frac{\theta}{\sqrt{2\alpha}}\sqrt{1 - e^{-2\alpha(t-s)}}. \tag{9.9}$$

Since other estimators of this interval are inherently more complicated and the length of this individualized interval is much smaller than the population interval, only the ML estimator

$$\hat{\zeta}_p(s,t|Y(s)) = \hat{\mu} + e^{-\hat{\alpha}(t-s)}(Y(s) - \hat{\mu}) \pm \sqrt{\chi_1^2(p)}\frac{\hat{\theta}}{\sqrt{2\hat{\alpha}}}\sqrt{1 - e^{-2\hat{\alpha}(t-s)}} \tag{9.10}$$

will be discussed. Just as with the usual population estimator of the reference limits, the parameters should be estimated using data other than the current observation $Y(t)$. A biologically significant change should be declared when the current observation is outside this interval. The clinical significance may require additional information.

A continuous time-invariant linear dynamic system is a system that changes in continuous time and space, can be characterized by a linear differential equation of any order, and has coefficients that are time-invariant [71, 72]. Such systems are ubiquitous in the engineering literature. Unfortunately, in most cases the systems are deterministic and the system parameters are known. In addition, most differential equations of order higher than 2 have no analytical solutions. Stochastic systems are dynamic systems with random coefficients and/or random variables. In general, dynamic systems have memory, that is, they depend not only on the current observation time, but also previous observation times. Equation (9.5) is an example of a deterministic second-order dynamic system and (9.6) is an example of a first-order dynamic system.

The OU process is typically modeled using state-space modeling techniques [71, 72]. State-space models are preferred in situations where the differential equations are of higher order or there are multiple inputs and outputs. The numerical calculations are very efficient relative to other approaches. States tend to be the underlying true stochastic process plus its true derivatives, all of which are unobservable. Using notation consistent with this chapter and an Itô representation, the state-space model is

$$d\mathbf{X} = \mathbf{A}(\mathbf{X} - \boldsymbol{\mu})dt + \boldsymbol{\Theta}d\mathbf{B}, \tag{9.11}$$

$$\mathbf{Y} = \mathbf{X} + \mathbf{E}, \tag{9.12}$$

where equation (9.11) is the state or transition equation and equation (9.12) is the space or measurement equation, $\mathbf{A}$ is a matrix called the system matrix, $\boldsymbol{\Theta}$ is a matrix (not necessarily square) called the noise gain matrix, $\mathbf{B}$ (in this case Brownian motion) is a vector that conforms to $\boldsymbol{\Theta}$, and $\mathbf{E}$ is a vector of measurement errors. This particular system model has no inputs and the vector $\mathbf{Y}$ represents the observed outputs of the underlying process vector $\mathbf{X}$. The estimation procedure for this particular model is called the Kalman–Bucy filter. In engineering applications, typically the dimension of $\mathbf{Y}$ is one. It is observed very frequently over a relatively long time interval and the dimension of $d\mathbf{X}$ is $k$, representing a system of $k$ differential equations. This allows good estimation using a single experimental unit.

The estimates can be updated at each observation time and, since all previous observations are used, the memory of the system does not need to be handled explicitly. For clinical situations, observations are generally few and far apart, requiring many patients to be observed over time in order to get good estimates of the parameters, and the system memory may have to be handled explicitly or ignored. In the clinical case, using the OU process, the dimension of $\mathbf{Y}$ is $n$ and the dimension of $d\mathbf{X}$ is $n$ since there is just one SDE per observation. For multivariate problems of dimension $r$, $r$ sets of equations are stacked, giving a dimension of $nr$.

Oravecz and Tuerlinckx [73] found that the state-space model estimation and the mixed-effects model estimation of the OU model are equivalent in many situations, in particular for the model of liver homeostasis presented in this section. They used the SDE solution

$$X(t) = \mu + e^{-\alpha(t-s)}(X(s) - \mu) + \theta e^{-\alpha t} \int_s^t e^{\alpha u} dB$$

rather than the SDE as the state model, and

$$Y(t) = X(t) + \varepsilon$$

as the space model.

For estimation, the first equation can be plugged into the second, with some reparameterization, giving the regression model

$$y_i(t) = \mu(1 - e^{-\alpha(t-s)}) + e^{-\alpha(t-s)} y_i(s) + \eta_i + \varepsilon_i$$

for the $i$th subject. Converting to a linear model representation gives

$$y_i(t) = \beta_0 + \beta_1 y_i(s) + \varepsilon_i^*$$

where the residuals (combined biological and analytical variation) are independent with

$$\varepsilon_i^* \sim \mathrm{N}\left(0, \frac{\theta^2}{2\alpha}\left(1 - e^{-2\alpha(t-s)}\right) + \sigma_\varepsilon^2\right). \tag{9.13}$$

The ML estimates for equally spaced observations and $\sigma_\varepsilon^2$ sufficiently small can be obtained as follows:

$$\widehat{\alpha} = -\frac{1}{t-s} \log(\widehat{\beta}_1),$$

$$\widehat{\mu} = \frac{\widehat{\beta}_0}{1 - e^{-\widehat{\alpha}(t-s)}},$$

$$\widehat{\theta} \approx \widehat{\sigma}_{\varepsilon^*}\sqrt{\frac{2\widehat{\alpha}}{1 - e^{-2\widehat{\alpha}(t-s)}}}. \tag{9.14}$$

The measurement variance can only be partitioned out if each blood sample is measured at least twice or if the laboratory provides it. For the analytes in this chapter, it is probably negligible. An overestimate of $\theta$ should still be better than current methods for determining abnormality.

## 9.5.2    OU data analysis

The nlme package of R was used for data analysis [74]. Four models were applied to the liver data and are compared below. Laboratories and subjects within laboratory in these models are treated as random effects. Models 1 and 2 are linear mixed-effects models using the approach of Oravecz and Tuerlinckx [73] and lme() in R [51]. All random effects are assumed to be independent and normally distributed.

Model 1 is just a linear model of the laboratory effect and subject effect without regard to autocorrelation:

$$y_{ij}(t_k) = \mu + \beta_{0i} + \beta_{1j} + b_0 + b_1 + \varepsilon_{ijk}^* \tag{9.15}$$

where $\mu$ is the fixed analyte mean, $\beta_{0i}$ is the fixed mean effect of the $i$th laboratory, $\beta_{1j}$ is the fixed mean effect of the $j$th subject within the $i$th laboratory, $b_0$ is the random laboratory effect with mean zero and variance $\sigma_0^2$, $b_1$ is the random subject effect with mean zero and variance $\sigma_1^2$, and $\varepsilon_{ijk}^*$ is the random residual effect of the $k$th time point of the $j$th subject within the $i$th laboratory with mean zero and variance $\sigma_{\varepsilon*}^2$. For simplicity of notation, the subscripts have not been subscripted as they should be with nested effects. The R code for this model is given below:

```
AST.OU.lme.1 <- lme(AST ~ 1,
                random = ~ 1 | lab / studysubject,
                method = 'ML',
                na.action = 'na.omit')

mu.est   <- fixef(AST.OU.lme.1)
mu.sd    <- sqrt(diag(AST.OU.lme.1$varFix))
varLab   <- as.numeric(VarCorr(AST.OU.lme.1)[2, 1])
varSubj  <- as.numeric(VarCorr(AST.OU.lme.1)[4,1])
varRes   <- as.numeric(VarCorr(AST.OU.lme.1)[5,1])
varTot   <- varLab + varSubj + varRes
```

The ML estimates of $\mu$, $\sigma_0^2$, $\sigma_1^2$, and $\sigma_{\varepsilon*}^2$ are obtained from mu.est, varLab, varSubj, and varRes, respectively.

For Model 2, a built-in R function corCAR1() was applied to Model 1. This function requires that equally spaced times are assumed. An example for the R code for this model is given below:

```
AST.OU.lme.2 <- update(AST.OU.lme.1,
                correlation = corCAR1(form = ~ day |
                    lab/studysubject))

mu.est     <- fixef(AST.OU.lme.2)
mu.sd      <- sqrt(diag(AST.OU.lme.2$varFix))
phi.est    <- coef(AST.OU.lme.2$modelStruct$corStruct,
               unconstrained = FALSE)
alpha.est <- -log(phi.est)
theta.est <- AST.OU.lme.2$sigma *
sqrt(2 * alpha.est / (1 - exp(-2 * alpha.est)))
anova(AST.OU.lme.1, AST.OU.lme.2)
```

The corCAR1() function estimates an additional parameter $\phi = e^{-\alpha}$, which represents the autocorrelation. The R code above shows how to retrieve the ML estimate of $\phi$. From this $\alpha$ can be estimated using equation (9.14). With the assumption that the time spacing is one unit and the measurement error is small, $\theta$ can be calculated as well using (9.14). The $p$-value for comparing Model 1 to Model 2 comes from the anova() function.

In order to account for the unequal time spacing of the liver data, Model 3 uses the R function nlme() and the conditional mean from equation (9.8). The parameter gamma appears in this model because it is used in Model 4 for comparison. Here it is set to a constant one. An example for the R code for this model is given below:

```
cond.mean <- function(ys, alpha, gamma, mu, t, s){
             deltaT <- (t - s)^gamma * (gamma > 0)
             expt   <- (alpha > 0) * exp(-alpha * (alpha > 0) * deltaT)
             func   <- mu + (deltaT > 0) * expt * (ys - mu)
             return(func)}

AST.OU.nlme.3 <- nlme(AST ~ cond.mean(AST0, alpha, gamma = 1, mu,
                 day, day0),
          fixed   = list(mu ~ 1, alpha ~ 1),
          random  = mu ~ 1 | lab/studysubject,
          start   = list(fixed = c(mu = mean(AST, na.rm = TRUE),
                 alpha = 0.01)),
          method  = 'ML', na.action = 'na.omit',
          control = nlmeControl(pnlsMaxIter = 50))
beta.est  <- fixef(AST.OU.nlme.3)
beta.sd   <- sqrt(diag(AST.OU.nlme.3$varFix))
theta.est <- AST.OU.nlme.3$sigma * sqrt(2 * beta.est['alpha'] *
          sum(!is.na(AST)) / sum(1 - exp(-2 * beta.est['alpha'] *
          (day - day0)), na.rm = TRUE))
```

In this model, $\mu$ in equation (9.15) is replaced by the conditional mean of the OU process in equation (9.8). The term AST0 is the previous observation taken at day 0. From equation (9.13), assuming that all $n$ residuals are independent and distributed as $N\left(0, \frac{\theta^2}{2\alpha}\left(1 - e^{-2\alpha(t-s)}\right)\right)$, the average variance can be used to estimate $\theta$ such that

$$V[\varepsilon_{ijk}^*] = \frac{1}{n}\sum_{\ell=1}^{n}\frac{\theta^2}{2\alpha}(1 - I\{t_\ell > 0\}e^{-2\alpha(t_\ell - t_{\ell-1})}),$$

$$\hat{\theta} \approx \hat{\sigma}_{\varepsilon^*}\sqrt{\frac{2n\hat{\alpha}}{\sum_{\ell=1}^{n}(1 - I\{t_\ell > 0\}e^{-2\hat{\alpha}(t_\ell - t_{\ell-1})})}},$$

where the observations are ordered by time within a subject and the first observation of the subject is at $t_\ell = 0$, and $I\{\cdot\}$ is the indicator function. The starting values for the nonlinear parameters may need to be varied to obtain convergence.

Apparent time variation in $\alpha$ and $\theta$ was observed to be removed when the autocorrelation terms in the multivariate OU models for liver analytes were replaced by the multivariate version of $e^{-\alpha\sqrt{t-s}}$ [50], but this finding is hard to justify theoretically. Since a nonlinear approach was used in Model 3, Model 4 could be applied univariately with a general exponent $\gamma$ just to explore this issue. This model assumes the regression model has the structure

$$y_i(t) = \mu(1 - e^{-\alpha(t-s)^\gamma}) + e^{-\alpha(t-s)^\gamma} y_i(s) + \eta_i + \varepsilon_i.$$

It is easy to show that $E[Y(t_2)|Y(t_1)]$ for $t_1 < t_2$ has this structure but, in general, the residuals are not independent and may have a very long memory. An example for the R code for Model 4 is given below:

```
AST.OU.nlme.4 <- nlme(AST ~ cond.mean(AST0,alpha,gamma,mu,day,day0),
            fixed  = list(mu ~ 1, alpha ~ 1, gamma ~ 1),
            random = mu ~ 1 | lab/studysubject,
            start  = list(fixed = c(mu = mean(AST, na.rm = TRUE),
                    alpha = 0.01, gamma = 0.25)), method = 'ML',
            na.action = 'na.omit',
            control = nlmeControl(pnlsMaxIter = 50, pnlsTol = 1e-6))
```

The parameter estimators are the same as Model 3 with the addition of gamma. In this model, convergence was more difficult to achieve for several of the analytes and, along with varying the starting values, the pnlsTol value had to be increased until convergence was achieved. In one case, ALP, convergence was not achieved satisfactorily. The estimator for theta was modified accordingly

$$\hat{\theta} \approx \hat{\sigma}_{\varepsilon*} \sqrt{\frac{2n\hat{\alpha}}{\sum_{\ell=1}^{n}(1 - I\{t_\ell > 0\}e^{-2\hat{\alpha}(t_\ell - t_{\ell-1})^{\hat{\gamma}})}}},$$

although this modification had little effect on the estimate. Again a $p$-value comparing Models 3 and 4 was obtained using the R function anova().

The modeling results for all four models are shown in Table 9.3. The choice of model made little difference in the estimates of the population means $\mu$ and residual variances $\sigma_{\varepsilon*}^2$. For all analytes except ALP and bilirubin, Model 2 was significantly different from Model 1 assuming equally spaced times. It is unclear why these two analytes would appear to have no autocorrelation. This time structure may have been destroyed by the lack of standardization in the laboratory methods, which may apply especially to ALP due to different assay temperatures and several chemical analysis methods. These methods may actually be measuring something different and may not be poolable. For bilirubin, clinicians insist on dropping all the decimals places but one, causing a noticeable discretization effect in the left tail of the distribution, which may also impact the autocorrelation.

Model 3 takes the unequal time spacing into account, making the estimates of $\alpha$ and $\theta$ more believable and the preferred model. The estimates of these parameters do vary between Models 2 and 3, although they may not be statistically significant. If convergence cannot be achieved with Model 3, Model 2 would not be a bad substitute. The estimates of $\gamma$ in Model 4 vary considerably among the analytes, making them difficult to interpret. Several are close enough to one to suggest that the OU model is a good fit, although the $p$-values may suggest otherwise. Overall Model 3 is probably the best of the four, with Model 4 being a stepping stone for additional research.

The components of variance for the four models are shown in Table 9.4. There are essentially no differences among the four models. The between-laboratory variation ranges

**Table 9.3**  Parameter estimates for the four models of the analyte processes and selected standard errors (se).

| Analyte | Model | $\hat{\mu}$ (se) | $\hat{\alpha}$ (se) | $\hat{\theta}$ | $\hat{\gamma}$ | $\hat{\sigma}_{\varepsilon^*}$ | p-value |
|---|---|---|---|---|---|---|---|
| AST | 1 | 3.039 (0.038) | | | | 0.201 | |
| | 2 | 3.041 (0.038) | 0.685 | 0.288 | | 0.213 | <0.0001 |
| | 3 | 3.041 (0.038) | 1.337 (0.144) | 0.402 | 1 | 0.202 | |
| | 4 | 3.041 (0.038) | 1.346 (0.153) | 0.404 | 0.989 (0.441) | 0.202 | 0.35 |
| ALT | 1 | 3.008 (0.043) | | | | 0.239 | |
| | 2 | 3.010 (0.043) | 0.896 | 0.366 | | 0.249 | <0.0001 |
| | 3 | 3.008 (0.043) | 3.374 (1.169) | 0.751 | 1 | 0.240 | |
| | 4 | 3.012 (0.044) | 1.141 (0.108) | 0.446 | 0.942 (0.312) | 0.241 | <0.0001 |
| GGT | 1 | 2.827 (0.059) | | | | 0.286 | |
| | 2 | 2.829 (0.059) | 1.463 | 0.507 | | 0.288 | 0.0008 |
| | 3 | 2.839 (0.053) | 2.173 (0.693) | 0.546 | 1 | 0.296 | |
| | 4 | 2.851 (0.053) | 1.231 (0.221) | 0.406 | 0.554 (0.262) | 0.288 | <0.0001 |
| ALP | 1 | 4.243 (0.025) | | | | 0.101 | |
| | 2 | 4.243 (0.025) | 1.463 | 0.255 | | 0.101 | 0.34 |
| | 3 | 4.245 (0.025) | 1.012 (0.077) | 0.175 | 1 | 0.100 | |
| | 4 | 4.242 (0.025) | 3.916 (2.047) | 0.331 | 1.110 (24.87) | 0.098 | NA |
| LD | 1 | 5.168 (0.073) | | | | 0.173 | |
| | 2 | 5.173 (0.074) | 1.463 | 0.247 | | 0.180 | <0.0001 |
| | 3 | 5.170 (0.076) | 1.378 (0.170) | 0.289 | 1 | 0.183 | |
| | 4 | 5.171 (0.076) | 1.130 (0.157) | 0.264 | 2.214 (2.070) | 0.183 | 0.0005 |
| Bilirubin | 1 | −0.479 (0.049) | | | | 0.298 | |
| | 2 | −0.479 (0.049) | 3.878 | 0.833 | | 0.299 | 0.63 |
| | 3 | −0.480 (0.049) | 2.974 (0.748) | 0.865 | 1 | 0.295 | |
| | 4 | −0.469 (0.049) | 2.582 (0.476) | 0.803 | 0.437 (0.602) | 0.294 | <0.0001 |
| Protein | 1 | 7.273 (0.037) | | | | 0.329 | |
| | 2 | 7.278 (0.037) | 1.024 | 0.512 | | 0.334 | <0.0001 |
| | 3 | 7.286 (0.038) | 1.598 (0.260) | 0.658 | 1 | 0.335 | |
| | 4 | 7.287 (0.038) | 1.515 (0.264) | 0.641 | 1.200 (0.672) | 0.335 | 0.23 |
| Albumin | 1 | 4.463 (0.033) | | | | 0.216 | |
| | 2 | 4.468 (0.033) | 0.918 | 0.325 | | 0.220 | <0.0001 |
| | 3 | 4.473 (0.034) | 1.032 (0.107) | 0.346 | 1 | 0.219 | |
| | 4 | 4.474 (0.034) | 0.799 (0.104) | 0.308 | 1.632 (0.349) | 0.219 | 0.004 |

**Table 9.4**  Components-of-variance estimates and their percentages (%).

| Analyte | Model | Laboratory | Subject | Residual | Total |
|---|---|---|---|---|---|
| AST | 1 | 0.0634 (41) | 0.0494 (32) | 0.0402 (26) | 0.153 |
|  | 2 | 0.0641 (42) | 0.0441 (29) | 0.0453 (30) | 0.153 |
|  | 3 | 0.0641 (42) | 0.0475 (31) | 0.0407 (27) | 0.152 |
|  | 4 | 0.0641 (42) | 0.0475 (31) | 0.0407 (27) | 0.152 |
| ALT | 1 | 0.0756 (27) | 0.144  (52) | 0.0572 (21) | 0.277 |
|  | 2 | 0.0758 (27) | 0.138  (50) | 0.0622 (23) | 0.276 |
|  | 3 | 0.0756 (27) | 0.143  (52) | 00574 (21) | 0.276 |
|  | 4 | 0.0762 (28) | 0.141  (51) | 0.0580 (21) | 0.275 |
| GGT | 1 | 0.0572 (18) | 0.176  (56) | 0.0818 (26) | 0.316 |
|  | 2 | 0.0569 (18) | 0.174  (55) | 0.0832 (26) | 0.314 |
|  | 3 | 0.0452 (15) | 0.178  (57) | 0.0876 (28) | 0.312 |
|  | 4 | 0.0436 (14) | 0.182  (59) | 0.0831 (27) | 0.308 |
| ALP | 1 | 0.0247 (26) | 0.0591 (63) | 0.0102 (11) | 0.0939 |
|  | 2 | 0.0247 (26) | 0.0590 (63) | 0.0103 (11) | 0.0939 |
|  | 3 | 0.0244 (26) | 0.0600 (64) | 0.0100 (11) | 0.0944 |
|  | 4 | 0.0247 (26) | 0.0601 (64) | 0.0097 (10) | 0.0945 |
| LD | 1 | 0.168  (76) | 0.0215 (10) | 0.0300 (14) | 0.219 |
|  | 2 | 0.170  (77) | 0.0187 (8) | 0.0322 (15) | 0.221 |
|  | 3 | 0.178  (77) | 0.0187 (8) | 0.0334 (15) | 0.230 |
|  | 4 | 0.182  (78) | 0.0182 (8) | 0.0334 (14) | 0.234 |
| Bilirubin | 1 | 0.102  (37) | 0.0867 (31) | 0.0891 (32) | 0.278 |
|  | 2 | 0.102  (37) | 0.0864 (31) | 0.0894 (32) | 0.277 |
|  | 3 | 0.101  (36) | 0.0902 (32) | 0.0873 (31) | 0.270 |
|  | 4 | 0.101  (36) | 0.0909 (33) | 0.0865 (31) | 0.279 |
| Protein | 1 | 0.0502 (18) | 0.118  (43) | 0.1083 (39) | 0.277 |
|  | 2 | 0.0501 (18) | 0.115  (42) | 0.1117 (40) | 0.277 |
|  | 3 | 0.0512 (18) | 0.113  (41) | 0.1124 (41) | 0.277 |
|  | 4 | 0.0512 (18) | 0.113  (41) | 0.1124 (41) | 0.277 |
| Albumin | 1 | 0.0446 (35) | 0.0349 (28) | 0.0466 (37) | 0.126 |
|  | 2 | 0.0427 (34) | 0.0332 (27) | 0.0482 (39) | 0.124 |
|  | 3 | 0.0459 (36) | 0.0331 (26) | 0.0479 (37) | 0.127 |
|  | 4 | 0.0452 (36) | 0.0333 (26) | 0.0478 (38) | 0.126 |

from about 15% to 75% of the total variation. Anyone serious about drug safety should be concerned about this and should be working diligently to remove this analytical variation from drug safety data. For liver tests, this is probably largely due to lack of standardization in assay temperatures and chemical methods, both of which can be fixed, or at least improved, by better protocol standards. The between-subject variation ranges from about 10% to 65% of the total. This is biological population variation that cannot be removed. Unfortunately this variation is large enough to mask liver toxicity signals in a population-based analysis, which is currently the norm. The within-subject (residual) variation accounts for about 10–40% for the total. Over 95% of this variation is an effect of the individual biological system and the rest is measurement error.

Overall, the estimates of $\alpha$ and $\theta$ produced by lme() and nlme() are not very good. Other references, one of which used essentially the same data as are presented here [50], and one which used a completely independent data set [75], were in general agreement on the magnitude of the estimates and gave much smaller estimates of $\alpha$, implying much stronger autocorrelations.

## 9.5.3    OU model applied to reference limits

It is apparent from Table 9.5 that the biological variation is about 50% between-individual and 50% within-individual. By removing the laboratory variation and using individualized statistical methods, it should be possible to improve the sensitivity and specificity of these common liver tests, lessening the need for new and expensive biomarkers. This means that each subject has personal reference limits for detecting toxicity signals, whose calculation may not be straightforward [70].

From equation (9.9), it is obvious that observations taken at short time intervals have relatively narrow reference limits, while those taken at long time intervals expand to an asymptotic boundary and are essentially independent. In this table $\hat{\alpha}$ was taken from [50], Table 3 and the other parameters estimates were taken from Model 3 in Table 9.3 of this chapter. The percentages show that for a one-day follow-up measurement, the interval length is only about one third of the population interval. A seven-day follow-up is still only 90–95% of the population internal. ALP seems to have a much longer time frame for reaching the population limits. These calculations were based on $\gamma = 1$ while the calculations in the other work used $\gamma = 0.5$. The half-life values for the autocorrelation were much longer in the latter case and seemed

**Table 9.5**    Autocorrelation half-life (days) and associated estimates of variation.

| Analyte | $\hat{\alpha}$ | $\hat{t}_{1/2}$ | $\hat{\sigma}_{\varepsilon*}(1)$ | $\hat{\sigma}_{\varepsilon*}(7)$ | $\hat{\sigma}_{\varepsilon*}(28)$ |
|---------|------|------|-----------|-----------|-----------|
| AST | 0.242 | 2.9 | 0.160 (38) | 0.403 (97) | 0.417 (100) |
| ALT | 0.164 | 4.2 | 0.205 (28) | 0.658 (90) | 0.732 (100) |
| GGT | 0.141 | 4.9 | 0.258 (25) | 0.904 (86) | 1.049 (100) |
| ALP | 0.046 | 15.1 | 0.096 (9) | 0.516 (47) | 1.004 (92) |
| LD | 0.192 | 3.6 | 0.152 (32) | 0.444 (93) | 0.477 (100) |
| Bilirubin | 0.195 | 3.6 | 0.244 (32) | 0.707 (93) | 0.756 (100) |
| Protein | 0.199 | 3.5 | 0.276 (33) | 0.790 (94) | 0.842 (100) |
| Albumin | 0.171 | 4.1 | 0.185 (29) | 0.582 (91) | 0.640 (100) |

more realistic. These autocorrelation results suggest that if data are not collected at sufficiently small time intervals, no information is available about the autocorrelation structure. It may also mean that highly correlated data collected too frequently when the autocorrelation is already known may be a waste of money. Overall it appears that the lme()/nlme() functions used in Models 2–4 are not suitable in their present form for OU estimation of $\alpha$ and $\theta$ using clinical laboratory data.

Besides the difficulties in estimating the parameters of the stochastic process, several other problems need to be addressed. The first of these is when parameter estimates (reference limits) from the laboratory should be used. It is customary to use laboratory-supplied reference limits for drug clinical trials. Unfortunately, these can be grossly inadequate both in data source and sample size [56]. When contracting for central laboratory services, it is important to verify the source of reference-limit data and the size of the sample for each limit. If either of these is inadequate, then another laboratory may need to be identified or a solution to improve the estimates may need to be pursued. If these criteria are met and the estimates are based on normal distributions, then an estimate of the population mean and standard deviation can be derived algebraically. The other estimates that the laboratory needs to supply are the analytical variance and bias, if any, for each analytical method. Central laboratories seem to be reluctant to supply these data but a good laboratory should be happy to prove the quality of its work. The key missing, and not readily available, estimates are the cross-correlations and autocorrelations. This is an area where industry needs to contribute, either by sponsoring research or by encouraging the central laboratories to do the work. It is entirely possible that these correlation parameters are laboratory-invariant and may be largely biologically invariant. If this is the case, the work will only need to be done once. However, this will probably require better estimation algorithms for these correlation parameters before spending the money to obtain the estimates.

The next question is which mean should be used for an individual. It is probably not reasonable to use individualized estimates of variance or covariance, due to the difficulty in obtaining enough data to get good estimates. This is entirely consistent with the current use of laboratory-supplied limits. However, the key individualizing parameter besides the time between measurements is the mean of the subject's stochastic process path, otherwise known as the equilibrium fixed point. When electronic health records are readily available, each subject should have a good set of data for estimating his/her mean for each common analyte and maybe the other parameter estimates can come from there as well. Until then we need another approach. Three obvious options are to use the population mean at each evaluation time, use the population mean and apply a Bayesian-type update as additional observations occur for the individual, or use the last observation(s) to compute a sample mean for the individual. The between-individual variance is also important.

Once all the estimation problems have been addressed, how will a toxicity signal be detected? Currently a hepatic toxicity signal occurs when one or more of the liver analytes crosses a boundary such as $3 \times ULN$, which is a population criterion. As said above, a signal occurs when the observed value exceeds the limits of randomness, which is a combination of analytical and biological variation. The most immediate way to detect a signal in an individual is to compare the current observation with the last one. This is equivalent to replacing $\hat{\mu}$ with $Y(s)$ in equation (9.10) and is essentially a test of non-random motion. Sequential methods could be applied here to control the Type I error with an alpha-spending function [68]. Comparison could be made with the baseline observation as well or instead. Another comparison might be where the individual reference limits for the current observation do not overlap the population limits. It may be possible to construct tests for each of the parameters individually or jointly to detect changes over time, but this may have to be a population approach to get enough data for estimation. The same may apply to a measure of acceleration, since an OU model assumes no acceleration.

## 9.6  Summary

In an attempt to improve the statistician's general knowledge of the liver and how it is affected by such drugs, this chapter reviews the biology, chemistry, and pathology of the liver so that this can be a simplified reference for understanding the basis for liver test measurements. Eight liver tests are discussed.

The use of central laboratories in drug clinical trials has helped remove some of the noise in laboratory data by reducing the between-laboratory variability. However, it is evident from the properties reviewed in Section 9.2.3 that many, if not all, of the liver test values decrease over time during transport and storage. This contributes to dampening the liver toxicity signal. With the advent of point-of-care (POC) technology, if every clinical site in a drug protocol or drug project used the same standardized POC device(s), then not only would the between-laboratory variation be reduced but also the stability and storage issues would diminish or disappear, and the lag time between sample collection and the availability of the results to the provider and the sponsor would almost vanish. If a toxicity signal were detected in real time, then the tests could be repeated or samples for toxicity follow-up tests could be obtained with little delay and inconvenience to the investigator or the subject. It may even be feasible for the subjects to have a POC device at home so that toxicity testing frequency could be increased without much additional cost or time consumption. It is also important that the statistician be intimately involved in the choice of laboratory and laboratory methods so that liver safety data can be analyzed in a meaningful way.

With the development of statins and the discovery of acetaminophen toxicity, DILI has become a major safety concern. Unfortunately, the quality and quantity of liver toxicity data are not optimal. DILIN was formed to help alleviate this problem but it is not likely to be enough. It would help if the pharmaceutical industry or the FDA pooled data across drug development programs to address some of the statistical issues presented in this chapter. It is not likely a single company or academic institution can do this alone. The FDA has provided a guidance document for the assessment of pre-marketing liver toxicity, but it suffers from the non-quantitative thinking of the clinical establishment.

Section 9.4 describes some of the current quantitative approaches to the detection of hepatic toxicity signals. Unfortunately, these are rather blunt instruments. The use of the ULN is archaic and helps to obscure the signal. This effect is even worse when a logarithmic transformation is not applied when it is needed. When all clinical decisions were made in the same setting using the same laboratory, the ULN provided a reasonable internally consistent benchmark for accessing the health status of a patient. With multicenter clinical trials and highly mobile patients, who may be accessing an electronic health record from multiple providers at multiple locations using multiple laboratories, these crude measures for probability distributions should be replaced with properly standardized measurements across laboratories and properly derived models and estimators for signal detection and classification.

The OU process is reviewed and proposed as a starting point for liver test modeling in Section 9.5. A good model of liver homeostasis (normalness) is needed before good signal detection algorithms can be proposed and evaluated. Mixed-effects models are used to illustrate how to remove the between-laboratory effects and the between-subject effects. Unfortunately, the particular algorithms used did not provide good estimates of the key OU parameters. More research needs to be done on this estimation problem with better data. Normally this author would be strongly advocating the use of multivariate methods for the analysis of liver tests. However, these ideas have yet to gain traction among clinicians and statisticians. It is probably more important to find the best univariate model that incorporates the autocorrelation before spending too much effort on the cross-correlations.

Hepatic toxicity is a very important issue for the safe use of pharmaceuticals. Currently toxicity signals can be dampened or hidden by lack of laboratory standardization, by shipping and storage of blood samples, by the use of multiples of the ULN, by inadequate protocol designs with respect to liver testing, by the lack of a model for individualized biological dynamic equilibrium, and by the lack of models in laboratory test space for describing liver pathology. All of these issues are complicated and there has been little or no effort to provide satisfactory resolutions. However, these issues need to be resolved for the well-being of patients.

# References

[1] Crawford, J.M. and Chen, L. (2010) Liver and biliary tract, in *Robbins and Cotran Pathologic Basis of Disease*, 8th edn, Chapter 18 (eds V. Kumar, A.K. Abbas, N. Fausto and J. Aster), Saunders, Philadelphia.

[2] Pincus, M.R. and Shaffner, J.A. (1996) Assessment of liver function, in *Clinical Diagnosis and Management by Laboratory Methods*, 19th edn, Chapter 12 (ed J.B. Henry), W. B. Saunders, Philadelphia.

[3] Lindblom, P., Rafter, I., Copley, C. *et al.* (2007) Isoforms of alanine aminotransferases in human tissues and serum – Differential tissue expression using novel antibodies. *Archives of Biochemistry and Biophysics*, **466**, 66–77.

[4] Trost, D.C. and Freston, J.W. (2008) Vector analysis to detect hepatotoxicity signals in drug development. *Drug Information Journal*, **42**, 27–34.

[5] Roberts, R.A., Ganey, P.E., Ju, C. *et al.* (2007) Role of the Kupffer cell in mediating hepatic toxicity and carcinogenesis. *Toxicological Sciences*, **96**, 2–15.

[6] Garcia-Tsao, G. (2012) Cirrhosis and its sequelae, in *Goldman's Cecil Medicine*, 24th edn, Chapter 156 (eds L. Goldman and A.I. Schafer), Elsevier Saunders, Philadelphia.

[7] Wedemeyer, H. and Pawlotsky, J.M. (2012) Acute viral hepatitis, in *Goldman's Cecil Medicine*, 24th edn, Chapter 150 (eds L. Goldman and A.I. Schafer), Elsevier Saunders, Philadelphia.

[8] Pawlotsky, J.M. and McHutchison, J. (2012) Chronic viral and autoimmune hepatitis, in *Goldman's Cecil*, 24th edn, Chapter 151 (eds L. Goldman and A.I. Schafer), Elsevier Saunders, Philadelphia.

[9] Ghany, M. and Hoofnagle, J.H. (2012) Approach to the patient with liver disease, in *Harrison's Principles of Internal Medicine*, 18th edn, Chapter 301 (eds D.L. Longo, A.S. Fauci, S.L. Hauser *et al.*), McGraw-Hill, New York.

[10] Henry, J.B. (1996) *Clinical Diagnosis and Management by Laboratory Methods*, 19th edn, W. B. Saunders, Philadelphia.

[11] Bacon, B.R. (2012) Inherited and metabolic disorders of the liver, in *Goldman's Cecil Medicine*, Chapter 153 (eds L. Goldman and A.I. Schafer), Elsevier Saunders, Philadelphia.

[12] Powell, L.W., Leggett, B.A. and Crawford, D.H.G. (1999) Hemochromatosis and other iron storage disorders, in *Shiff's Diseases of the Liver*, 8th edn, Chapter 44 (eds E.R. Schiff, M.F. Sorrell and W.C. Maddrey), Lippincott Williams & Wilkins, Philadelphia.

[13] Perlmutter, D.H. (1999) Alpha-1-antitrypsin deficiency, in *Shiff's Diseases of the Liver*, 8th edn, Chapter 45 (eds E.R. Schiff, M.F. Sorrell and W.C. Maddrey), Lippincott Williams & Wilkins, Philadelphia.

[14] Kyle, R.A. and Gertz, M.A. (1999) Amyloidosis of the liver, in *Shiff's Diseases of the Liver*, 8th edn, Chapter 49 (eds E.R. Schiff, M.F. Sorrell and W.C. Maddrey), Lippincott Williams & Wilkins, Philadelphia.

[15] Moyer, K.D. and Balistreri, W.F. (2011) Liver disease associated with systemic disorders, in *Nelson Textbook of Pediatrics*, 19th edn, Chapter 352 (eds R.M. Kleigman, J.W. Stanton, J.W. St Geme *et al.*), Elsevier Saunders, Philadelphia.

[16] Afdhal, N.H. (2012) Diseases of the gallbladder and bile ducts, in *Goldman's Cecil Medicine*, 24th edn, Chapter 158 (eds L. Goldman and A.I. Schafer), Elsevier Saunders, Philadelphia.

[17] Polson, J. and Lee, W.M. (2005) AASLD position paper: the management of acute liver failure. *Hepatology*, **41**, 1179–1197.

[18] Keeffe, E.G. (2012) Hepatic failure and liver transplantation, in *Goldman's Cecil Medicine*, 24th edn, Chapter 157 (eds L. Goldman and A.I. Schafer), Elsevier Saunders, Philadelphia.

[19] O'Grady, J.G., Alexander, G.J.M., Hyllar, K.M. *et al.* (1989) Early indicators of prognosis in fulminant hepatic failure. *Gastroenterology*, **97**, 439–445.

[20] Krebs, H.A. (1950) Chemical composition of blood plasma and serum. *Annual Review of Biochemistry*, **19**, 409–430.

[21] Moss, D.W. and Henderson, A.R. (1999) Clincal enzymology, in *Tietz Textbook of Clinical Chemistry*, Chapter 22 (eds C.A. Burtis and E.R. Ashwood), W. B. Saunders, Philadelphia.

[22] Pincus, M.R., Zimmerman, H.J. and Henry, J.B. (1996) Clinical enzymology, in *Clinical Diagnosis and Management by Laboratory Methods*, 19th edn, Chapter 12 (ed J.B. Henry), W. B. Saunders, Philadelphia.

[23] Tietz, N.W. (1995) *Clincal Guide to Laboratory Tests*, 3th edn, W. B. Saunders, Philadelphia.

[24] Tolman, K.G. and Rej, R. (1999) Liver function, in *Shiff's Diseases of the Liver*, 8th edn, Chapter 33 (eds E.R. Schiff, M.F. Sorrell and W.C. Maddrey), Lippincott Williams & Wilkins, Philadelphia.

[25] Johnson, A.M., Rohlfs, E.M. and Silverman, L.M. (1999) Proteins, in *Tietz Textbook of Clinical Chemistry*, Chapter 20 (eds C.A. Burtis and E.R. Ashwood), W. B. Saunders, Philadelphia.

[26] Trost, D.C., Hu, M., Brailey, A.G. and Hoffman, J.M. (2002) Probability-based construction of reference ranges for ratios of log-Gaussian analytes. *American Journal of Clinical Pathology*, **117**, 851–856.

[27] Poller, L. (2004) International normalized ratios (INR): the first 20 years. *Journal of Thrombosis and Haemostatis*, **2**, 849–860.

[28] Zimmerman, H.J. (1999) *The Adverse Effects of Drugs and Other Chemicals on the Liver*, 2nd edn, Lippincott Williams & Wilkins, Philadelphia.

[29] Bernal, W. (2003) Changing patterns of causation and the use of transplantation in the United Kingdom. *Seminars in Liver Disease*, **23**, 227–237.

[30] Lee, W.M. (2000) Drugs and acute liver failure, in *New Directions in Drug-Induced Liver Injury: Mechanisms and Test Systems*, National Institutes of Health, Bethesda, MD.

[31] Lee, W.M. (2003) Acute liver failure in the United States. *Seminars in Liver Disease*, **23**, 217–225.

[32] U.S. Food and Drug Administration FDA Drug Safety Communication: Prescription Acetaminophen Products to be Limited to 325 mg Per Dosage unit, Boxed Warning Will Highlight Potential for Severe Liver Failure, U.S. Food and Drug Administration, http://www.fda.gov /Drugs/DrugSafety/ucm239821.htm (accessed 24 June 2014).

[33] Lee, W.M. (2003) Drug-induced hepatotoxicity. *New England Journal of Medicine*, **349**, 474–485.

[34] Abboud, G. and Kaplowitz, N. (2007) Drug-induced liver injury. *Drug Safety*, **30**, 277–294.

[35] Senior, J.R. (2009) Monitoring for hepatotoxicity: what is the predictive value of liver "function" tests? *Clinical Pharmacology and Therapeutics*, **85**, 331–334.

[36] Suzuki, A., Andrade, R.J., Bjornsson, E. *et al.* (2010) Drugs associated with hepatotoxicity and their reporting frequency of liver adverse events in VigiBase. *Drug Safety*, **33**, 503–522.

[37] U.S. Food and Drug Administration Drug-induced Liver Injury: Premarketing Clinical Evaluation, U.S.Food and Drug Administration, http://www.fda.gov/downloads/Drugs /GuidanceComplianceRegulatoryInformation/Guidances/ucm174090.pdf (accessed 24 June 2014).

[38] Watkins, P.G., Seligman, P.J., Pears, J.S. *et al.* (2008) Using controlled clinical trials to learn more about acute drug-induced liver injury. *Hepatology*, **48**, 1680–1689.

[39] Fontana, R.J., Watkins, P.B., Bonkovsky, H.L. *et al.* (2009) Drug-induced liver injury network (DILIN) prospective study. *Drug Safety*, **32**, 55–68.

[40] Zimmerman, H.J. (1999) Drug-induced liver disease, in *Shiff's Diseases of the Liver*, 8th edn, Chapter 40 (eds E.R. Schiff, M.F. Sorrell and W.C. Maddrey), Lippincott Williams & Wilkins, Philadelphia.

[41] Wanless, R. (1999) Physioanatomic considerations, in *Shiff's Diseases of the Liver*, 8th edn, Chapter 1 (eds E.R. Schiff, M.F. Sorrell and W.C. Maddrey), Lippincott Williams & Wilkins, Philadelphia.

[42] Chalasani, N.P. (2012) Alcoholic and nonalcoholic steatohepatitis, in *Goldman's Cecil Medicine*, 24th edn, Chapter 155 (eds L. Goldman and A.I. Schafer), Elsevier Saunders, Philadelphia.

[43] Tandra, S., Yh, M.M., Brunt, E.M. *et al.* (2011) Presence and significance of microvesicular steatosis in nonalcoholic fatty liver disease. *Hepatology*, **55**, 654–659.

[44] Kaplowitz, N. (2005) Idiosyncratic drug hepatotoxicity. *Drug Discovery*, **4**, 489–499.

[45] Lee, W.M. (2012) Toxin- and drug-induced liver disease, in *Goldman's Cecil Medicine*, 24th edn, Chapter 152 (eds L. Goldman and A.I. Schafer), Elsevier Saunders, Philadelphia.

[46] Amacher, D.E. (2010) The discovery and development of proteomic safety biomarkers for the detection of drug-induced liver toxicity. *Toxicology and Applied Pharmacology*, **245**, 134–142.

[47] Davis, C.E. (1976) The effect of regression to the mean in epidemiologic and clinical studies. *American Journal of Epidemiology*, **104**, 493–498.

[48] Bond, G.R., Ho, M. and Woodward, R.W. (2012) Trends in hepatic injury associated with unintentional overdose of paracetamol (acetaminophen) in products with and without opioid. *Drug Safety*, **35**, 149–157.

[49] Schildcrout, J.S., Jenkins, C.A., Ostroff, J.H. *et al.* (2008) Analysis of longitudinal laboratory data in the presence of common selection mechanisms: a view toward greater emphasis on pre-marketing pharmaceutical safety. *Statistics in Medicine*, **27**, 2248–2266.

[50] Trost, D.C., Overman, E.A., Ostroff, J.H. *et al.* (2010) A model for liver homeostasis using modified mean-reverting Ornstein-Uhlenbeck process. *Computational and Mathematical Methods in Medicine*, **11**, 27–47.

[51] R Development Core Team (2014) *R: A Language and Environment for Statistical Computing*, http://www.R-project.org, Vienna, R Foundation for Statistical Computing.

[52] Sarkar, D. (2008) *Lattice: Multivariate Data Visualization with R*, Springer, New York. The reference manual for the use of the lattice graphical display system implemented in R.

[53] International FEDERATION of Clinical Chemistry and the International Committee for Standardization in Haematology (1986) Approved recommendations on the theory of reference values. Part 1. The concept of reference values. *Journal of Clinical Chemistry and Clinical Biochemistry*, **25**, 337–342.

[54] Boyd, J.C. and Lacher, D.A. (1982) The multivariate reference range: an alternative interpretation of multi-test profiles. *Clinical Chemistry*, **28**, 259–265.

[55] Solberg, H.E. (1983) The theory of reference values. Part 5. Statistical treatment of collected reference values: determination of reference limits. *Journal of Clinical Chemistry and Clinical Biochemistry*, **21**, 749–760.

[56] Trost, D.C. (2006) Multivariate probability-based detection of drug-induced hepatic signals. *Toxicological Reviews*, **25**, 37–54.

[57] Chew, V. (1966) Confidence, prediction, and tolerance regions for the multivariate normal distribution. *Journal of the American Statistical Association*, **61**, 605–617.

[58] Wellek, S. (2011) On easily interpretable multivariate reference regions of rectangular shape. *Biometrical Journal*, **53**, 491–511.

[59] Anderson, T.W. (1984) *An Introduction to Multivariate Statistical Analysis*, 2nd edn, John Wiley & Sons, Inc., New York.

[60] Huang, J.-Y., Chen, L.-A. and Welsh, A.H. (2010) A note on reference limits, in *Nonparametrics and Robustness in Modern Statistical Inference and Time Series Analysis: A Festschrift in Honor of Professor Jana Jurečková* (eds J. Antoch, M. Huskova and P.K. Sen), Institute of Mathematical Statistics, Beachwood, OH.

[61] Lipid Research Clinics Program (1984) The Lipid Research Clinics Coronary Primary Prevention Trial results I: Reduction in incidence of coronary heart disease. *Journal of the American Medical Association*, **251**, 351–364.

[62] Lipid Research Clinics Program (1984) The Lipid Research Clinics Coronary Primary Prevention Trial results II: The relationship of reduction in incidence of coronary heart disease to cholesterol lowering. *Journal of the American Medical Association*, **251**, 365–374.

[63] Seeff, L.B. (2000) Hyman J. Zimmerman, MD – obituary. *Journal of the American Medical Association*, **283**, 812–812.

[64] Watkins, P.B., Desai, M., Berkowitz, S.D. *et al.* (2011) Evaluation of drug-induced serious hepatotoxicity (eDISH): Application of this data organization approach to Phase III clinical trials of rivaroxaban after total hip or knee replacement surgery. *Drug Safety*, **34**, 243–252.

[65] Durrett, R. (1996) *Stochastic Calculus*, CRC Press, Boca Raton, FL.

[66] Karatzas, I. and Shreve, S.E. (1991) *Brownian Motion and Stochastic Calculus*, 2nd edn, Springer, New York.

[67] Oksendal, B. (2000) *Stochastic Differential Equations: An Introduction with Applications*, 5th edn, Springer, New York.

[68] Proschan, M.A., Lan, K.K.G. and Wittes, J. (2006) *Statistical Monitoring of Clinical Trials*, Springer, New York.

[69] Brockwell, P.J. and Davis, R.A. (1991) *Time Series: Theory and Methods*, Springer-Verlag, New York.

[70] Solberg, H.E. (1995) Subject-based reference values. *Scandinavian Journal of Clinical Laboratory Investigation*, **55**, 7–10.

[71] Bar-Shalom, Y., Li, X.-R. and Kirubarajan, T. (2001) *Estimation with Applications to Tracking and Navigation*, John Wiley & Sons, Inc., New York.

[72] Gajic, Z. (2003) *Linear Dynamic Systems and Signals*, Pearson Education, Upper Saddle River, NJ.

[73] Oravecz, Z. and Tuerlinckx, F. (2011) The linear mixed model and the hierarchical Ornstein–Uhlenbeck model: some equivalences and differences. *British Journal of Mathematical and Statistical Psychology*, **64**, 134–160.

[74] Pinheiro, J., Bates, D., DebRoy, S., and Sarkar, D. (2013) nlme: Linear and Nonlinear Mixed Effects Models. R package version 3.1-117., http://cran.r-project.org/package=nlme

[75] Rosenkranz, G.K. (2009) Modeling laboratory data from clinical trials. *Computational Statistics and Data Analysis*, **53**, 812–819.

# 10

# Neurotoxicity

## A. Lawrence Gould
*Merck Research Laboratories, 770 Sumneytown Pike, West Point, PA, 19486, USA*

## 10.1    Introduction

Neurotoxic events, which can be biochemical, anatomical, physiological, or behavioral, reflect adverse effects on the structure or function of the central or peripheral nervous system following exposure to a chemical, physical, or biological agent [1, 2]. Neurobehavioral effects include adverse changes in somatic/autonomic, sensory, motor, or cognitive function. They can be reversible or irreversible. However, even reversible effects can reflect damage to the organism [3].

The potential neurotoxicity of a compound can be evaluated in various ways. The general term "neurotoxicity" applies here to any event affecting neurological function, including effects on behavior, neurochemistry, neurophysiology, and neuropathology. At a basic level, treatments in a clinical trial or in a designed experiment can be compared with respect to the incidence of neurological signs and symptoms, including the timing, frequency of recurrence, or intensity of the reported or observed events. The assessment of this information proceeds for neurological events as for any other class of adverse events as described elsewhere in this book, so is not pursued further here.

Potential neurotoxicity can be evaluated at other than basic levels. Neurotoxicity screening can be based on a battery of measurements and observations such as the functional observational battery that has been in use for a number of years [4]. Many, if not most, of the elements of this (and similar) batteries would be especially appropriate to preclinical evaluations carried out in animals in the early stages of product development for determining maximum tolerable doses, or for screening potentially toxic chemicals from an environmental perspective. We

*Statistical Methods for Evaluating Safety in Medical Product Development*, First Edition.
Edited by A. Lawrence Gould.
© 2015 John Wiley & Sons, Ltd. Published 2015 by John Wiley & Sons, Ltd.

focus here (Section 10.2) on statistical methods for assessing this information, which generally consists of sequences of multivariate measurements over time, taking account of possible dose effects and evolution of risk with exposure.

Electroencephalograms (EEGs) that provide a picture of the brain's electrical activity present yet another level of complexity. These measurements provide the possibility of detecting subtle changes in neurological function soon enough to identify and address potential toxicity before it becomes disabling or irreversible. EEG data present important challenges for the analyst, including multiplicity, data complexity and volume, and contamination of electrical signals by artifacts such as eye movement. Methods for analyzing EEG data comprise examples of a more general class of methods falling under the paradigm of functional data analysis.

This chapter outlines briefly some statistical approaches that may be useful for the evaluation of neurological toxicity, especially as manifested in changes in EEG recordings, in the context of clinical trials. Although there is a substantial literature on ways to analyze EEG recordings, not all of these currently lend themselves to "routine" application of data from clinical trials, typically because of the lack of readily available software for carrying out complex calculations, and the difficulty in communicating the clinical meaning and implication of differences between treatment groups that the calculations may reveal. Consequently, the focus here is on methods that can be implemented in a practical way for "routine" evaluation of neurotoxicity assessments obtained in the course of clinical trials. The volume and complexity of the data used for neurological assessments preclude including specific worked-out examples here, although details are provided in the publications describing the particular methods. The software used for the calculations is either very specialized or fairly routine, so specific code (with some exceptions) is also not provided.

## 10.2   Multivariate longitudinal observations

Zhu [5, 6] describes a family of nonlinear mixed effect models for expressing the effects of exposure (or dose), time, and other covariates included in a neurotoxicity panel. The covariates can be continuous, categorical, or binary. The objective is to characterize the longitudinal effects of exposure on outcome more precisely than conventional methods that employ simple longitudinal analyses of variance. This approach clearly is not limited to the exploration of neurotoxicity, but can be applied to any collection of measurements expressing aspects of toxicity. The family of mathematical functions considered for modeling is defined by the relationship

$$h(d,t) = A(t) + f(d,t), \tag{10.1}$$

where $h(d,t)$ is the expected value of the neurological outcome at time $t$ for subjects having exposure $d$. The component $A(t)$ describes the spontaneous longitudinal trajectory if there is no exposure, that is, a reference trajectory for a control group. As a matter of convention, the "baseline" state is represented by the value of $A(0)$, which can be used to adjust for marginal individual effects. If the time span for the trial or experiment is relatively short, then $A(t)$ should be representable by a simple polynomial or some other simple relationship. The second component, $f(d,t)$, represents the effect of the initial exposure intensity and duration of observation. Since these effects can be assumed absent at the outset of observation before the exposure, this component satisfies the restriction

$$f(0,t) = f(d,0) = 0.$$

The development in [5] focuses on functions $f(d,t)$ of the form

$$f(d,t) = \frac{tB(d,t)}{1 + tC(d,t)} \,. \tag{10.2}$$

These are similar to Michaelis–Menten functions except that the functions $B$ and $C$ can depend on time and exposure. A toxico-diffusion model based on one-compartment kinetics is a particular example of equation (10.2),

$$f(d,t) = \frac{tdB\,e^{-K_e t}}{1 + tdCe^{-K_e t}} \,. \tag{10.3}$$

The parameters $B$ and $C$ can depend on attributes other than exposure and time of observation, at least in principle, although this possibility is not addressed directly in [5]. The function $f(d,t)$ in (10.3) reaches its maximum value (peak effect) at time $t_{PE} = 1/K_e$, usually referred to as the time of peak effect (TOPE) that is independent of the exposure $d$. Special cases of (10.3) include the linear-exponential model obtained by setting $C = 0$ and the complementary-exponential model obtained by replacing $(1 + tdCe^{-K_e t})^{-1}$ with a first-order Maclaurin expansion of $(1 + tdCe^{-K_e t})^{-1}$ with respect to $d$. Another variation is a diffusion model,

$$f(d,t) = \frac{Bdt}{1 + t^r e^{dC}} \,,$$

whose TOPE depends on the exposure $d$,

$$t_{PE} = \left( \frac{e^{-dC}}{r-1} \right)^{-1} .$$

Models with $r > 1$ describe transient events because the effect of exposure diminishes as the duration increases. Models with $r < 1$ do not have a positive TOPE, so that the effect of the exposure increases with time.

Random effects can be incorporated in a natural way, which Zhu [5] illustrates in terms of model (10.3). More specifically, suppose that $Y_{ij}$ represents the observation of subject $i$ at occasion $j$, and that

$$Y_{ij} = \mu(\mathbf{x}_{ij}, \boldsymbol{\theta}_i) + \varepsilon_{ij} \,, \tag{10.4}$$

where $\boldsymbol{\theta}_i$ denotes a vector of fixed and subject-specific (random) parameters,

$$\boldsymbol{\theta}_i = \mathbf{A}_i \boldsymbol{\beta} + \mathbf{B}_i \mathbf{b}_i \,,$$

where $\mathbf{A}_i$ and $\mathbf{B}_i$ are design matrices, $\boldsymbol{\beta}$ denotes the "fixed" effects that are the same for all subjects at all times, $\mathbf{b}_i$ denotes subject-specific random components, $\mathbf{x}_{ij}$ denotes a vector of covariates (typically time and exposure level), and $\varepsilon_{ij}$ denotes random measurement error.

A mixed-effects version of (10.3) therefore might be

$$\mu(\mathbf{x}_{ij}, \boldsymbol{\theta}_i) = A + a_i + \frac{t_{ij} d_{ij} (B + b_i)\, e^{-K_e t_{ij}}}{1 + t_{ij} d_{ij} C e^{-K_e t_{ij}}} \,, \tag{10.5}$$

assuming scalar parameters and allowing for exposure to change with time. If the exposures do not change with time, then $d_{ij}$ would be replaced with $d_i$, the exposure (dose) administered to the $i$th individual. The analysis can be carried out using conventional methods for nonlinear mixed-effects models, for which software is readily available, for example, the nlme package in the R system [7] or the NLMIXED procedure in SAS®. The random effects to include in the model need to be chosen judiciously: too many random effects can lead to excessive inter-correlation, especially when parameters really are nearly the same for all subjects. Different models can be fitted to a set of data to ascertain where subject-specific variation of parameters would be appropriate and where constant parameter values would be adequate.

Expression (10.4) would be appropriate for continuous outcomes, possibly after a transformation so that, for example, $Y_{ij}$ could denote the logarithm of the quantities actually observed. Expression (10.5) also can be used for categorical and mixed models by using generalized mixed models. For example, if the response is binary, then one might define $\mu(\mathbf{x}_{ij}, \boldsymbol{\theta}_i)$ as the logit of the true event rate corresponding to the observation at time $j$ on subject $i$. The actual likelihood for the data would be binomial with the true event rates as the parameters; standard methods could be used in this case as well. Software for carrying out the calculations is available both in the R system [8–11] and via the NLMIXED and GLIMMIX procedures in SAS®. Also, at least in principle, model (10.5) could be extended to vector outcomes by making the various parameters vectors instead of scalars, and recognizing that the residual error $\varepsilon_{ij}$ in (10.4) is a vector with possibly correlated components.

The calculations can be carried out using Bayesian methods without assuming normality or asymptotic properties, although this is not described in [5], nor does it appear to have been described explicitly elsewhere. The likelihood for any of the models considered here can be written out explicitly, and incorporation of the random effects is straightforward. For example, the following OpenBUGS [12] code fragment could be used to carry out the Markov chain Monte Carlo (MCMC) calculations for model (10.5). This code fragment assumes that values of the $A$ and $C$ parameters must be positive, so parameterizes the model in terms of their logarithms. This example uses one mathematical definition of the expected response, but other definitions can be accommodated by suitably modifying the code.

```
A <- exp(log.A)
C <- exp(log.C)
Ke <- exp(log.Ke)
for (j in (1:ntimes)) { xtime[j] <- time[j]*exp(-Ke*time[j])
for (i in (1:nsub))
{                                           # likelihood
  log(a[i]) ~ dnorm(log.A,tau.A)
  log(b[i]) ~ dnorm(log.B,tau.B)
  for (j in 1:ntimes)
  {
    x[i,j] <- xtime[j]*dose[i]                # One of a number of
    mu[i,j] <- a[i] + (x[i,j]*b[i])/(1+C*x[i,j])  # possible model
    y[i,j] ~ dnorm(mu[i,j],tau.eps)           # definitions.
  }
}
}
```

The values of $A$, $B$, $C$, and $K_e$ are "population" values. The random effects are $a$ and $b$ (suitably subscripted). The parameters do not have to have normal distributions; central $t$

distributions could be used to allow for heavier tails than the normal distribution provides. The distributions do not have to be symmetric, either, but the log transformation often will lead to symmetric distributions. A hierarchy of submodels can be obtained by omitting some of the random effects and using the "population" values instead, and judgments about the necessity of any of the random effects can be based on the divergence information criterion that the software provides. The MCMC software produces a set of realizations from the joint posterior distribution of all of the parameters. Depending on additional code steps, it also can produce realizations of functions of the parameters, and predictions about outcomes from future subjects.

Zhu [5] compared the effects of fitting various models to data on the effect of various doses of a neurotoxic agent, triethyltin (TET), on hindlimb grip strength of rats and found for those data that a model like (10.5) with a random intercept (the $a_i$) provided the best fit. However, Figure 3a from that paper suggests that a simpler model may work as well. In particular, consider the following model for a rat's change in grip strength from baseline:

$$Y_{ij} = \mathbf{x}_i'\mathbf{d} + a_1 \log(t_j) + a_2 \log (t_j)^2 + \alpha_i + \varepsilon_{ij} , \qquad (10.6)$$

where $\mathbf{d}$ denotes effects corresponding to the dosages used (0, 0.75, 1.5, 3, and 6 mg/kg), $\mathbf{x}_i = (x_{i1}, \ldots, x_{i5})'$ with $x_{ik} = 1$ if rat $i$ received dose $k$, $\alpha_i$ is the effect of rat $i$, and $t_j$ is the hour at which the measurement is made. The terms involving log $(t_i)$ are omitted for the baseline observations, corresponding to hour 0. Alternatively, one could model each rat's change from baseline. The analysis using both approaches is easy, and illustrated below. This model separates the effects of dosage and time, so that the zero dosage group could have a non-zero trajectory of change values. Separate effects are fit for each dosage, like in a conventional ANOVA model. The model includes a random rat effect to capture the intraclass correlation due to the fact that repeated measurements were made on each rat. Table 10.1 provides digitized hindlimb grip strength values of rats following a single exposure to one of five doses of TET from [5, Figure 4]. Appendix 10.A provides OpenBUGS [12] code for the calculations.

The results of the analysis are displayed in Table 10.2 and Figure 10.1. The message conveyed seems fairly clear, at least for these data: grip strength decreases as dosage increases, the effect increases initially, then resolves eventually, although perhaps not as quickly in the highest dose.

The data that motivated the development in [5] consist of a collection of outcomes that are analyzed separately. This raises an issue of interpretation that, unfortunately, remains even if multivariate analyses are carried out, namely what the findings based on the analyses of a collection of outcomes say about potential neurotoxicity. This is the same issue as the interpretation of safety implications from a collection of comparisons of adverse event reports among treatments groups, and can be addressed in the same way by categorizing the components of the screening panel as "Tier 1" or "Tier 2" (see Chapter 11 for further details).

## 10.3   Electroencephalograms (EEGs)

### 10.3.1   Special considerations

EEGs are recordings of the electrical activity of the brain detected by a set of electrodes (channels) applied to a subject's or patient's scalp. Clinical and pharmacologic applications of EEGs

**Table 10.1**  Hindlimb grip strength of rats (kg) following a single exposure to TET (digitized from Figure 4 of [5]).

| Dose (mg/kg) | Hour | Rat 1 | Rat 2 | Rat 3 | Rat 4 | Rat 5 | Rat 6 | Rat 7 | Rat 8 | Rat 9 | Rat 10 |
|---|---|---|---|---|---|---|---|---|---|---|---|
| 0 | 0 | 0.69 | 0.78 | 0.80 | 0.81 | 0.82 | 0.91 | 1.01 | 1.02 | 1.14 | 1.16 |
|  | 2 | 1.14 | 0.74 | 0.85 | 1.09 | 0.91 | 1.03 | 1.39 | 1.35 | 0.76 | 0.77 |
|  | 24 | 1.03 | 0.45 | 0.87 | 0.88 | 0.69 | 0.93 | 0.87 | 0.96 | 1.02 | 0.78 |
|  | 168 | 1.02 | 0.60 | 0.76 | 1.25 | 1.12 | 0.93 | 0.59 | 0.90 | 0.83 | 0.91 |
| 0.75 | 0 | 0.83 | 0.83 | 0.83 | 0.93 | 0.96 | 0.96 | 0.97 | 1.01 | 1.04 | 1.27 |
|  | 2 | 0.61 | 0.61 | 0.91 | 1.14 | 1.07 | 0.81 | 0.76 | 0.50 | 0.70 | 0.89 |
|  | 24 | 0.68 | 0.66 | 0.87 | 0.97 | 0.67 | 0.80 | 0.82 | 1.05 | 0.68 | 0.80 |
|  | 168 | 0.99 | 0.74 | 0.79 | 0.86 | 0.74 | 0.73 | 0.79 | 0.99 | 0.78 | 1.01 |
| 1.5 | 0 | 0.58 | 0.77 | 0.82 | 0.83 | 0.85 | 0.88 | 0.88 | 0.95 | 1.01 | 1.06 |
|  | 2 | 0.39 | 0.70 | 0.66 | 0.50 | 0.78 | 0.85 | 0.33 | 0.63 | 0.73 | 0.69 |
|  | 24 | 0.43 | 0.52 | 0.77 | 0.38 | 0.77 | 0.70 | 0.42 | 0.59 | 0.76 | 0.81 |
|  | 168 | 0.63 | 0.77 | 0.84 | 0.93 | 1.02 | 0.67 | 0.50 | 0.73 | 0.77 | 0.61 |
| 3 | 0 | 0.48 | 0.65 | 0.67 | 0.68 | 0.76 | 0.78 | 0.81 | 0.88 | 1.03 | 1.06 |
|  | 2 | 0.46 | 0.35 | 0.32 | 0.54 | 0.50 | 0.62 | 0.54 | 0.65 | 0.47 | 0.60 |
|  | 24 | 0.65 | 0.54 | 0.54 | 0.48 | 0.64 | 0.57 | 0.64 | 0.59 | 0.43 | 0.61 |
|  | 168 | 0.82 | 0.76 | 0.78 | 0.68 | 0.83 | 0.66 | 0.64 | 0.76 | 0.88 | 1.39 |
| 6 | 0 | 0.57 | 0.62 | 0.71 | 0.84 | 0.85 | 0.87 | 0.96 | 0.98 | 1.06 | 1.10 |
|  | 2 | 0.35 | 0.72 | 0.48 | 0.34 | 0.52 | 0.45 | 0.40 | 0.40 | 0.48 | 0.46 |
|  | 24 | 0.35 | 0.50 | 0.55 | 0.37 | 0.52 | 0.39 | 0.46 | 0.35 | 0.55 | 0.53 |
|  | 168 | 0.56 | 0.81 | 0.32 | 0.30 | 0.67 | 0.48 | 0.30 | 0.30 | 0.32 | 0.50 |

**Table 10.2**  Medians and 95% credible intervals for the parameters in model (10.6) applied to the data in Table 10.1.

| Parameter | Actual values | | | Changes from baseline | | |
|---|---|---|---|---|---|---|
|  | LB | Median | UB | LB | Median | UB |
| $E(\alpha_i)$ | 0.93 | 1.00 | 1.08 | −0.12 | 0.01 | 0.14 |
| $sd(\alpha_i)$ | 0.004 | 0.05 | 0.09 | 0.12 | 0.16 | 0.21 |
| $d_{0.75}$ | −0.15 | −0.06 | 0.03 | −0.31 | −0.14 | 0.03 |
| $d_{1.5}$ | −0.29 | −0.20 | −0.11 | −0.36 | −0.20 | −0.03 |
| $d_3$ | −0.33 | −0.24 | −0.16 | −0.31 | −0.14 | 0.02 |
| $d_6$ | −0.45 | −0.35 | −0.27 | −0.56 | −0.39 | −0.23 |
| $a_1$ | −0.20 | −0.15 | −0.10 | −0.12 | −0.06 | 0.01 |
| $a_2$ | 0.02 | 0.03 | 0.04 | 0.001 | 0.01 | 0.02 |
| $sd(\varepsilon_{ij})$ | 0.16 | 0.17 | 0.20 | 0.14 | 0.16 | 0.18 |

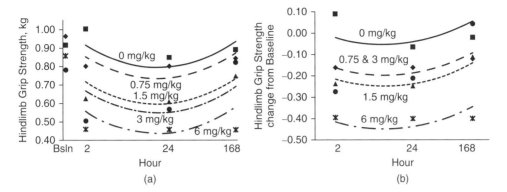

**Figure 10.1**   (a) Observed mean values and (b) changes from baseline of hindlimb grip strength at each time for rates treated with single doses of TET at various concentrations, along with fitted trajectories of a simple mixed effects longitudinal model expressing grip strength as a quadratic function of log hour.

have been studied since their description by Berger over 80 years ago (5 years after his initial discovery) [13]. Pharmaco-EEG is concerned with the evaluation of drug-induced effects on human EEGs, and arose as a scientific discipline about 60 years ago. Research findings since then have suggested that EEGs could be valuable central nervous system biomarkers, and could be useful for assessing pharmacodynamic effects following administration of drugs typically targeted toward the nervous system.

EEG recording durations vary from a few minutes to hours. Recordings may be made under various conditions, for example, following some intervention or event (such as a seizure), or during sleep. The data from an individual's EEG recording session, of which there may be more than one, consist of a collection of time series (or, alternatively, of a time series whose realization at any time point is a vector) that may or may not be stationary and, in practice, include perturbations due to artifacts caused (for example) by contractions of periorbital or scalp muscles.

Each EEG record consists of many numbers. The EEG data from a clinical trial consist of recordings from several recording sessions conducted during each of several periods or visits by each patient in the trial that together generate tens of gigabytes of numbers because each recording contains signals from several EEG channels containing thousands of numbers recorded over minutes or hours, at different brain locations. EEG data for a trial consequently are very voluminous, so that processing and analyzing EEG recordings historically has been computationally intensive and expensive. However, the increasing availability of inexpensive hardware and the development of signal processing methods for processing EEG data, combined with the non-invasive nature of EEGs and their simplicity of implementation, have made EEGs increasingly attractive as a component of the clinical development process. This is important because routine reduction of the thousands of numbers in each EEG channel by sophisticated signal processing methods to one, or a few, values is necessary to make EEGs practical as a means of evaluating neurotoxicity on a large scale [14, 15].

Key issues for EEG analyses include data reduction, accounting for potential correlations across time and among channels, and non-stationarity. Data reduction leads to metrics that are functions of the EEG series such as power within specific frequency ranges, measures of fractal properties from a nonlinear dynamic expression of the EEGs, or parameters of hierarchical statistical models for the EEGs allowing for the possibility of time-dependent covariance structures.

The complexities arising from the presence of multiple channels can be handled in different ways. The expected value of the reduced metric corresponding to each channel can be expressed as a function of the spatial position of the corresponding electrodes [16]. Alternatively, the entire suite of measurements can be analyzed as a multivariate time series using models that explicitly incorporate covariances among channels and among time points [17–22]. Reducing the time series to a manageable number of biologically meaningful focuses the analyses on the important biological questions.

Quantitative EEG information has been used to obtain clinical insight. For example, Hornero *et al.* compared various metrics based on nonlinear methods applied to EEGs and MEGs (magnetoencephalograms) with respect to their ability to distinguish between 11 normal patients and 11 patients with Alzheimer's disease and found that measures of entropy that did not require stationarity could in fact distinguish between the two kinds of patients [23]. As another example, brain symmetry indices that are functions of standardized ratios of differences between the power spectra of corresponding channels on the left and on the right side of the head have been shown in limited sets of patients to be reproducible measures of differences of electrical activity between the two sides of the brain that correlate with clinical severity of acute ischemic stroke [24, 25]. Metrics derived from EEGs also may be useful for detecting potentially elevated stroke risk [26] and as additional regressors may improve the accuracy of logistic models for identifying dementia and mild cognitive impairment [27].

All (or most) analysis strategies start by applying conventional signal processing techniques to remove perturbations and other recognizable discrete influences. The subsequent analyses become simpler if the refined series is stationary, or nearly so. Stationary series can be described as weighted sums of sine waves corresponding to various frequencies and can be summarized in terms of the power spectral density (PSD) representing the power or weight corresponding to each frequency. The areas under the spectral density for specified frequency ranges or bands are common data reduction strategies. The frequency bands chosen are those that are known or believed to have clinical or biological significance.

There are, however, other ways to characterize EEGs. Non-stationary series can be characterized in principle like stationary series by using different basis functions. The basis functions for stationary series amount to trigonometric functions via the Fourier transform. The basis functions for nonstationary series amount to a set of basis functions in a smooth localized complex exponential (SLEX) collection [20, 28–30]. These can be used to estimate spectral quantities that can be incorporated in analyses. EEGs also can be characterized as fractal processes or nonlinear dynamic systems [31]. Metrics characterizing these processes can be calculated and also incorporated in subsequent analyses [32–35]. The point is that appropriate metric(s), once obtained, can be incorporated into analyses like any other scalar or vector observation, either as an outcome or as a covariate.

The International Pharmaco-EEG Society (IPEG) published a guideline on EEG data statistical analysis for pharmacodynamic trials in 1999 that recommended using nonparametric methods such as the Mann–Whitney test and the Kruskal–Wallis ANOVA for a parallel group study design, and the Wilcoxon signed-rank test and Friedman ANOVA for a crossover study design [36].

Ma *et al.* [16] surveyed a number of recently published medical research papers presenting EEG results from various clinical trials. The most popular treatment effect analysis methods used in those papers were either Student's $t$ test, or parametric repeated measures ANOVA [37, 38]. Most of these analyses were applied separately to each channel ignoring within-subject correlations of findings between different channels. Some, for example, [39], used Hotelling's $T^2$ test applied to the vector of endpoints from the various channels to determine if there was an overall treatment effect. Such methods present identifiability problems when, as often is the case, there are fewer subjects than channels. In short, the statistical methods that often have been used to assess EEG findings after the reductive signal processing steps have been for the most part fairly conventional. There is room for improvement.

## 10.3.2    Mixed effect models

The fact that each subject provides a vector of observations corresponding to the channels associated with each of the electrodes used to obtain the EEG reading suggests that the vectors of observations within subjects are likely to be correlated because they are provided by the same subject. Mixed effect models provide a way to avoid the potential identifiability issues with multivariate analyses while accounting for possible correlation among the data from the various channels provided by each subject in a trial. In fact, the channels (or, more precisely, the electrodes that are used to obtain the signals) do not simply supply a vector of measurements. The electrodes are placed on the surface of a human head at specific locations, and so are spatially related to each other in (conceptually) the same way that a sequence of measurements obtained over time would be temporally related. The nature of the relationship provides an opportunity to obtain increased precision or sensitivity for estimating treatment effects by incorporating the spatial relationship information into the analyses explicitly. Ma *et al.* [16] described a method for incorporating this spatial information into mixed effect models. A brief overview of their method follows.

The observations in general consist of measurements $y_{ijk}$ on subject $i = 1, \dots, N_s$ on treatment $j = 1, \dots, N_t$ derived from EEG signals recorded on channel $i = 1, \dots, N_c$. The findings from two crossover trials were used to illustrate the analyses. There were two recording sessions for each subject at each visit, one before receiving treatment and the other afterwards. The data consisted of the recordings from 27 electrodes (channels) obtained from a 3-minute eye-closed EEG segment at each session. The $y_{ijk}$ values were the log-transformed averages of the power spectra over the gamma band (frequencies 24–60 Hz). This transformation reduced the hundreds/thousands of numbers recorded for each channel to single values.

A conventional mixed-effects linear model for the outcomes can be written as

$$y_{ijk} = \alpha_k + \beta_j + (\alpha\beta)_{jk} + b_i + a_{ik} + e_{ijk}$$

$$= (\text{channel})_k + (\text{treatment})_k + (\text{channel} \times \text{trt})_{jk}$$

$$+ (\text{subject})_i + (\text{sub} \times \text{channel})_{ik} + (\text{residual}). \tag{10.7}$$

The channel, treatment, and channel $\times$ treatment effects are assumed fixed, that is, the same for all subjects. The other effects allow for random variation among subjects. These effects usually are assumed to have independent normal distributions with zero means and effect-specific variances, $V(b_i) = \sigma_1^2$, $V(a_{ik}) = \sigma_2^2$, and $V(e_{ijk}) = N(0, \sigma^2)$. The independence assumption within each subject may not be justified because the channels are spatially related. If so, then the assumptions about the variances need to be replaced with specifications of correlation matrices. IPEG Society guidelines [36] recommended the inclusion of baseline information in the analysis, which can be accommodated using the constrained longitudinal data analysis method [40] by a simple modification of (10.7),

$$y_{ijk} = \alpha_k + \widetilde{\beta}_j + (\alpha\widetilde{\beta})_{jk} + b_i + a_{ik} + e_{ijk},\tag{10.8}$$

where $j$ refers to treatment $j$ if $j = 1, \ldots, N_t$, or to the baseline effect if $j = N_t + 1$. Models (10.7) and (10.8) do not appear (as of this writing) to have been used previously in published analyses. The computations for both models can be carried out with readily available software such as the nlme procedure in R [7]. Omitting the terms corresponding to channel effects $(\alpha_k, (\alpha\beta)_{jk}, a_{ik})$ from models (10.7) and (10.8) leads to simple repeated measures models applied separately to each channel that ignore channel effects and include only treatment effects.

These analyses also can be carried out using Bayesian methods that do not require assuming that the random effects are normally distributed. The following OpenBUGS code fragment illustrates how this might be done for model (10.7).

```
tau.eps ~ dunif(0,100)
for (i in (1:nsub))
   subj[i] ~ dnorm(0.0,1.0E-6)
for (i in (1:ntrt))
   alpha[i] ~ dnorm(0.0,1.0e-6)
for (i in (1:nchan))
{
   beta[i] ~ dnorm(0.0,1.0e-6)
   for (j in (1:ntrt)) alpha.beta[i,j] ~ dnorm(0.0,1.0e-6)
   for (j in (1:nsub)) chan.sub[i,j] ~ dnorm(0;0,1.0e-6)
}
df <- 3
for (i in (1:nobs))
{
   mean.sub[i] <- alpha[trt[i]] + beta[chan[i]]
                  + alpha.beta[trt[i],chan[i]] + subj[sub[i]]
                  + chan.sub[chan[i],sub[i]]
   y[i] ~ dt(mean.sub[i],tau.eps,df)
}
```

Prior distributions – normality here is a convenient way to define diffuse, nearly non-informative prior distributions

Allow for heavy tails by using a $t$ distribution with 3 d.f.

This simple example does not explicitly model the multivariate correlative structure of the parameters and, in fact, assumes that the parameters have independent prior distributions. The correlation structure can be modeled explicitly [41]. However, the joint posterior distribution of the parameters generally will demonstrate a correlation structure even if it is not explicitly modeled.

This example uses a $t$ distribution with a small number of degrees of freedom for the distribution of the observations to allow for the possibility that the data distribution may be more heavy-tailed than the normal distribution. It is not necessary to fix the degrees of freedom: the actual degrees of freedom also could be a random parameter. The prior distributions for the parameters are specified as very diffuse normal distributions. The normality assumption should have little impact here but, if it is a critical issue, the priors could as well be assumed to arise from uniform distributions over ranges of likely values of the parameters. As usually is the case with Bayesian analyses, the sensitivity of the inferences to the prior assumptions can be assessed by carrying out the calculations with different prior distributions.

### 10.3.3   Spatial smoothing by incorporating spatial relationships of channels

Models (10.7) and (10.8), incorporate random effects and potential intraclass correlation effects due to the fact that multiple measurements are made on each subject, but do not account for the spatial relationship of the channels. Ma *et al.* [16] propose incorporating the spatial relationship in the following way, under the assumption that the locations of the channel electrodes on a human head can be approximated by their locations on a sphere, expressed in spherical coordinates with the *x*-axis pointing outward from the front of the face and the *z*-axis pointing upward, so that the coordinates are the azimuth (left-right angular orientation) and the zenith (angular displacement from vertical).

An EEG signal in any channel is a combination of two signals: a signal representing electrical activity in the brain, that is, a true EEG, and a non-EEG signal reflecting artifacts caused by the movement of muscles such as the ocular muscles that affects the channels differently. For example, artifacts due to ocular muscle movement would affect channels close to the front of the head more than channels at the back of the head. One way to mitigate the effect of non-EEG signals is by means of spatial smoothing. It is reasonable to assume that the true EEG signal varies spatially in a smooth way because of the filtering effect of the skull and scalp [42]. Consequently, it should be possible to approximate the pattern of variation of the true EEG signal across the head by some smoothly varying function. This is similar in principle to a model for longitudinal observations over time: instead of requiring that the model contain a separate parameter for the effect of each time point, one might assume a functional relationship between time and its effect such as linearity (effect $= \alpha \times$ time) or quadratic (effect $= \alpha_1 \times$ time $+ \alpha_2 \times$ time$^2$) so that the effect of time is captured in one or two parameters ($\alpha_1$ or $\alpha_1$ and $\alpha_2$) instead of as many parameters as there are distinct time points. The smoothly varying function, the components of which are called basis functions, can be chosen in a number of ways. Ma *et al* use spherical harmonic functions (SPHARM) [42] which are functions of the azimuth and zenith angles that are represented by associated Legendre functions. The SPHARM of degree *h* and order m is defined as

$$
s_h^m(\theta, \varphi) = \begin{cases}
\sqrt{\dfrac{(2h+1)(h-|m|)!}{2\pi(h+(|m|)!}}\, P_h^{|m|} \cos\theta \sin(|m|\varphi) & -h \le m \le -1 \\[3ex]
\sqrt{\dfrac{2h+1}{4\pi}}\, P_h^0 \cos\theta & m = 0 \\[3ex]
\sqrt{\dfrac{(2h+1)(h-|m|)!}{2\pi(h+(|m|)!}}\, P_h^{|m|} \cos\theta \cos(|m|\varphi) & 1 \le m \le h
\end{cases}
\tag{10.9}
$$

where $\theta$ denotes the zenith angle and $\varphi$ denotes the azimuth angle, and $P_h^m$ denotes the associated Legendre function of degree *h* and order *m*. The position of any channel electrode can be expressed by the combination of the zenith and azimuth angles on the surface of a unit sphere. The location (zenith, azimuth) of any channel and a set of degrees and orders defines a set of covariates that applies to the channels. To illustrate, suppose that the model uses

**Table 10.3** Comparisons of model fits when baseline is included or ignored, and when smoothing is and is not applied to the channel effects.

Ignoring baseline

|         |        | Simple model | Model (10.6) | Smoothed model (10.6) | Model (10.7) | Smoothed model (10.7) |
|---------|--------|--------------|--------------|-----------------------|--------------|-----------------------|
| Trial 1 | LogLik | −1148        | −1162        | −707                  | −2009        | −1685                 |
|         | AIC    | 2566         | 2541         | 1616                  | 4453         | 3772                  |
| Trial 2 | LogLik | −1416        | −1463        | −777                  | −2546        | −1804                 |
|         | AIC    | 3157         | 3197         | 1806                  | 5419         | 3910                  |

The simple model is the same as model (10.6) with the terms pertaining to channel omitted (from [16], Table 2).

$K$ SPHARMs, characterized by the known values of $h$ and $m$, $s_{h_k}^{m_k}$, $k = 1, \dots, K$. Let $(\theta_{ij}, \varphi_{ij})$ denote the zenith and azimuth angles corresponding to the $j$th channel for the $i$th subject. If $x_{ijk} = s_{h_k}^{m_k}(\theta_{ij}, \varphi_{ij})$ denotes the value of the covariate corresponding to the $k$th SPHARM evaluated at the $j$th channel for the $i$th subject, then the model representation of an observation corresponding to the $j$th channel for the $i$th subject is

$$ y_{ij} = \sum_{k=1}^{K} \beta_k x_{ijk}, $$

which depends on $K$ parameters. The contributions of all the channels then would be expressed by the values of $\beta_1, \dots, \beta_K (K < N_c)$ instead of $N_c$ (e.g., $N_c = 27$) parameters corresponding to the individual channels that would be needed if the spatial relationship of the channels were ignored. Conventional regression techniques can be applied for inference. This approach does not require a standard placement of EEG electrodes because equation (10.9) depends on where there electrodes actually are, rather than where a standard placement strategy says they should be.

Table 10.3 summarizes the findings for the calculations carried out by Ma *et al.* [16]. The key finding is that incorporating smoothing substantially improved the model fits, as indicated by the increases of the log likelihood and the decreases of the AIC values. Augmenting the simple model by including separate effects for each channel (model (10.7)) did not appear to lead to a consistent improvement in model fit: the simple model had a larger log likelihood and a larger AIC for trial 1, and a larger log likelihood, but smaller AIC for trial 2.

### 10.3.4     Explicit adjustment for muscle-induced (non-EEG) artifacts

The smoothing resulting from the SPHARM basis function approach described above adjusts for the effect of non-EEG artifacts implicitly. However, the presence of muscle artifacts still hinders the correct interpretation of EEG recordings, and there is a pressing need to correct for the effects of the artifacts without compromising the quality of the recordings [43]. A number of corrective techniques have been described. The most common approach adjusts the filter settings to attenuate higher frequency components of the signal. However, some neuropathologies, for example, seizures, are manifested in terms of higher frequency components of the

EEG, so there is value in not filtering out this part of the signal [44–46]. Component-based analysis methods decompose the EEG signal so that muscle artifacts can be identified and removed, after which the signals are reconstituted without the artifacts.

Ma et al. [47] presented a method for automatically identifying muscle artifact components when the data consist of a large amount of multichannel continuous EEG recordings, specifically when the recording length of each channel (signal duration × sampling rate) is greater than 10 times the number of channels. An earlier paper on the reduction of ocular artifacts [48] described an important special case of the more general method, of which an outline follows. This artifact reduction method is used on the raw EEG signals to produce a set of cleaner EEG endpoints that can be analyzed using the statistical modeling method just described.

An $N$-channel EEG signal $\mathbf{x}(t)$ is decomposed into $N$ independent components using the Infomax independent component analysis (ICA) algorithm [49],

$$\mathbf{x}(t) = \mathbf{A}\,\mathbf{s}(t) + \mathbf{n}(t), \quad \mathbf{A} = (\mathbf{a}_1, \dots, \mathbf{a}_N), \ \mathbf{s}(t) = (s_1(t), \dots, s_N(t))',$$

where $s_i(t)$, called the activation, describes how the signal for component $i$, $i = 1, \dots, N$, varies over time and $\mathbf{a}_j = (a_{i_1}, \dots, a_{iN})$, called the spatial vector, describes how the power of component $i$ changes across the channels. The term $\mathbf{n}(t)$ denotes a vector of random noise elements. The elements $s_i(t)$ of $\mathbf{s}(t)$ are vectors of observations obtained at a sequence of time points, and typically will have many elements. A muscle artifact-free signal is obtained by setting the components of $\mathbf{s}(t)$ corresponding to the muscle artifacts equal to zero. The problem lies in deciding which components of $\mathbf{s}(t)$ correspond to muscle artifacts. Human visual inspection has been, and for the most part remains, the most common way to identify muscle artifacts, but often is inadequate and inefficient, [50] and is not practical on a large scale. This is the problem addressed by Ma et al. [47].

Assume that a sufficient amount of EEG recording data is available, and that simple automatic pre-processing procedures have removed large peak artifacts and strong power-line frequency interference to reduce the number of signal components identified as muscle activity contaminants in the subsequent analysis steps [51, 52]. Ma et al. [47] propose synthesizing realistic muscle-contaminated recordings $\mathbf{x}_{N \times 1}^{\lambda,p}$ from pure EEG signals and muscle activities using the relationship

$$\mathbf{x}_{N \times 1}^{\lambda,p} = \mathbf{b}_{N \times 1}(t) + \begin{bmatrix} \beta_1^{(p)} & & \\ & \ddots & \\ & & \beta_N^{(p)} \end{bmatrix} \mathbf{m}_{N \times 1}(t) \tag{10.10}$$

where $\mathbf{b}_{N \times 1}(t)$ denotes pure muscle-free $N$-channel EEG signals, $\mathbf{m}_{N \times 1}(t)$ denotes $N$ muscle signals randomly selected from a pool of representative muscle signals and scaled to equal the power of the EEG signal at channel Pz in $\mathbf{b}_{N \times 1}(t)$, and $\beta_1^{(p)}, \dots, \beta_N^{(p)}$ are independent Bernoulli $(p)$ variates ($\beta = 0$ or $1$, $p$ in $(0, 1)$). Large values of $p$ imply that there are more muscle-contaminated channels in $\mathbf{x}_{N \times 1}^{\lambda,p}$. Large values of $\lambda$ (in $(0, 1)$) imply stronger muscle contamination signals. The use of equation (10.10) still requires human intervention to identify signals. However, if there are enough data, then the signals might be identified without human intervention. This is not part of the method itself, though.

It turns out that some high-frequency segments of the PSD of muscle artifact components remain flat or even increase at frequency ranges above 40 Hz, while EEG component PSDs decrease above 40 Hz. In other words, the components of the EEG signal corresponding to electrical activity of the brain tend to consist primarily of low-frequency signals, while the components of (some) muscle artifacts tend to be consist primarily of high-frequency signals. This provides an opportunity to differentiate muscle artifact components using what is called a spectral ratio (SR) feature. The strategy described by Ma *et al.* [47] entails first decomposing the signal using ICA, and then identifying the muscle artifact components using the SR feature described below in equation (10.11).

Let $S_i(f)$ denote the power spectrum of the activation $s_i(t)$ for component $i$ at frequency $f$, let

$$H(S_i(f)) = \sum_{f \in [40,60]} S_i(f)/\#(f \in [40, 60])$$

denote the average power spectrum for component $i$ over the (high) frequency range from 40 to 60 Hz, and let

$$L(S_i(f)) = \min_{f \in [4,30]} F_{smooth}(S_i(f))$$

denote the smallest value of a smoothed version of $S_i(f)$ over a (low) frequency range from 4 to 30 Hz. The function $F_{smooth}$ is a moving average smoothing filter (see [47] for details) Then component $i$ is or is not a muscle artifact component accordingly as

$$\log\left(\frac{H(S_i(f))}{L(S_i(f))}\right) \begin{cases} \leq \Delta & \to \text{ not muscle} \\ > \Delta & \to \quad \text{muscle.} \end{cases} \tag{10.11}$$

Expression (10.11) is called the spectral ratio feature; $\Delta$ is a prespecified non-negative parameter.

The performance of the approach is expressed in terms of mean squared errors (MSEs). Let

$$MSE(\Delta) = MSE_m(\Delta) + MSE$$

where

$$MSE_m(\Delta) = \frac{1}{n|T|} \sum_{t \in T, i=1}^{N} m_i(\mathbf{b}_i(t) - \widehat{\mathbf{b}}_i(t))^2$$

denotes the MSE between the muscle-free EEG signal and the muscle-reduced signal for muscle-contaminated channels, and

$$MSE_c(\Delta) = \frac{1}{(N-n)|T|} \sum_{t \in T, i=1}^{N} (1 - m_i)(\mathbf{b}_i(t) - \widehat{\mathbf{b}}_i(t))^2$$

denotes the MSE between the muscle-free EEG signal and the muscle-reduced signal for non-contaminated channels. $T$ denotes the time duration of the recording, $|T|$ denotes the number of time points in $T$, $M = (m_1, \ldots, m_N)$ with $m_i = 1$ if channel $i$ is muscle-contaminated or 0 if not, and $n = \sum m_i$ denotes the number of muscle-contaminated channels.

Figure 10.2 displays the results of a simulation study carried out to evaluate the performance of the method and the effect of varying $\lambda$ and $p$. It is clear from Figure 10.2 that the effect of $\Delta$ on the MSE depended on whether the channels were muscle-contaminated or not. The MSE increased with $\Delta$ for the contaminated channels, and decreased for the non-contaminated channels. Small values of $\Delta$ imply that more signal components are identified as muscle components for removal, leading to cleaner definitions of the muscle-contaminated channels and smaller values of $MSE_m$. Setting $\lambda = 0.5$ led (for $\Delta < 0.4$) to smaller values of $MSE_m$ and MSE than did setting $\lambda = 0.9$, and the difference for $MSE_c$ was quite small. Since $MSE_m$ was much greater than $MSE_c$, setting $\lambda = 0.5$ would seem to be preferable. Setting $p = 0.08$ led to uniformly smaller MSE values regardless of the value of $\Delta$ or $\lambda$. Therefore, setting $\Delta = 0.2$, $p = 0.08$, and $\lambda = 0.5$ may represent a good compromise. Ma *et al.* in fact suggest that $\lambda = 0.5$, $p = 0.5$, and $\Delta = 0.08$ should be the default, but this may be a minor typo because the MSE for $p = 0.5$ always exceeded the MSE for $p = 0.08$.

Finally, even though the method appeared to work reasonably well, Ma *et al* recommended that the final processed results undergo human review. This is not unreasonable, since a post-analysis review is much easier than an initial review of raw signals.

### 10.3.5    Potential extensions

The methods described above use spectral power over fixed frequency ranges as the fundamental analysis measure. However, there are some other possibilities that are worth mentioning and possibly exploring, although doing so is beyond the scope of this chapter. For example, EEGs can be regarded as realizations of fractal processes that can be analyzed using nonlinear dynamic methods that yield a variety of potentially useful metrics. Fractal processes can be self-similar or scale-invariant, that is, demonstrate approximately similar patterns at different scales or degrees of magnification. These processes can be monofractal or multifractal. The scale invariance properties of monofractal objects can be characterized by a single scaling exponent, typically a quantity referred to as the Hurst parameter. Multifractal objects consist of a combination of monofractal objects and are characterized by a collection of different exponents. Fractal analysis methods provide an opportunity to characterize complex brain function expressed by EEG records. Weiss *et al.* [34, 35] provide extensive bibliographies and methods for estimating the Hurst parameter, a measure of self-similarity, and the range of fractal spectra, useful for assessing the degree to which self-similarity actually holds, and apply these methods to the evaluation of sleep stages measured via EEGs.

## 10.4    Discussion

This chapter has outlined briefly some statistical approaches that may be useful for the evaluation of neurological toxicity, especially as manifested in changes in EEG recordings, in the context of clinical trials. The focus has been on methods that can be implemented in a practical way for "routine" evaluation of neurotoxicity assessments obtained in the course of

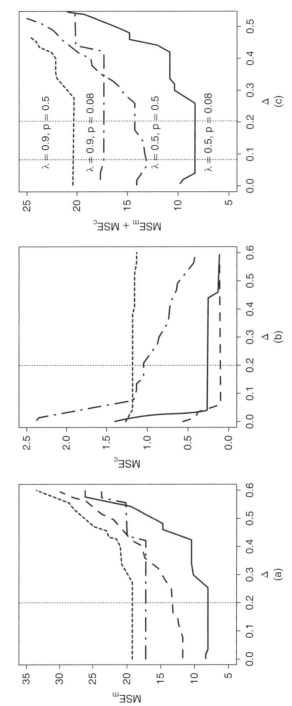

**Figure 10.2** Mean squared errors between the true muscle-free EEG signal and the muscle-reduced signal (a) for channels that were muscle-artifact contaminated ($MSE_m$), (b) for channels that were not contaminated ($MSE_c$) and (c) for all channels (MSE). Vertical lines are at $\Delta = 0.2$ and, for total MSE, at 0.08. From Ma *et al.* [47].

clinical trials. There is a substantial literature covering a greater variety of ways to analyze EEG recordings, but not all of these currently lend themselves to "routine" application of data from clinical trials, typically because of the lack of readily available software for carrying out complex calculations, and the difficulty in communicating the clinical meaning and implication of differences between treatment groups that the calculations may reveal. Nonetheless, the methods that are described represent substantial advances in methodology for analyzing and interpreting complex neurological data.

The potential neurotoxicity of a compound can be evaluated in various ways. Treatments in a clinical trial or in a designed experiment can be compared with respect to the incidence of neurological signs and symptoms, including the timing, frequency of recurrence, or intensity of the reported or observed events. The assessment of this information proceeds for neurological events as for any other class of adverse events, so does not need special consideration here.

There are, however, other dimensions to the evaluation of neurotoxicity. Neurotoxicity screening typically is carried out in animals in the early stages of product development for determining maximum tolerable doses, or for screening potentially toxic chemicals from an environmental perspective, using a battery of measurements and observations such as the functional observational battery that has been in use for a number of years [4]. This information generally consists of sequences of multivariate measurements over time, and statistical methods for assessing this information often rely on nonlinear random-effects models to account for possible dose effects and evolution of risk with exposure. Although the evaluation of the results of neurotoxicity screening experiments employs standard nonlinear regression techniques, it is a key element of safety evaluation in product development and therefore worth separate consideration.

EEGs represent the most complex measures of central neurological function and present what appears to be the most promising for identifying potential centrally manifested neurotoxicity. There is an enormous literature on the subject, and the diagnostic value of EEGs for characterizing neurologic pathologies has been demonstrated in a number of applications. However, although EEGs are relatively easy to measure and capture, they generate a very large amount of information and their analysis is complicated. Exploiting this technology for routine evaluation of potential toxicity of new products is currently a major challenge, but progress is being made. The key issues are data processing, removal of artifacts to the brain signals due to muscle movements, and reduction of the mass of data to a small number of relevant summary measures that convey clinical insight. The papers by Ma *et al.* provide paths forward to resolving these issues and should be helpful in developing standard operating procedures and protocols for evaluating neurotoxicity.

# Appendix 10.A  OpenBUGS code

The following OpenBUGS code provides the calculations producing Table 10.2 and Figure 10.1. The analyses of actual values and changes from baseline are carried out simultaneously.

```
model
{
  A ~ dt(0.0, 0.4, 1)
  A.diff ~ dt(0.0, 0.4, 1)
  for (i in 1:2) {
    b.hour[i] ~ dt(0.0, 0.4, 1)
    b.hour.diff[i] ~ dt(0.0, 0.4, 1)
  }
```

Prior distributions for the parameters using Cauchy densities as suggested by Gelman *et al.* [53]

```
  sigma.A ~ dunif(0.0, 100)
  sigma.eps ~ dunif(0.0, 100)
  sigma.A.diff ~ dunif(0.0, 20)
  sigma.eps.diff ~ dunif(0.0, 20)
```

Uniform prior densities for the standard deviations

```
  for (i in 1:4) {
    b.dose[i] ~ dt(0.0, 0.4, 1)
    b.dose.diff[i] ~ dt(0.0, 0.4, 1)
  }
  for (i in 1:4) {
    bb.dose[i + 1] <- b.dose[i]
    bb.dose.diff[i + 1] <- b.dose.diff[i]
  }
  bb.dose[1] <- 0.0
  bb.dose.diff[1] <- 0.0
```

There are four real doses, so create a dummy parameter (bb.dose[1], bb.dose.diff[1]) for the 0 mg/kg group

```
  tau.A <- 1/pow(sigma.A, 2)
  tau.eps <- 1/pow(sigma.eps, 2)
  tau.A.diff <- 1/pow(sigma.A.diff, 2)
  tau.eps.diff <- 1/pow(sigma.eps.diff, 2)
  for (j in 1:ntimes) {
    indHour[j] <- step(Hour[j] - 1)
    xHour[j] <- indHour[j] *
        Hour[j] + 1 - indHour[j]
    logHour[j] <- log(xHour[j])
  }
```

Transformations – OpenBUGS works with precisions rather than variances or s.d.s

```
  for (i in 1:nsub) {
    dosecat[i] <-1 +
    step(Dose[i]-0.5) + step(Dose[i]-1) + step(Dose[i]-2)
                  + step(Dose[i]-4)
    a[i] ~ dnorm(A, tau.A)
    a.diff[i] ~ dnorm(A.diff, tau.A.diff)
    for (j in 1:ntimes) {
      mu[i, j] <- a[i] + bb.dose[dosecat[i]] + b.hour[1]*logHour[j]
                  + b.hour[2] * pow(logHour[j], 2)
      Resp[i, j] ~ dnorm(mu[i, j], tau.eps)
    }
```

Likelihood for actual values

```
    for (j in 1:(ntimes - 1)) {
      Diff[i, j] <- Resp[i, j + 1] - Resp[i, 1]
      mu.diff[i, j] <- a.diff[i] + bb.dose.diff[dosecat[i]]
                  + b.hour.diff[1] * logHour[j + 1]
                  + b.hour.diff[2] * pow(logHour[j + 1], 2)
      Diff[i, j] ~ dnorm(mu.diff[i, j], tau.eps.diff)
    }
  }
}
```

Likelihood for changes from baseline

# References

[1] Office of Technology Assessment (1990) *Neurotoxicity: Identifying and Controlling Poisons of the Nervous System (OTA-BA-436)*, U.S. Government Printing Office, Washington, DC.

[2] Tilson, H.A. (1990) Neurotoxicology in the 1990s. *Neurotoxicology and Teratology*, **12**, 293–300.

[3] U.S. Environmental Protection Agency (1998) Guidelines for neurotoxicity risk assessment. *Federal Register*, **63**, 26926–26954.

[4] McDaniel, K.L. and Moser, V.C. (1993) Utility of a neurobehavioral screening battery for differentiating the effects of two pyrethroids, permethrin and cypermethrin. *Neurotoxicological Teratology*, **15**, 71–83.

[5] Zhu, Y. (2005) Dose-time-response modeling of longitudinal measurements for neurotoxicity risk assessment. *EnvironMetrics*, **16**, 603–617.

[6] Zhu, Y., Wessel, M.R., Liu, T. and Moser, V.C. (2005) Analyses of neurobehavioral screening data: dose-time-response modeling of continuous outcomes. *Regulatory Toxicology and Pharmacology*, **41**, 240–255.

[7] Pinheiro, J., Bates, D., DebRoy, S., and Sarkar, D. (2013) nlme: Linear and Nonlinear Mixed Effects Models. R package version 3.1-117., http://cran.r-project.org/package=nlme

[8] Berridge, D.M. and Crouchley, R. (2011) *Multivariate Generalized Linear Mixed Models Using R*, CRC Press, Boca Raton, FL.

[9] Lindsey, J. (2011) Generalized Nonlinear Regression Models, http://www.commanster.eu/rcode/gnlm.zip (accessed 23 June 2014).

[10] Lindsey, J. (2011) Non Normal Repeated Measurements Models, http://www.commanster.eu/rcode/repeated.zip (accessed 23 June 2014).

[11] Turner, H. and Firth, D. (2012) Generalized Nonlinear Models in R: An Overview of the gnm Package (R package version 1.0-6), http://CRAN.R-project.org/package=gnm (accessed 23 June 2014).

[12] Lunn, D., Spiegelhalter, D., Thomas, A. and Best, N. (2009) The BUGS project: evolution, critique, and future directions (with discussion). *Statistics in Medicine*, **28**, 3049–3082.

[13] Berger, H. (1929) Über das elektrenkephalogramm des menschen. *Archiv für Psychiatrie*, **87**, 527–570.

[14] Lopes da Silva, F. (2005) Computer-assisted EEG diagnosis: pattern recognition and brain maping, in *Electronecephalography: Basic Principles, Clinical Applications, and Related Fields*, 5th edn (eds E. Nidermeyer and F. Lopes da Silva), Lippincott Williams & WIlkins.

[15] Lopes da Silva, F. and Van Rotterdam, A. (2005) Biophysical aspects of EEG and magnetoecephalogram generation, in *Electronecephalography: Basic Principles, Clinical Applications, and Related Fields*, 5th edn (eds E. Nidermeyer and F. Lopes da Silva), Lippincott Williams & WIlkins.

[16] Ma, J., Wang, S., Raubertas, R. and Svetnik, V. (2010) Statistical methods to estimate treatment effects from multichannel electroencephalography (EEG) data in clinical trials. *Journal of Neuroscience Methods*, **190**, 248–257.

[17] Carvalho, C.M. and West, M. (2007) Dynamic matrix-variate graphical models. *Bayesian Analysis*, **2**, 69–98.

[18] Krafty, R.T., Hall, M. and Guo, W. (2011) Functional mixed effects spectral analysis. *Biometrika*, **98**, 583–598.

[19] Krystal, A.D., Prado, R. and West, M. (1999) New methods of time series analysis of non-stationary EEG data: eigenstructure decompositions of time varying autoregressions. *Clinical Neurophysiology*, **110**, 2197–2206.

[20] Ombao, H., von Sachs, R. and Guo, W. (2005) SLEX analysis of multivariate nonstationary time series. *Journal of the American Statistical Association*, **100**, 519–531.

[21] Prado, R., West, M. and Krystal, A.D. (2001) Multichannel electroencephalographic analyses via dynamic regression models with time-varying lag-lead structure. *Applied Statistics*, **50**, 95–109.

[22] Prado, R., Molina, F. and Huerta, G. (2006) Multivariate time series modeling and classification via hierarchical VAR mixtures. *Computational Statistics and Data Analysis*, **51**, 1445–1462.

[23] Hornero, R., Abasolo, D., Escudero, J. and Gomez, C. (2009) Nonlinear analysis of electroencephalogram and magnetoencephalogram recordings in patients with Alzheimer's disease. *Philosophical Transactions of the Royal Society A: Mathematical Physical and Engineering Sciences*, **367**, 317–336.

Nonlinear methods have been applied to study the EEG and MEG background activity in patients with Alzheimer's disease and control subjects: approximate entropy, sample entropy, multiscale entropy, auto-mutual information, and Lempel–Ziv complexity. The same databases of EEG and MEG recordings were used to compare the performance of these methods. EEG and MEG background activities in patients with Alzheimer's disease turned out to be less complex and more regular than in healthy control subjects, suggesting that nonlinear analysis techniques could be useful in diagnosis of Alzheimer's disease.

[24] Sheorajpanday, R.V.A., Nagels, G., Weeren, A.J.T.M. *et al.* (2009) Reproducibility and clinical relefance of quantitative EEG parameters in cerebral ischemia: a basic approach. *Clinical Neurophysiology*, **120**, 845–855.

This paper defines a revised version of van Putten BSI. Suppose $M$ frequencies from Fourier analysis of EEG and $N$ channels, and let $R(i,f)$ and $L(i,f)$ denote power at frequency $f$ for right-hand channel $i$ and left-hand channel $i$. The modified BSI = average value of $|R(i,f) - L(i,f)|/(R(i,f) + L(i,f))$. This is applied to the EEGs of 31 patients with subacute ischemic cardiovascular disease and 10 age-matched controls. The modified BSI was sensitive to asymmetry in various models, with good reproducibility, and correlated well with NIH Stroke Scale score. It also could differentiate between patients with stroke and normals or those with transient ischemic attack.

[25] van Putten, M.J.A.M. and Tavy, D.L.J. (2004) Continuous quantitative EEG monitoring in hemispheric stroke patients using the brain symmetry index. *Stroke*, **35**, 2489–2492.

This paper defines an index of bilateral brain symmety. On the basis of a spectral (Fourier) decomposition of an EEG signal, let $R(i,f)$ denote the power at frequency $f$ (assume $M$ such frequencies) for channel $i$ on the right-hand side of the brain and let $L(i,f)$ denote the corresponding power for the left channel. Take the sum of the ratios $(R(i,f) - L(i,f))/(R(i,f) + L(i,f))$ over the channels (which gives $M$ ratio values). Then the Brain Symmetry Index (BSI) is the average of these sums over the collection of $M$ frequencies. The measure was applied to the EEGs of 21 patients, and showed a positive correlation (0.86) between the BSI and the NIH Stroke Scale.

[26] Friedman, D. and Claassen, J. (2010) Quantitative EEG and cerebral ischemia. *Clinical Neurophysiology*, **121**, 1707–1708.

[27] Snyder, S.M., Hall, J.R., Cornwell, S.L. and Falk, J.D. (2011) Addition of EEG improves accuracy of a logistic model that uses neuropsychological and cardiovascular factors to identify dementia and MCI. *Psychiatry Research*, **186**, 97–102.

This paper evaluates the improvement in diagnostic properties of a logistic model for identifying dementia and mild cognitive impairment (MCI) in a sample of 111 individuals (78 normal, 33 with dementia or MCI) that was realized by including summary measures obtained from EEG recordings, including power spectrum components and fractal dimension (complexity). Including EEG information (especially complexity) along with information from neuropsychological testing (ADAS-Cog score) and cardiovascular history and risk factors improved the accuracy of the predictions. This was a small study, so its generalizability is limited.

[28] Böhm, H., Ombao, H., von Sachs, R. and Sanes, J. (2010) Classification of multivariate non-stationary signals: the SLEX-shrinkage approach. *Journal of Statistical Planning and Inference*, **140**, 3754–3763.

[29] Ombao, H., Raz, J.A., von Sachs, R. and Guo, W. (2002) The SLEX model of a non-stationary random process. *Annals of the Institute of Statistical Mathematics*, **54**, 171–200.

[30] Ombao, H.A., Raz, J.A., von Sachs, R. and Malow, B.A. (2001) Automatic statistical analysis of bivariate nonstationary time series. *Journal of the American Statistical Association*, **96**, 543–560.

[31] Stam, C.J. (2005) Nonlinear dynamical analysis of EEG and MEG: review of an emerging field. *Clinical Neurophysiology*, **116**, 2266–2301.
    This paper provides an extensive guide to the literature (∼ 500 references) on nonlinear dynamical system (chaos theory) analysis of EEG and MEG (magnetoencephalogram) data. It includes review of various applications, including sleep, coma/anesthesia, seizure prediction, psychopharmacology, mental states, and cognition.

[32] Alonso, J.F., Mañanas, M.A., Romero, S. *et al.* (2010) Drug effect on EEG connectivity assessed by linear and nonlinear couplings. *Human Brain Mapping*, **31**, 487–497.
    This paper evaluates the pharmacologic effect of a dose of alprazolam on wakeful brain connectivity using linear and nonlinear reductions of EEG signals in a double-blind placebo-controlled crossover trial with nine subjects. Channels were analyzed separately and then compared pairwise. Alprazolam induced changes in EEG connectivity measured using cross-conditional entropy between channels, corresponding to scalp regions.

[33] Alonso, J.F., Mañanas, M.A., Romero, S. *et al.* (2012) Cross-conditional entropy and coherence analysis of pharmaco-EEG changes induced by alprazolam. *Psychopharmacology*, **221**, 397–406.

[34] Weiss, B., Clemens, Z., Bódizs, R. *et al.* (2009) Spatio-temporal analysis of monofractal and multifractal properties of the human sleep EEG. *Journal of Neuroscience Methods*, **185**, 116–124.

[35] Weiss, B., Clemens, Z., Bódizs, R. and Halász, P. (2011) Comparison of fractal and power spectral EEG features: effects of topography and sleep stages. *Brain Research Bulletin*, **84**, 359–375.
    This paper provides a comprehensive empirical evaluation of the relationship between measures of fractality (Hurst coefficient, range of fractal spectra) and conventional measures (band powers and spectral edge frequencies) calculated from EEGs across different sleep stages and topographic locations based on sleep studies carried out on two successive nights with 22 subjects. Extensive literature citations are given. The key finding is that fractal features provide additional useful information about EEG signals, and that a multifractal approach (range of fractal spectra) may be more helpful for modeling complex brain activities.

[36] Ferbera, G., Abth, K., Fichter, K. and Luthringerd, R. (1999) IPEG guideline on statistical design and analysis for pharmacodynamic trials. *Neuropsychobiology*, **39**, 92–100.

[37] Yamada, K., Isotani, T., Irisawa, S. *et al.* (2004) EEG global field power spectrum changes after a single dose of atypical antipsychotics in health volunteers. *Brain Topography*, **16**, 281–285.

[38] Yoshimura, M., Koenig, T., Irisawa, S. *et al.* (2007) A pharmaco-EEG study on antipsychotic drugs in healthy volunteers. *Psychopharmacology*, **191**, 995–1004.

[39] John, E.R., Prichep, L.S., Fridman, J. and Easton, P. (1988) Neurometrics: computer-assisted differential diagnosis of brain dysfunction. *Science*, **239**, 162–169.

[40] Liu, W., Tao, J., Shi, N.Z. and Tang, M.L. (2009) Model selection in toxicity studies. *Statistica Neerlandica*, **63**, 418–431.

[41] Congdon, P. (2001) *Bayesian Statistical Modelling*, John Wiley & Sons, Ltd, Chichester.

[42] Nunez, P.L. and Srinivasan, R. (2006) *Electric Fields of the Brain: The Macrophysics of EEG*, 2nd edn, Oxford University Press, New York.

[43] Bautista, R.E.D. (2012) Eliminating muscle artifacts from EEG recordings: a necessary imperative. *Clinical Neurophysiology*, **123**, 1481–1482.

[44] Andrade-Valenca, L.P., Dubeau, F., Mari, F. *et al.* (2011) Interictal scalp fast oscillations as a marker of the seizure onset zone. *Neurology*, **77**, 524–531.

[45] Bragin, A., Engle, J. Jr., and Staba, R.J. (2010) High-frequency oscillations in epileptic brain. *Current Opinion in Neurology*, **23**, 151–156.

[46] Jacobs, J., LeVan, P., Chatillon, C.E. *et al.* (2009) High frequency oscillations in intracranial EEGs mark epileptogencity rather than lesion type. *Brain*, **132**, 1022–1037.

[47] Ma, J., Tao, P., Bayram, S. and Svetnik, V. (2012) Muscle artifacts in multichannel EEG: characteristics and reduction. *Clinical Neurophysiology*, **123**, 1676–1686.

[48] Ma, J., Bayram, S., Tao, P. and Svetnik, V. (2011) High-throughput ocular artifact reduction in multichannel electroencephalography (EEG) using component subspace projection. *Journal of Neuroscience Methods*, **196**, 131–140.

[49] Bell, A.J. and Sejnowski, T.J. (1995) An information-maximisation approach to blind separation and blind deconvolution. *Neural Computation*, **7**, 1129–1159.

[50] Fatourechi, M., Bashashati, A., Ward, R.K. and Birch, G.E. (2007) EMG and EOG artifacts in brain computer interface systems: a survey. *Clinical Neurophysiology*, **118**, 480–494.

[51] Anderer, P., Semlitsch, H.V., Saletu, B. and Barbanoj, M.J. (1992) Artifact processing in topographic mapping of electroencephalographic activity in neuropsychopharmacology. *Psychiatric Research*, **45**, 79–93.

[52] Anderer, P., Roberts, S., Schlögl, A. *et al.* (1999) Artifact processing in computerized analysis of sleep EEG -- a review. *Neuropsychobiology*, **40**, 150–157.

[53] Gelman, A., Jakulin, A., Pittau, M.G. and Su, Y.S. (2008) A weakly informative default prior distribution for logistic and other regression models. *Annals of Applied Statistics*, **2**, 1360–1383.

# 11

# Safety monitoring

## Jay Herson

*Johns Hopkins Bloomberg School of Public Health, Baltimore, MD 20815 USA*

## 11.1   Introduction

This chapter will deal with statistical methods used in safety monitoring. The latter will be defined as those activities that take place during a clinical trial. Hence, the methods to be described will be those that are used to capture safety signals of a clinical trial in progress rather than to summarize the entire safety profile of a completed trial or integrate the safety data of a particular trial with those of other trials in the same clinical program. Some of the statistical methods used will be the same as or similar to those used at trial completion, but the objectives will differ. While the statistical methods used in final safety analysis often appear in the publication of trial results, the many analyses that take place during the trial are not published, so that statistical best practices in safety monitoring are not widely known. We concentrate here on statistical methods for safety monitoring in randomized controlled Phase 3 confirmatory trials. Most of what is presented can be generalized to Phase 2 and single-arm trials.

Statistical monitoring of safety has the objective of bringing up potential signals for clinical discussion. There are many who think that the sole objective of safety monitoring is to discover serious and severe adverse event (AE) signals. This is an important function, but common low-grade AEs observed in the limited follow-up of clinical trials could develop into serious adverse events (SAEs) in long-term use post market. Safety suspicions raised in pre-market trials can be used to create an efficient post-market surveillance plan.

During the conduct of the trial many issues will arise for clinical evaluation from clinicians concerned with observed levels of AEs regardless of statistical significance. For example,

*Statistical Methods for Evaluating Safety in Medical Product Development*, First Edition.
Edited by A. Lawrence Gould.
© 2015 John Wiley & Sons, Ltd. Published 2015 by John Wiley & Sons, Ltd.

if three cases of renal failure are reported in the experimental treatment group and none in the control group of a trial in rheumatoid arthritis, there will be reason for concern even though that difference may not be of statistical significance. Thus, unlike efficacy analysis, statistical calculations are not the main analytic force in safety analysis. As a result, the safety data collected do not go through the intensive adjudication that efficacy endpoints endure. The grading of some AEs is somewhat subjective, thus leading to variation among investigators. In addition, safety monitoring analyses are made in the absence of information on efficacy, so that risk–benefit considerations are rare. Edwards *et al.* [1] presented sophisticated analysis of safety data as it existed at that point in time. This chapter will update the methodology they describe in the area of safety monitoring.

We first describe some useful steps for the planning for safety monitoring. Next the statistical methodology will be discussed in two parts: methods used by the sponsor and those employed by the data monitoring committee (DMC). The reason for this dichotomy is that the sponsor staff is masked to treatment, while the DMC is at least partially unmasked. We focus on a "bottom line" of what statistical methods and operations are most essential for safety monitoring, yet encourage experimentation with methods such as evidential likelihood and Bayesian methods. The chapter concludes with a discussion of the challenges of emerging issues such as adaptive designs, real-time SAE reporting via the internet, the anticipated merger of healthcare delivery and clinical trials, and the high-tech future of drug safety.

## 11.2  Planning for safety monitoring

The Safety Planning, Evaluation and Reporting Team (SPERT) [2] and the CIOMS Working Group VI [3] have both recommended that a program safety analysis plan (PSAP) be formulated at the start of the first phase II trial of a clinical program and amended as the research progresses. The PSAP provides the details of safety data definition, collection, and analysis. The document should contain both analytic methods for both the monitoring phase as well as the final report phase of the program. See also [4] for further applications of the SPERT recommendations. Table 11.1 displays the key statistical elements of a PSAP.

The PSAP should indicate how data will be collected and validated. The dictionary to be used for AE classification by body system and preferred term should be specified. The Medical Dictionary for Regulatory Activities (MedDRA) [5] is the choice of most regulatory agencies but some oncology trials use the Common Terminology Criteria for Adverse Events (CTCAE) [6]. Rules must be established for how terms from these dictionaries are to be combined into common AE terminology such as nausea, vomiting, and dizziness. Some combinations will cross body systems such as the definition of stroke or congestive heart failure. The care taken to make these definitions will reduce the "granularity" in AE definitions, that is, sparse tables with many cells containing zero or one counts. In addition, a system for grading the severity of the AEs should also be specified.

Modern safety analysis divides AEs into three tiers [2, 7, 8]. Tier 1 is a list of AEs for which specific hypotheses and analysis methods are described before the trial begins. Typically these will be AE types for which there is concern due to the experience of previous human or animal studies and which are critical to the safety profile for the new compound. In Tier 2 we place those AEs that were not prespecified but have become apparent during safety monitoring in the trial and where there are sufficient number events for data analysis. Tier 3 events are infrequent events that do not lend themselves to statistical analysis but description, perhaps

**Table 11.1**    Statistical elements of a program safety analysis plan.

1. Specification of adverse event dictionary to be used during the trial (e.g., MedDRA and CTCAE)

2. Designation of Tier 1 adverse events

3. Rules for combining preferred terms to minimize granularity

4. Computation of assay sensitivity of sample size to detect adverse events of varying incidences

5. Decide if adverse event collection will be spontaneous or solicited

6. Design of tables, listings, and graphs to be provided to sponsor staff (masked to treatment) and to the data monitoring committee (unmasked or partially unmasked to treatment)

merely listings, will be supplied. Description of statistical methods in this chapter will be with regard to the three tiers.

Tier 1 events represent prespecified statistical hypotheses. Hence there should be some analysis in the protocol to demonstrate that the sample size chosen for efficacy considerations will deliver the required power for assessing treatment differences in these events. More will be said about this under "assay sensitivity" in Section 11.4.3. In response to the recent controversy over cardiovascular risk among Type II diabetes mellitus patients treated with rosiglitazone [9], the US Food and Drug Administration issued a guidance calling for all Type II diabetes protocols to provide statistical evidence that the sample size for the trial is sufficient to detect cardiovascular effects [10]. Ibrahim *et al.* [11] subsequently proposed using Bayesian meta-analysis to assess the adequacy of a clinical program to evaluate cardiovascular risk. Bayesian borrowing is used to incorporate data from clinical trials outside the current development program.

A useful "rule of thumb" for assessing program sensitivity to find AEs is the rule of $3000/n$. If $n$ represents the total number of patients exposed to an experimental treatment in a clinical program then $3000/n$ is an estimate of the rate per 1000 that this program is likely to yield at least one event of that type. Thus with 3000 patients exposed we are likely to find at least one case of an AE occurring with the incidence of $1/1000$. Conversely, if we wanted to find at least one case of a Tier 1 AE that has an estimated incidence of $1/10\,000$, a total of 30 000 patients would have to be exposed. This calculation relates to case ascertainment only, and not to power to detect treatment differences. AEs that are likely to be drug-related occur early after treatment start, those that are caused by allergy to the drug some time after that, and those that are caused by carcinogenicity years or decades later [1]. This is a broad generalization, but it is good to keep this in mind when considering the sensitivity of a program to AEs.

At the outset of the trial it should be decided whether AE data will be collected as spontaneous or solicited. In spontaneous collection the patient is asked on each clinic visit to describe the AEs he/she has had since the previous visit. In solicited collection the patient is asked to respond to a predefined list of AEs. Solicited lists are preferred when there is a long time interval between visits and/or when certain AEs are potentially embarrassing, such as sexual dysfunction. In many trials some AEs will be solicited and the rest spontaneous with the former usually consisting of the Tier 1 events. Wernicke *et al.* [12] studied three randomized placebo-controlled trials where both methods were employed and found that reporting rates were higher in solicited collection compared with spontaneous, but the latter method was more effective in distinguishing treatment differences (i.e., experimental vs placebo).

Laboratory values will be part of the final safety analysis for the trial, but researchers must decide at the outset what role these data will play in safety monitoring. A general rule is that laboratory values out of the normal range or those with extreme changes should be reported as AEs (e.g., hypercalcemia and hypokalemia) and the dynamics will be analyzed through these AEs. Extreme value modeling methods have been applied to relate laboratory values to the prediction of severe AEs [13].

It is assumed that unmasked or partially unmasked safety data will be reviewed periodically by an independent DMC [14, 15]. The term "partially unmasked" means that the DMC will review the safety data with treatments identified only as A and B or some other symbol. The DMCs usually have the right either to be unmasked at any time to a particular patient's treatment group because of a safety concern or to be completely unmasked to treatment identity for all patients. Many DMCs elect to be completely unmasked from the start of the trial because they feel it is the only way they can properly fulfill their stewardship responsibilities. DMC members usually cannot avoid guessing treatment identity as AE reports arrive but, if masked, they could guess incorrectly and this could adversely affect their decision-making throughout the trial.

A major effort in the PSAP would be the design of the tables, listings, and graphs to be used for safety monitoring. Generally the sponsor staff will review the same tables, listings, and graphs as the DMC, with the difference being that the sponsor version will be pooled over treatment groups and the DMC version will present data by treatment group even if coded by letter (partially masked). The term "listings" above refers to line listings of patient safety data. This is an important component of safety monitoring, but it does not lend itself to statistical analysis so it will not be discussed further in this chapter.

The types of tables and graphs useful in safety monitoring will vary according to the drug and indication but the following would usually be included:

- Cumulative distribution of patient exposure to drug

- Reason for discontinuation

- Treatment emergent AEs by body system, usually sub-classified by grade/severity or preferred terms describing events within body system

- Same for treatment-emergent SAEs

- Laboratory values listing, flagging those patients outside of normal range.

Some sponsors prepare tables sub-classifying AEs by individual investigators' classification of relatedness to study drug. It is widely considered best practice to exclude these tables from routine use. The relatedness classification is subjective, and it is better to be conservative and assume all AEs are drug-related. In addition to providing the number of patients randomized to each treatment and overall, the number of patient-years of follow-up by treatment and overall should be reported. This will allow for quick ascertainment of differential exposure among treatment groups. Further use of exposure data will be discussed below. The tables and graphs enumerated above would normally be produced for routine use by both the masked sponsor protocol team and the DMC. The only difference will be that the sponsor staff will receive the data pooled over treatment groups, while the tables sent to the DMC will be generated by treatment group.

There are ad hoc tables, listings, and graphs that may be requested by the DMC for just one meeting or for all future meetings. These tables will be requested in response to safety issues that arise in the course of the trial. All tables provided to the DMC will be created by the data analysis center (DAC), a group separate from the sponsor protocol team. The non-voting statistician who represents the DAC at DMC closed sessions will be responsible for preparing these reports. He/she is sometimes referred to as the "reporting statistician."

## 11.3    Safety monitoring-sponsor view (masked, treatment groups pooled)

Sponsor staff can review pooled safety data (i.e., both treatment groups combined) as often as they like. Multiplicity is usually not of concern, although some statistical analysis is performed even though treatment groups are not compared. The most likely analysis time will be just prior to a DMC meeting. However, sponsor staff can perform ad hoc analyses of particular AE types of interest more frequently. The objective of sponsor analysis will be to find types of AEs that have higher frequencies than expected. These would normally be serious and severe treatment-emergent AEs not easily controlled by drug treatment (e.g., pain controlled by non-steroidal anti-inflammatory drugs, antibiotics to treat infection). Analysis will usually be performed with respect to the three tiers as described above.

Sponsors also should periodically review the characteristics of patients as they are enrolled in the trial to identify high-risk safety attributes, such as history of heart or kidney disease and smoking habits. This can be a signal for vigilance when reviewing reports of related AEs.

### 11.3.1    Frequentist methods for masked or pooled analysis

Periodic analysis will usually begin with analysis of individual SAE reports and analysis of frequency of the treatment-emergent SAEs by body system and preferred term. This table will be sparse, but sponsor staff will look for any SAEs noted in individual reports and Tier 1 SAEs. When SAE frequencies of interest are found they can be compared to frequencies from previous trials of this drug in the current clinical program and those found for already approved drugs of the same therapeutic class. It must be kept in mind that while the sponsor staff sees only the SAE frequencies for both treatments combined, previous trials provide frequencies for the experimental drug. Taking the current trial's control group into account, sponsor staff would nevertheless have in mind an incidence level that would be of concern if observed.

Sponsors might first look at incidence rates for AE types of interest together with the 95% confidence interval. Although normal approximation confidence intervals are still used, the "exact" Clopper–Pearson binomial confidence interval [16] is becoming more common because it can easily be retrieved from statistical software commonly in use. Sponsors would use these data to see if the pooled incidence is in an acceptable or unsurprising range.

The incidence calculation does not take exposure to the treatment into account. A low rate of an SAE might be observed only because patients have dropped out of the trial for efficacy failure or some other AE and have not been exposed to the drug long enough to experience the AE. O'Neill [17] describes the importance of taking exposure into account and some inferential problems in ignoring exposure.

A preferable way to look at incidence would be to examine the rate of an AE per 100 patient-years of exposure. This is calculated by dividing the observed number of events by the total patient-years and multiplying this ratio by 100. This measure takes exposure into account. The reference distribution for the rate per 100 patient-years is the Poisson distribution. Herson [15] describes both a normal and binomial approximation to the confidence interval for this rate. Methods for constructing confidence intervals for the difference between both binomial and Poisson rates are reviewed in [18].

Once an AE type of concern is identified sponsors might want to make a Kaplan–Meier life table graph of the accumulation of AEs over time [19]. This analysis will provide "landmark" estimates of incidence at various time points post treatment start (e.g., 6 and 12 months). The graph will also show the pattern of incidence over time, that is, whether the events occur within the first month of treatment and then level off or whether the events occur late, for example, after 12 months of treatment. Sponsors may also want to investigate if certain subsets of patients are experiencing the AE types of interest. It is not recommended that statistical hypothesis testing be used for identifying subsets. The identification of a subset is merely for future safety surveillance and suggestions of protocol modification.

## 11.3.2   Likelihood methods for masked or pooled analysis

The methods discussed above come under the general category of frequentist statistical methods. These methods use deductive inference by deriving the underlying statistical foundation for inference from imaginary repeated sampling from a specified probability distribution. Methods such as likelihood methods and Bayesian methods are inductive because they derive their inferential foundation conditional on the data observed rather than repeated sampling. The likelihood methods adhere to the likelihood principle which is the foundation for statistical inference. A number of authors have described both the theoretical and applied aspects of what are becoming known as evidential likelihood methods [15, 20–22]. We will just use the term "likelihood" to mean evidential likelihood in what follows.

One goal of likelihood inference is to derive a support interval for an unknown parameter, that is, an interval of values for the parameter that are supported by the accumulated data [23]. A common support interval would be those values of the unknown parameter that have likelihoods at least 1/8 that of the maximum likelihood. Likelihood statisticians justify the 1/8 support interval by reasoning that if one were to observe three heads in three tosses of a coin (probability 1/8) one might begin to think there is lessening support that the coin is fair. Sponsors would use this interval to determine the relative likelihoods of values of safety parameters that are not acceptable and take action if necessary. Herson [15] describes the computational details and provides examples of the 1/8 support interval for the rate per 100 patient-years. Figure 11.1 shows a graphical depiction of a support interval for a Poisson rate per 100 patient-years. The data come from the Adenomatous Polyp Prevention on Vioxx (APPROVe) clinical trial [24]. This trial was designed as a label extension study to compare rofecoxib with placebo for the prevention of recurrent neoplastic polyps after 3 years of treatment. However, concern developed over the frequency of thrombotic AEs that were observed in the rofecoxib arm. The pooled analysis for the rate of adjudicated treatment-emergent thrombotic events included a total of 2586 patients, 6386 patient-years of follow-up, and 72 events. The pooled Poisson rate for thrombotic events is 1.13 per 100

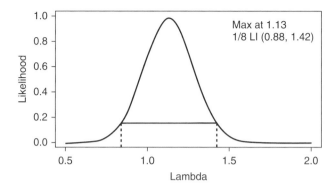

**Figure 11.1** The 1/8 support interval for lambda, the Poisson rate per 100 patient-years of adjudicated treatment-emergent thrombotic events in the APPROVe clinical trial.

patient-years. Figure 11.1 shows that the likelihood ratio for the Poisson rate is maximized at 1 (by definition) and occurs at the maximum likelihood estimate, 1.13. The latter rate is the best supported value for rate but values close on either side are well supported. Support decreases on either side of the maximum. The horizontal line depicts the 1/8 support interval for the pooled Poisson rate, (0.88, 1.42). Sponsors would compare this interval to what they might expect for a pooled rate. This would be a disappointing result if they expected the pooled rate to be no more than 0.50 per 100 patient-years. For comparison, the frequentist 95% confidence interval for this rate using the normal approximation would be (0.87, 1.39). Agreement of the type is not unusual. In fact for the normal distribution likelihood 1/6.7 support limits correspond to the frequentist 95% confidence interval. For more on agreement, see the next subsection on masked analyses.

Unmasked analysts, like DMC members, could apply this methodology to each treatment group and to the Poisson rate ratio. Herson [15] presents an extensive likelihood analysis of the APPROVe thrombotic event data.

### 11.3.3  Bayesian methods for masked or pooled analysis

Bayesian statistical methods allow for the incorporation of prior information into inference. Like the likelihood methods just described, Bayesian methods allow for inference conditional on the observed data while incorporating the prior information. The prior information comes in the form of probability distributions for the unknown parameters of the reference distribution for the data. When the prior distribution is combined with the reference distribution the resulting distribution is called the posterior distribution. This distribution carries data from the prior and the reference distribution and is conditional on the data observed. The Bayesian approach uses the posterior distribution to calculate the probability that the null hypothesis is true. This is a metric that cannot be derived from frequentist methods. The analog to the frequentist confidence interval is the credible interval also derived from the posterior distribution. The interpretation of the 95% credible interval is that the probability of the unknown parameter lying in the interval is 0.95. This is an interpretation that many non-statisticians naïvely and incorrectly apply to the frequentist confidence interval. The interpretation of the latter is merely that if researchers were to perform the experiment repeatedly and computed the confidence intervals using the frequentist methods then 95% of the intervals so calculated would contain the true parameter. It is strictly a repeated sampling paradigm. The Bayesian posterior credible interval with a uniform prior often has favorable frequentist properties in terms of coverage (see Chapter 6). This method of confidence interval construction is "exact" in the sense that it does not require approximations. Severini has written about the theoretic relationship between Bayesian and frequentist interval estimation [25, 26]. Casella and Berger [27] and Berger and Sellke [28] have written about the relationship between Bayesian and frequentist hypothesis testing.

Proposals for basing the final efficacy analysis of the primary endpoint in confirmatory trials raise concerns among by regulators because of the possibility that sponsors could choose a prior distribution in a way that may skew the results in a favorable direction. As a result Bayesian methods have not been used often for drug or biologic submissions at the FDA; there have been some submissions for medical devices [29], but even here priors based on objective information are required [30]. Bayesian methods have been used for drugs and biologics in exploratory trials where the sponsor generally has more analytic freedom than in confirmatory trials. However, because the prior distribution is considered a means to summarize prior information in a personal way there is no reason why the sponsor could not use Bayesian methods to review pooled safety data. For safety screening the Bayesian methods are merely a tool that biostatisticians use to call possible safety signals to the attention of the clinical staff. Hence there is less of a need to teach the clinical staff the details of Bayesian methods for safety than there might be for efficacy analysis.

Typical prior and reference distribution combinations are the normal prior for the normal reference distribution, resulting in a normal posterior distribution. When the posterior distribution is the same distribution as the prior and reference distribution the prior is called a conjugate prior. Another popular combination is the beta distribution prior for the binomial reference distribution, resulting in a beta-binomial posterior. For survival data the priors for the exponential reference distribution often are drawn from the gamma distribution family, resulting in a gamma posterior distribution.

Sponsors review safety data pooled over treatment groups, but the Bayesian credible interval can be applied to incidence rates in a manner similar to the support interval for likelihood methods described above. With knowledge of the rate for an AE expected in both experimental treatment and control groups, a prior distribution could be constructed for the AE incidence in the combined group. The reference distribution might be binomial and the prior beta with parameters based on prior knowledge. The credible interval for incidence would then incorporate both prior and current data on the combined groups.

Closely related to the *classical* Bayesian methods described above are the *empirical* Bayesian methods. While the classical Bayesian specifies a prior with fixed parameters, the empirical Bayesian specifies a family of priors (e.g., gamma family) and estimates the parameters of the prior using method of moments or maximum likelihood estimation from marginal distributions of data collected in the trial. Large sample sizes usually are needed to do this, as illustrated by DuMouchel [31] in his analysis of the FDA post-marketing MEDWATCH reports. Classical Bayesians can address many of the concerns of empirical Bayesians about the arbitrariness of the choice of priors for classical Bayesian analyses through sensitivity analysis, that is, assessing how different assumptions of prior distribution parameters would affect the conclusions. Classical Bayesians do not consider empirical Bayes methods to be Bayesian at all. They feel that empirical Bayesians are merely using Bayesian machinery to carry out a frequentist analysis. The classical Bayesian prior is independent of the data collected during the trial, as they feel it must be. The empirical Bayes prior is based on data collected during the trial, so it cannot be independent.

It would be interesting if sponsors would experiment with Bayesian methods during the long period when they review only pooled safety data but, to the author's knowledge, this is rarely done.

## 11.4 Safety monitoring-DMC view (partially or completely unmasked)

### 11.4.1 DMC data review operations

The DMC members review accumulating safety data periodically. Their job is to protect patient safety by reviewing tabular and graphical displays of safety data as well as narrative summaries of AE experiences prepared by investigators. The DMC members are looking for early safety signals. These signals would usually arrive in the form of a difference in incidence or rate per 100 patient-years between experimental treatment and control groups. The DMC members are especially aware of the Tier 1 AEs. As data accumulate the DMC may compile a Tier 2 AE list and possibly a Tier 3 list. DMC meetings will typically have an open and closed session. The open session is attended by sponsor staff and DMC members. Sponsor staff report study progress and pooled AE data at these open sessions. The closed sessions are attended by the DMC members. There are two biostatisticians at these meetings – the voting and the non-voting. The voting biostatistician is appointed to the DMC at the same time the clinical members are appointed. The non-voting biostatistician is employed by the DAC, the group responsible for preparing reports to the DMC, and it is the non-voting biostatistician (sometimes called the reporting biostatistician) who will present the reports during the meeting. DMC members will initially be partially masked to treatment identity but, as indicated above, they may become completely unmasked at any time and this is considered preferable by many DMC members.

### 11.4.2 Types of safety data routinely reviewed

Just prior to each DMC meeting the members will receive safety data in the form of tables, listings, and possibly graphs. These data come in the form of a table of frequency of treatment-emergent AEs classified by body system and event types within body system. Additional frequency tables classify the AEs by grade/severity and investigator judgment of relatedness to study drug. As indicated above, the latter table is not generally considered useful. These tables are repeated separately for SAEs. The term SAE is a regulatory term which applies to an AE that results in death, is life-threatening, requires inpatient hospitalization or prolongation of existing hospitalization, results in persistent or significant disability/incapacity, or is a congenital anomaly/birth defect [32]. While this subgroup is certainly worthy of attention, many DMC members also prefer to review frequency tables of patients of AEs and SAEs of moderate or worse severity. Severity is usually classified as none, mild, moderate, severe, or life-threatening. A typical definition of these grades is provided by Herson [15].

The AE tables will have a column for each treatment group. It is typical for the sample size for each group to appear under the treatment group identity on all AE tables. Although not often done, as indicated above, it is highly recommended that, for each table, under the sample size the column should display the number of patient-years of exposure. We will make frequent use of patient-years in this chapter. The AE data may be summarized by incidence, rate per 100 patient-years or time to event via a Kaplan–Meier graph. In frequentist analyses treatment group differences may be summarized as follows: incidence by the odds ratio, rate per 100 patient-years by the Poisson rate ratio, and time to event by the hazard ratio. Herson [15] provides details and examples for these computations.

The DMC members might be interested in descriptive statistics of the experimental treatment group regardless of the corresponding rate in the control group. In these cases methods discussed in Section 11.3.3 on masked analyses will apply even though the DMC members are unmasked to treatment.

Between-treatment group tests of statistical significance for evaluating safety do not have the drama that they have in efficacy analysis. Statistical significance testing for Tier 2 events will usually be unplanned and thus will be used to suggest to the DMC that further consideration may be necessary. The PSAP may indicate planned statistical significance testing for Tier 1events, and the consequences of statistically significant treatment effects should be noted in the PSAP or the protocol. Of course statistical significance does not imply clinical significance of the magnitude of the treatment effect. That is a matter for discussion among DMC members.

Most of the safety information reviewed by DMCs has been presented traditionally in tabular form. Graphical displays have recently come into use and have facilitated the finding of treatment differences. Figure 11.2 (see Chapter 2), an extension of a display described by Amit *et al.* [33], displays treatment differences in AE incidence by treatment group along with 95% confidence intervals for the relative risks. Volcano plots originally used in microarray research also may prove informative [34].

### 11.4.3   Assay sensitivity

Before summarizing various ways that statistical significance might be tested, it is important to introduce the concept of assay sensitivity. The assay sensitivity of a statistical comparison seeks to clarify what differences the current sample size had the desired power to find statistically significant. It also addresses what power the current sample size provides for detecting the treatment difference that the protocol specified as clinically significant and for which the trial sample size was derived [35]. Table 11.2 displays the assay sensitivity for various scenarios in a hypothetical clinical trial. We assume that cardiovascular events were placed in Tier 1 and the protocol specified an expected 2.0% incidence in the placebo group. With that assumption the protocol might have specified a sample size of 1290 patients in each group to yield a power of 0.80 to detect a 3.6% rate on experimental therapy. This rate would likely be chosen because it would be considered a clinically significant difference from the placebo rate. If the trial is now at the point where there are 600 patients in each treatment group then the statistical test has a power of 0.80 to detect an experimental rate of 4.6% and the power to detect the clinically significant 3.6% is only 0.51. If there were only 300 patients in each group an experimental treatment rate of 6.0% would have a power of 0.80 of detection while the power for the 3.6% rofecoxib rate of interest would be only 0.32. The DMC should be presented with a table such as Table 11.2 for all Tier 1 AE comparisons as well as Tier 2 AE types that emerge during the trial. This is vital so that all members understand the limitations of the current sample size to find differences of interest. Assay sensitivity should always be

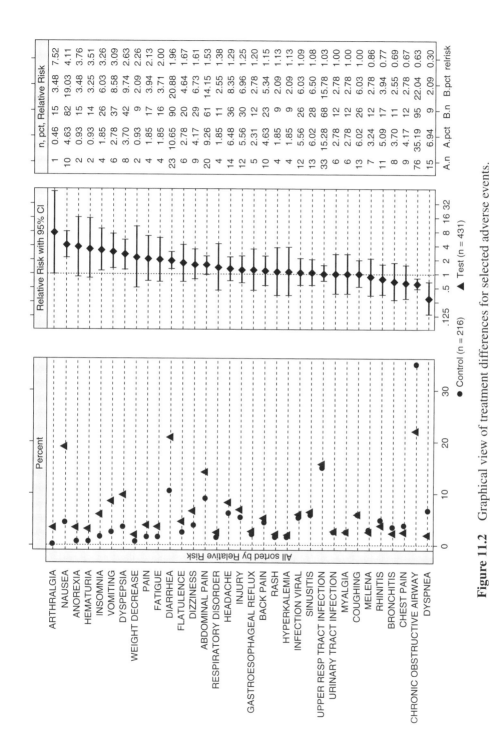

**Figure 11.2** Graphical view of treatment differences for selected adverse events.

**Table 11.2**    Assay sensitivity: analysis of experimental treatment vs placebo assuming the incidence of cardiovascular events in the placebo group is 2.0%.

| Sample size in each group | Experimental group incidence (%) | Power to detect the experimental rate in previous column |
| --- | --- | --- |
| 1290 | 3.6 | 0.80 |
| 600 | 4.6 | 0.80 |
| – | 3.6 | 0.51 |
| 300 | 6.0 | 0.80 |
| – | 3.6 | 0.32 |

computed when trials are terminated early for efficacy. This would be to avoid the naïve (and incorrect) conclusion that sufficient evidence for concluding efficacy implies that the evidence for concluding safety also is sufficient. The lack of treatment differences in safety could, in fact, be due to the smaller sample size. Many trials will continue to treat patients at least on the experimental treatment in these cases to do a better job in assessing safety. Including this type of follow-up in the protocol would be a good issue for the DMC biostatistician to bring up before the trial begins. Absence of evidence is not evidence of absence. This is especially true in safety analysis.

## 11.4.4    Comparing safety between treatments

### 11.4.4.1    Frequentist methods

Statistical significance between treatments can be tested in various ways. For count data the common chi-square test can be used. The question now arises as to how biostatisticians might help find early signals of AEs to place in Tier 2, that is, possible weak signals of safety parameters to follow. An informative method for DMC use is computation of the odds ratio and its 95% confidence interval. The odds ratio is a measure of relative risk of AEs between treatment groups. An odds ratio of 1 would indicate no association between events and treatment group. The odds ratio is the non-centrality parameter of the chi-square distribution and its confidence interval is computed from this distribution, although several methods are commonly used [36–39]. The confidence interval is easily computed using readily available computer software. DMC members will want to consider the upper limits of these confidence intervals, but it must be emphasized that early in the trial the confidence intervals will be wide due to the small sample sizes and not because the upper limit of the odds ratio, which could be in double digits during the progress of the trial, is really a plausible measure of risk.

The relative risk is a statistic that is closely related to the odds ratio. The relative risk is the ratio of the incidence of an event in the experimental group to its incidence in the control group. If $r_E$ of $n_E$ subjects in the experimental group and $r_C$ of $n_C$ subjects in the control group demonstrate an event, then the incidence in the experimental group, $p_E$, is estimated by $\hat{p}_E = r_E/n_E$ and the incidence in the control group, $p_C$, is estimated by $\hat{p}_C = r_C/n_C$. The relative risk, $R = p_E/p_C$, is estimated by $\hat{R} = \hat{p}_E/\hat{p}_C$. A confidence interval for $R$ can be computed assuming that $\log(\hat{R})$ is approximately normally distributed with mean $m = \log(R)$ and variance

$$s^2 = \frac{n_E - r_E}{n_E r_E} + \frac{n_C - r_C}{n_C r_C}.$$

The 95% confidence interval for $R$ is calculated as $\exp(m \pm 1.96s)$.

Epidemiologists favor the relative risk over the odds ratio because of its intuitive appeal and because they consider it appropriate for cohort studies. Although epidemiologists associate the odds ratio with case–control studies, biostatisticians favor using the odds ratio in clinical trial safety analyses because of its extension to logistic regression analysis that often is used to adjust for factors other than treatment that may affect safety. In addition, the odds ratio is the non-centrality parameter of the chi-square distribution and the minimal sufficient statistic of the multinomial likelihood, which ensures efficient estimation and hypothesis testing.

At the beginning of a clinical trial the DMC members might specify that they want odds ratios and 95% confidence intervals computed for all AEs which have been observed with some minimal frequency, say 10. Upon receiving the reports the biostatistician should scan the reports of SAEs for odds ratios greater than some cutoff, maybe 3 or 5, regardless of statistical significance and bring these events to the physician members of the committee. In many cases the physician members will indicate that there is no clinical concern, but the biostatistician is fulfilling his/her role by calling these potential signals to the attention of the full committee.

Of course the odds ratio using incidence does not take exposure into account. This could lead to some problems in decision-making because exposure could be less in one treatment group than in another due to dropouts, deaths, or treatment failures. We thus consider the ratio of Poisson rates of events per 100 patient-years. The 95% confidence interval for the Poisson rate ratio can be calculated using either a normal or binomial approximation, with the latter being preferred when the total number of events is less than 50; see [15] for computational details. A ratio of unity indicates no difference in rate between treatment groups. A rate of 2 would indicate that the risk per unit time of an event in the experimental group is twice that for the control group.

As stated previously, the best way to consider exposure for the sponsor safety review is with Kaplan–Meier life table analyses. For each AE type of interest a time to first occurrence of that event is computed with a separate Kaplan–Meier (cumulative incidence over time) curve for each treatment group. Clinicians can see at what point after treatment start the treatment differences begin. This would be important for treatments that might be labeled for short-term use. These dynamics cannot be learned from the Poisson analysis. In efficacy analysis, such as survival time, it is common for the curves to be displayed monotonically non-increasing (going downward). For safety it is useful for the curves to be shown monotonically non-decreasing (going upward). This way one can look at a Kaplan–Meier graph and know if it is an efficacy or safety endpoint just by looking at the direction of curves. Statistical significance of the difference between Kaplan–Meier curves is tested by the log-rank test [40, 41] using Cox proportional hazards regression analysis [41]. The proportional hazards regression model also allows for the computation of the hazard ratio and its confidence interval. This ratio is analogous to the Poisson rate ratio. It provides the relative risk of AE per unit time. Its computation requires the assumption of proportional hazards which may not apply for some events. The Poisson rate ratio would have a similar assumption. The latter is sometimes called the poor man's hazard ratio. It is a quick way of getting at relative risk per unit time and is useful for routine safety monitoring regardless of what assumptions might be violated. The Kaplan–Meier curves also yield what are known as landmark estimates of cumulative incidence. The Kaplan–Meier life table provides estimates of, say, 12-month incidence of events as well as the standard error of the estimate. The Kaplan–Meier landmark estimate for a given time point is definitely superior to the naïve calculation of dividing the number of people with the AE at or before the time point of interest by a denominator that does not adequately account for those patients who are no longer at risk due to discontinuation. The DMC biostatistician would usually request Kaplan–Meier time to first occurrence curves only for those AEs of interest to the DMC. Some of these graphs will inevitably be produced after the DMC meeting where the particular AE type is discussed for the first time.

Researchers should be aware of the phenomenon of informative censoring when computing Kaplan–Meier curves and testing for statistical significance. The censored observations, sometimes called incomplete observations, are those follow-up times for patients who did not experience the AE of interest and whose time will be not time to event but just time to last follow-up. It is assumed that censoring occurs randomly, but for safety analysis patients may be censored for an AE type because they have dropped out of the trial for toxicity or lack of efficacy. The typical time-to-event analysis of safety is time to first episode of a particular AE type. Comparing treatment groups using a log-rank test is certainly informative but it must be kept in mind that this analysis ignores all other types of AEs or discontinuations. At times analyses of time to first SAE, time to first moderate or worse episode of nausea/vomiting, for example, might be requested. Censoring progression-free survival (PFS) in oncology trials at the time of drop-out due to toxicity could tend to make the efficacy analysis of PFS actually favor the more toxic and likely less efficacious treatment [41, 42].

It may be useful to look at the changes in the hazard ratio over time to see how the treatment-associated risks might vary over a treatment regimen. One way to view this would be to plot the hazard ratio and its 95% confidence interval over time corresponding to treatment eras – cycles, induction, maintenance, and so on. In addition to the log-rank test for treatment difference in time to event, there is the generalized Wilcoxon test [43]. The generalized Wilcoxon test puts greater weight on events that occur early in treatment, while the log-rank test puts equal weight over all possible time periods [44]. Finding that the generalized Wilcoxon test yielded a smaller $p$-value than the log-rank test when applied to a set of event times might be evidence that the treatment effect occurs early, which may be apparent from the shape of the Kaplan–Meier curves.

Once an AE type of interest is found, analyses of repeated episodes may be of interest. Use of statistical methods for recurrent events [41, 45] might not be applicable because those patients with the shortest gap times between events are likely to drop out of the trial, introducing informative censoring. Also, the extra scrutiny of reviewing whether events are really recurrences of a previous event or new events would introduce some inconsistency and would not likely be worth the time. Time to the most severe episode of a particular event type should also be avoided. That analysis is based on an order statistic the distribution of which depends on the number of episodes a patient has had and, taking censoring into account, would create a very complicated analysis and certainly the naïve Kaplan–Meier analysis ignoring this complication would be misleading. Useful software for analyzing recurrent events has recently been described [46].

After an AE type is selected for further study in a Kaplan–Meier analysis biostatisticians should lead discussions with clinicians on the timing, duration, and repeat episodes of this event.

### 11.4.4.2    Likelihood methods

The likelihood methods of support discussed above for the Poisson rate per 100 patient-years for both treatment groups combined also can be applied to the ratio of two Poisson rates. A 1/8 support interval can be computed for the ratio. The interval will always include the maximum likelihood estimate of the ratio and indicate relative support for different alternative ratios. In practice, due to asymptotic approximations, the 1/8 support intervals are often close to frequentist intervals. However, the support intervals adhere closely to the likelihood principle [22]. The inference is conditional on what is observed and not on repeated sampling of outcomes that will never be observed as is the case with frequentist inference. The fact that there is usually little difference in the inference between support and frequentist methods may be the reason why frequentist methods have stood the test of time. They are approximating methods that are derived from the likelihood principle. Royall [22] presents several methods for computing the support limits for the odds ratio. Similar methods can be derived for the risk ratio. Conditioning on nuisance parameters is necessary in both cases.

### 11.4.4.3    Bayesian methods

Bayesian methods would use various prior and reference distribution combinations as described above for the sponsor view of pooled treatment groups. The probability that the null hypothesis of no difference between the treatment groups is true could be calculated from the resulting posterior distribution. A credible interval could be generated from the posterior distribution using a random mixture model [47, 48]. This is described in the next section along with the advantage certain Bayesian models have in dealing with multiplicity.

   The choice of prior distribution for this type of analysis would be solely up to the DMC biostatistician in consultation with the clinical members. If the Bayesian analysis is the basis for a decision for protocol change or trial termination then the prior distribution would have to be defended when presented to the sponsor. The DMC would have to be prepared with sensitivity analyses showing that the conclusions are robust over a sufficiently wide range of priors.

   A meta-analysis of previous trials using the same drug would be one source of data to justify a prior distribution, but this is a major undertaking and it is doubtful that a DMC could carry out such an extensive project within the limitations of time and budget. Even if a meta-analysis already exists for the drug–AE combination under investigation, there are many potential pitfalls associated with the use of such data [15, 49]. Among them would be confounding dose and indication, that is, the drug might be used for both migraines and epilepsy at different doses, also different doses by gender, criteria for selection of trials to include, whether the control group was the same in all trials, whether some trials were analyzed by fixed effects and some random effects and, of course, publication bias. Even looking at a single past trial has its inferential pitfalls [50]. Recent attempts at meta-analysis for safety issues for rosiglitazone for Type II diabetes [9] and pediatric antidepressants [51] have caused considerable controversy but have created a new interest in developing statistical methods for safety applications of meta-analysis [52–55].

   Previous trials may have had different eligibility requirements, discontinuation rates may have been lower and exposure times longer in the past because fewer alternative treatments existed at that time, difference in use of spontaneous or solicited AE reporting, and so on. These issues should be kept in mind when considering comparisons with data in previous trials.

A useful checklist for content of meta-analysis of previous trials is found in the PRISMA statement [56] which identifies 27 items that should be present in a meta-analysis report (e.g., consistence of results across studies, sensitivity to subgroup analysis). PRISMA has become the standard for systematic review and meta-analysis reporting. Hammad *et al.* [57] reviewed a series of selected published meta-analyses and present the variation in percentage of the 27 items that are included. The results are disappointing but there was no attempt to weight the items by importance.

The problem of combining $2 \times 2$ tables for the same AE (columns for treatment, rows for event present or absent) for phase II and phase III trials is closely related to the inferential issues just described. Biostatisticians should be aware of Simpson's paradox in this case [2, 58]. This is the phenomenon where there may be a treatment effect in the two $2 \times 2$ tables separately but it disappears or is reversed when the tables are combined. When this occurs it is important to look for additional confounding factors that may be causing this paradox – for example, differing sample sizes and differing supportive care between the trials. Combining tables using the Mantel–Haenszel test [59] might be helpful in this case.

### 11.4.4.4  Dealing with multiplicity

Multiplicity in safety monitoring occurs because safety parameters are compared periodically during the lifetime of a trial and, at each DMC meeting, several different variables may be compared for a treatment difference. While this is a well-known and well-addressed concern in frequentist efficacy analysis, it does not present a major problem in safety monitoring. Performing statistical hypothesis testing in safety monitoring is just one way to call attention to potential safety signals. As was suggested above, computing odds ratios and looking further into those AE types that have odds ratios higher than a certain threshold regardless of statistical significance is a perfectly reasonable way to screen for early signals. It is considered better to be conservative and bring up more potential signals than to try to be parsimonious and ignore some, especially since so many potential signals brought to the attention of DMC clinicians by the biostatistician are dismissed for good clinical reasons.

Nevertheless several authors have dealt with multiplicity in safety analysis, although their approach was applied to, and might be more appropriate for, final analysis of a completed trial rather than for use in interim monitoring. Mehrotra and Heyse [8] use data from a clinical trial in children for a quadrivalent vaccine against measles, mumps, rubella, and varicella (henceforth referred to as the MH data). They begin by dividing the 40 observed Tier 2 AE types into 11 body systems. A false discovery rate (FDR) [60–63] is used for error control instead of the familiar Type I error, which is also called the familywise error rate. The FDR measures the proportion of tests of true hypotheses tests (i.e., no treatment effect) that are lead to rejection of the null hypothesis (i.e., declared statistically significant). The FDR is the proportion of all tests that are declared statistically significant where there was, in fact, no treatment difference in AE frequency. They create a two-step process called a double FDR where in the first step the method assesses if each body system has a representative AE to go to the next round on the basis of an adjusted $p$-value. In the second round those body systems who qualify for the second round have further adjustment to their individual AEs and finally those that qualify are reported as AE events that are free from multiplicity concerns. Only one AE type (irritability) emerged as statistically significant. Mehrotra and Adewale [64] recently extended the Mehrotra–Heyse method to create more favorable power for signal detection.

This approach is potentially problematic because many AE types are classified under different terms in different body systems. For example, congestive heart failure could be classified as dyspnea, fatigue, or orthopnea. Strokes could be classified under a cardiovascular or neurologic body system. Herson [15] suggests not using the body system-preferred term hierarchy at all but instead dividing AEs into four quadrants – those SAEs with high impact, SAEs with low impact, AEs with high impact, AEs with low impact – and applying the Mehrotra and Heyse [8] methodology to just these four quadrants instead of multiple body systems. Herson claims that there will be less overlap among quadrants as there is overlap using the body system-preferred term approach and quadrants can be defined with appropriate clinical input, but could not apply this method to the MH data because dividing AE types within the four quadrants would require consultation with the clinical team that worked on the clinical trial.

Berry and Berry [65] present a Bayesian three-level hierarchical mixed model approach to the MH data. The lowest level is AE type, followed by body system associated with the specific AE and, thirdly, the collection of all body systems. Their model allows for Bayesian borrowing of information within body system. This reduces the problem of an AE type being arbitrarily classified among several AE types within a body system. The results of this analysis are the same as that of Mehrotra and Heyse (irritability was the only AE found to have statistical significance), but the authors point out that they did not have access to the complete data set which might have allowed for the deployment of the full artillery of Bayesian borrowing and, perhaps, led to different results. A simulation study showed that the Bayesian approach had more frequentist power to detect AE differences under certain alternative hypotheses than the double FDR approach [66]. This is presumably due to the ability of Bayesian methods to model the relationship between AE types.

Bayesian random mixture models can be useful for safety monitoring [48]. These models apply a beta prior to a binomial reference distribution and compute the posterior probability that the event frequency is equal among the two treatment groups. This model can be applied to several event types and the random mixture feature automatically adjusts for multiplicity [67]. The random mixture model framework also permits direct evaluation of the diagnostic properties (sensitivity, specificity, FDR, and missed discovery rate) of the method. Application of this approach to the MH data indicated, consistently with other methods, that irritability is the sole AE type to flag for further consideration [48].

Bayesian methods offer much promise for incorporating prior information and for multiplicity correction. The modeling decisions would be solely in the hands of the DMC biostatistician in collaboration with the clinical DMC members and the reporting biostatistician. Resulting analyses would aid in DMC decision-making only. When the trial concludes it would be up to the sponsor to decide if such an analysis should be submitted to regulators at the time the product label is created.

For the likelihood approach to data analysis multiplicity is not as central as issue as is the case in frequentist analyses because, unlike in a frequentist analysis, the probability of misleading evidence due to actions like repeat support level assessments is bounded [21]. This is not the case in frequentist analysis. Repeat testing of safety data which is inherent in periodic data review is not an issue for likelihood or Bayesian approaches because these methods closely follow the likelihood principle which is invariant to the number of looks at the data.

Southworth and O'Connell [68] compare frequentist, support, evidential likelihood methods, Bayesian methods, and state-of-the-art data mining methods for data-guided review of clinical trial safety data. They also give useful software and graphical presentations.

### 11.4.4.5  Safety information in efficacy data

For some diseases a gray area exists between efficacy and safety. In oncology, for instance, death and progression are common efficacy endpoints but they may also be safety endpoints. Experimental treatment dosage could be related to a disproportionate number of these events in the experimental group. If the same imbalance occurs in trials where a known effective agent is serving as active control and the trial compares this active control alone with an arm consisting of the experimental treatment and active control combined, it is possible that the experimental treatment is interfering with the efficacy of the active control. In most oncology trials the number of deaths and progressions in each group would routinely be reported to the DMC for their periodic data review. It is very important that efficacy data be handled with care and that only protocol-specified interim analyses take place. However, the DMC may feel unable to ignore an imbalance of these events between treatment groups when it occurs.

DMC members should be mindful of the information time when these unexpected efficacy/safety concerns take place. For binary efficacy outcomes, such as complete response, information time is computed as the ratio of the number of patients enrolled to the anticipated total number of patients. For time-to-event efficacy analyses, such as survival time or PFS, the information time is computed as the ratio of the number of events number of events to the total expected event count regardless of number of patients enrolled. DMCs might want to wait until at least information time 0.50 to perform an unscheduled interim analysis. This analysis can be performed by the DMC biostatistical member: odds ratio for binary endpoints, Poisson rate ratio for time-to-event endpoints. If the DMC choose to terminate the trial on the basis of this analysis they must be firm in their convictions because they will be reporting to the sponsor an unplanned efficacy analysis which could compromise trial integrity. Usually an intermediate position would be to talk over the situation with sponsor staff who can unmask. This would usually be the pharmacovigilance staff, medical governance staff or high level clinical and biostatistical executives.

An important metric in making the case for termination on the basis of the safety information implied by an efficacy endpoint would be conditional power. The latter is a frequentist method for computing the power to reject the null hypothesis of the primary efficacy endpoint given the data accumulated under various assumptions of the future drift of the efficacy variable. A DMC with a safety concern of any type might ask for a conditional power calculation. Before calculation the DMC should decide on the value of conditional power for which they would approach the sponsor for termination. Values between 0.10 and 0.20 are common. If 0.10 is chosen the DMC would be saying that if there is less than a power of 0.10 to find a statistically significant difference at the end of the trial the trial it would be unethical to continue the trial due to the safety concern. It should be emphasized that conditional power for an efficacy parameter can be computed for any safety concern, for example, neutropenia, gastritis, not just for the efficacy/safety gray area concerns.

Conditional power is computed when a planned interim efficacy futility analysis is included in the trial protocol. This is done so that a trial might terminate early if there is little chance of concluding efficacy regardless of the existence of safety concerns. The Bayesian analog to conditional power is predictive power. Here Bayesians provide a prior distribution on the future efficacy data and use the posterior distribution to compute the probability that the null hypothesis will be rejected at the end of the trial. Several authors have discussed methods for conditional power, futility analysis, and predictive probability [69–71].

### 11.4.4.6   Granularity (sparse tables)

Granularity refers to the practice of generating AE tables with many preferred terms within each body system. This results in tables with many sparse cells. In addition, it is rarely clear to investigators how to choose a preferred term for a given AE since there are many AEs that can be arbitrarily classified in more than one preferred term. Indeed, spreading AEs among several plausible terms can keep important AE types off of the resulting product label due to all of the competing terms appearing to have low incidence. Bayesian borrowing for the multiplicity correction above has some promise here [65]. However, it is far better for the DMC biostatistician to meet the DMC physicians before the start of the trial and decide on groupings within body systems that make sense for the particular trial. Herson [15] gives several examples of how different strategies for grouping the nine preferred terms within eye disorders can yield different results. One grouping is by inflammation type, the other by the tissue type involved. These groupings are not independent, but they do yield information that is potentially useful for clinical judgment and should be considered. The use of preferred terms in the analyses should be driven by overall incidence [72]. Those body systems with small total incidence would either not be analyzed at all or only be considered in the aggregate over all body systems. For those body systems with some threshold incidence preferred terms can be considered and perhaps grouped. The DMC biostatistician can help in deciding this analysis policy before the start of the trial.

### 11.4.4.7   Competing risks

It is important to consider competing risks when comparing treatments with respect to safety. Suppose, for example, that halfway through a trial the DMC observes a lower frequency of cardiotoxicity on the experimental arm than on the active control. This could be a legitimate safety difference between treatments. Patients on the experimental treatment possibly might have discontinued the trial earlier than control patients due to severe vomiting/diarrhea, and so might not have been in the trial long enough to experience cardiotoxicity. "Competing risks" refers to the situation where multiple events are being followed and the occurrence of one can affect or preclude the occurrence of another. The possibility of competing risks underscores the necessity for taking exposure into account either with a Poisson analysis or Kaplan–Meier time-to-event analysis. The reasons for discontinuation table should always be consulted for treatment differences that might explain competing risks. Gray [73] presents a method for performing a time-to-event analysis correcting for competing risks when Kaplan–Meier analysis is undertaken. Crowder [74] and Pintilie [75] present overviews of competing-risk methodology. While the DMC biostatistician should always bring the possibility of competing risks to the attention of the committee, physician input regarding the actual AE types is very important.

### 11.4.4.8   Multiregional trials, stratification, and adjustment

There are several cases where a stratified analysis of AE treatment comparisons might be preferable. This is particularly the case in multinational trials where geographic differences may be factors in treatment differences in AE frequency. Diet and genetic differences among regions may affect treatment differences. There may be a differential propensity to self-report AEs among regions: patients in some regions tend to be more stoical than in other regions or more suspicious about sharing this type of information. In some countries the health systems provide financial incentives for patients to be hospitalized, that is, the health systems pay more when a patient is hospitalized for an AE than when he/she is treated as an outpatient. Hospitalization is part of the definition of an SAE so, in addition to a stratified analysis, the DMC might decide to down-classify some of these events for the purpose of safety monitoring only, not for regulatory submission. The reclassification would come about after DMC physicians read the individual AE narratives and conclude that reclassification is warranted. In some cases regions may differ in use of supportive care or surgical techniques. When active controls are used the same active control may not be approved in all countries or, if the active control drug is expensive, as is often the case in oncology, there may be little experience with the active control. In these cases odds ratios between treatments may be considerably affected. A similar situation would arise when the control group is standard care and the latter differs among countries. Regulatory agencies have long been aware of the heterogeneity involved in multinational trials. Ibia and Binkowitz [76] provide a summary of the important issues in multiregional clinical trials.

There are other cases where, instead of a stratified analysis, an analysis adjusted for confounding variables might be indicated. In comparing treatment groups, researchers may notice a difference in the distribution of baseline characteristics between groups – gender, diastolic blood pressure, serum creatinine, and so on. Adjustments for differences could be made using the classic Mantel–Haenszel test [59, 77], but multivariable adjustment for AE count data is implemented more frequently through logistic regression analysis [78] which adjusts odds ratios for differences in baseline data. Similarly, the Cox proportional hazards model [41] can be used to correct hazard ratios for baseline characteristics in time-to-event analysis. Poisson regression can be used to adjust rate ratios in a somewhat similar manner.

## 11.5   Future challenges in safety monitoring

### 11.5.1   Adaptive designs

The advent of adaptive clinical trial designs must be considered in any discussion of what changes in statistical methods for safety monitoring might need in the future [79, 80]. Adaptive designs use efficacy information accumulating in the trial to alter the design of the trial. The most common adaptive design is sample size re-estimation. Other types of adaptive designs include dropping a dose or treatment group, adaptive assignment to treatment group, changing objectives of the trial particularly changing from a superiority trial to a non-inferiority trial, seamless transition from a phase II to phase III trial, and changing the effect size of interest.

There are clearly safety implications in all of these changes. DMCs must avoid the situation where sponsors, who are masked to treatment, follow adaptive protocols for design changes based on efficacy alone without any knowledge of treatment differences in safety. Adaptation may require dropping a dose for efficacy reasons, but it may be the only dose where the DMC has no safety concern. In changing from superiority to a non-inferiority efficacy design, DMC clinicians may feel that the experimental treatment has already demonstrated itself as inferior on the basis of safety. Clearly there is a need for "white space" in the process whereby the DMC has the opportunity to decide if the adaptation should proceed on the basis of safety. If adaptation is to reduce the effect size of interest, as is the case when the sample size re-estimation methodology of Cui *et al.* [81] is employed, the DMC must be clear that if they are comfortable with the safety profile with the original effect size, on the basis of a risk–benefit consideration, they also must be comfortable with this safety profile if the effect size is to be reduced. An interim analysis sample size re-estimation method that does not require a decrease in effect size does not create a problem because the DMC would, presumably, recommend trial termination at this point. An overview of sample size re-estimation methods is provided in [82], the details of adaptive design challenges to safety monitoring by DMCs are discussed in [15], and a presentation of detailed issues for randomized phase II/III trials in oncology is provided in [83].

### 11.5.2    Changes in the setting of clinical trials

Califf *et al.* [84] predict that future clinical trials will be performed in a regular healthcare setting. Patients will be randomized to treatments in a clinical trial if they meet eligibility requirements and if they consent. Otherwise they will be treated as usual. This will allow for clinical trials to accrue more rapidly and to include patients over a broader spectrum of characteristics, making the patients more representative of those seen in practice. We might expect an increase in underreporting of some types of AEs if investigators are not in a clinical trial mode when they see patients because of the mix of outpatient and clinical trial patients. Also the broad spectrum of patients that will enter trials of this type might make it difficult to identify safety signals because there are insufficient patients of the type most vulnerable to AEs. This will leave it to post-marketing surveillance to discover these events. It is hoped that biostatisticians will join the discussion of this innovative way of conducting trials so that these types of problems will be minimized.

### 11.5.3    New technologies

Many of the new technologies for data collection and recording will be of benefit in post-marketing surveillance. However, some will generate large volumes of safety data for pre-market clinical trials. Electronic health records will allow for efficient submission of safety data to sponsors. Then there will be continuous reporting of safety data from wireless sensors in the home, nanoparticles in the drugs will send messages to the internet which will help to monitor compliance. There will be a continual analysis of urine from the toilet in the home and vital signs through wireless sensors and smartphone apps. Thus the database will be much larger than today. Biostatisticians will be an important part of the decision as to how much data to use in a safety analysis and in what manner. Some statistical methods that may be useful are being developed today in bioinformatics and in neurological imaging.

## 11.6    Conclusions

This chapter has indicated many ways that the sponsor and DMC biostatisticians are vital members of the safety monitoring team and how this role is becoming important today and will become increasingly important as new technologies provide more continuous safety data for analysis. Many statistical methods have been discussed. Table 11.3 summarizes typical biostatistical activities of both the sponsor staff and the DMC biostatisticians during a trial. It represents what is typically done today. However, biostatisticians are encouraged to experiment with likelihood and Bayesian methods and develop new methods to deal with new safety issues as they arise.

**Table 11.3**  Typical biostatistical activities in safety monitoring.

1. Sponsor biostatistical staff (masked to treatment)

   Participate in creation of the program safety analysis plan

   Monitor adverse event levels throughout trial, taking pooling of treatment groups into account – both incidence and rate per100 patient-years. Compute confidence intervals

   Compile Tier 2 and 3 adverse event lists as data accumulate

2. Data monitoring committee biostatistical member and reporting biostatistician (partially or completely unmasked)

   Comment on PSAP

   Help DMC decide between being partially vs completely unmasked during trial

   Assist clinical members on pooling preferred terms to avoid granularity in analyses

   Review assay sensitivity for sample size at each meeting

   Monitor adverse event incidence and rate/100 patient-years by treatment group – also for serious adverse events, moderate or worse adverse event levels

   Compare treatment groups – odds ratios and confidence intervals, Poisson rate ratio and confidence intervals. Call differences that appear extreme to attention of clinical members regardless of statistical significance

   Apply stratification and/or covariate adjustment methods when indicated, for example, in multiregional trials

   Compile Tier 2 and 3 adverse event lists

   Kaplan–Meier time to first occurrence and log-rank test for Tier 1 and 2 events

   Consideration of timing, duration, and reoccurrence of Tier 1 and 2 events

   Caution clinical members on multiplicity and competing risks

# References

[1] Edwards, S., Koch, G.G., Sollecito, W.A. and Peace, K.E. (1990) Summarization, analysis, and monitoring of adverse experiences, in *Statistical Issues in Drug Research and Development* (ed K.E. Peace), Marcel Dekker, New York, pp. 19–170.

[2] Crowe, B.J., Xia, H.A., Berlin, J.A. *et al.* (2009) Recommendations for safety planning, data collection, evaluation and reporting during drug, biologic and vaccine development: a report of the safety planning, evaluation, and reporting team. *Clinical Trials*, **6**, 430–440.

[3] CIOMS Working Group (2005) Management of Safety Information From Clinical Trials, Report of CIOMS Working Group VI.

[4] Xia, H.A., Crowe, B.J., Schriver, R.C. *et al.* (2011) Planning and core analyses for periodic aggregate safety reviews. *Clinical Trials*, **8**, 175–182.

[5] Brown, E.G., Wood, L. and Wood, S. (1999) The medical dictionary for regulatory activities (MedDRA). *Drug Safety*, **20**, 109–117.

[6] US National Cancer Institute. Common Terminology Criteria for Adverse Events, v 3.0, US National Cancer Institute, http://ctep.cancer.gov/protocolDevelopment/electronic_applications/docs/ctcaev3.pdf.

[7] Gould, A. L., Lydick, E., and Gruer, P. (1996) Evaluating Safety in Clinical Trials: Internal Merck Memorandum 1/18/1996.

[8] Mehrotra, D.V. and Heyse, J.F. (2004) Use of the false discovery rate for evaluating clinical safety data. *Statistical Methods in Medical Research*, **13**, 227–238.

[9] Nissen, S.E. and Wolski, K. (2007) Effect of rosiglitazone on the risk of myocardial infarction and death from cardiovascular causes. *New England Journal of Medicine*, **356**, 2457–2471.

[10] FDA Diabetes Mellitus Evaluating Cardiovascular Risk in New Antidiabetic Therapies to Treat Type 2 Diabetes: Guidance for Industry, Food and Drug Administration, http://www.fda.gov/downloads/Drugs/GuidanceComplianceRegulatoryInformation/Guidances/ucm071627.pdf (accessed 26 June 2014).

[11] Ibrahim, J.G., Chen, M.H., Xia, H.A. *et al.* (2012) Bayesian meta-experimental design: evaluating cardiovascular risk in new antidiabetic therapies to treat type 2 diabetes. *Biometrics*, **68**, 578–586.

[12] Wernicke, J.F., Faries, D., Milton, D. *et al.* (2005) Detecting treatment-emergent adverse events in clinical trials – a comparison of spontaneously reported and solicited collection methods. *Drug Safety*, **30**, 437–455.

[13] Southworth, H. and Hefferman, J. (2012) Extreme value modeling of laboratory safety data from clinical trials. *Pharmaceutical Statistics*, **11**, 361–366.

[14] Ellenberg, S.S. and Braun, M.M. (2002) Monitoring the safety of vaccines – assessing the risks. *Drug Safety*, **25**, 145–152.

[15] Herson, J. (2009) *Data and Safety Monitoring Committees in Clinical Trials*, Chapman & Hall/CRC Press, Boca Raton, FL.

[16] Clopper, C.J. and Pearson, E.S. (1934) The use of confidence or fiducial limits illustrated in the case of the binomial. *Biometrika*, **26**, 404–413.

[17] O'Neill, R.T. (1987) Statistical analyses of adverse event data from clinical trials: special emphasis on serious events. *Drug Information Journal*, **21**, 9–20.

[18] Liu, G.F., Wang, J.Y., Liu, K. and Snavely, D.B. (2006) Confidence intervals for an exposure adjusted incidence rate difference with applications to clinical trials. *Statistics in Medicine*, **25**, 1275–1286.

[19] Kaplan, E.L. and Meier, P. (1958) Nonparametric estimation from incomplete observations. *Journal of the American Statistical Association*, **53**, 457–480.

[20] Blume, J.D. (2002) Tutorial in biostatistics: likelihood methods for measureing statistical evidence. *Statistics in Medicine*, **38**, 1193–1206.

[21] Blume, J.D. (2008) How often likelihood ratios are misleading in sequential trials. *Communications in Statistics – Theory and Methods*, **37**, 1193–1206.

[22] Royall, R.M. (1997) *Statistical Evidence: A Likelihood Paradigm*, Chapman & Hall, London.

[23] Edwards, A.W.F. (1992) *Likelihood*, Johns Hopkins University Press, Baltimore, MD.

[24] Bresalier, R.S., Sandler, R.S., Quan, H. *et al.* (2005) Cardiovscular events associated with rofecoxib in a colorecal adenoma chemoprevention trial. *New England Journal of Medicine*, **352**, 1092–1102.

[25] Severini, T.A. (1991) On the relationship between Bayesian and non-Bayesian interval estimates. *Journal of the Royal Statistical Society, Series B*, **51**, 611–618.

[26] Severini, T.A. (1993) Bayesian interval estimates which are also confidence intervals. *Journal of the Royal Statistical Society, Series B*, **55**, 533–540.

[27] Casella, G. and Berger, R.L. (1987) Reconciling Bayesian and frequentist evidence in the one-sided testing problem. *Journal of the American Statistical Association*, **82**, 106–111.

[28] Berger, J.O. and Sellke, T. (1987) Testing a point null hypothesis: the irreconcilability of p-values and evidence. *Journal of the American Statistical Association*, **82**, 112–122.

[29] Campbell, G. (2011) Bayesian statistics in medical devices: innovation sparked by FDA. *Biopharmaceutical Statistics*, **21**, 871–887.

[30] Pennello, G. and Thompson, L. (2008) Experience with reviewing Bayesian medical device trials. *Journal of Biopharmaceutical Statistics*, **18**, 81–115.

[31] DuMouchel, W. (1999) Bayesian data mining in large frequency tables, with an application to the FDA spontaneous reporting system (Disc: p190–202). *American Statistician*, **53**, 177–190.

[32] ICH Expert Working Group Post-approval sfety data management: definitions and standards for expedited reporting E2D, http://www.ich.org/fileadmin/Public_Web_Site/ICH_Products /Guidelines/Efficacy/E2D/Step4/E2D_Guideline.pdf (accessed 27 June 2014). (2003)

[33] Amit, O., Heiberger, R.M. and Lane, P.W. (2008) Graphical approaches to the analysis of safety data from clinical trials. *Pharmaceutical Statistics*, **7**, 20–35.

[34] Zink, R.C., Wolfinger, R.D. and Mann, G. (2013) Summarizing incidence of adverse events using volcano plots and time intervals. *Clinical Trials*, **10**, 398–406.

[35] D'Agostino, R.B., Massaro, J.M. and Sullivan, L.M. (2003) Non-inferiority trials: design concepts and issues –the encounters of academic consultants in statistics. *Statistics in Medicine*, **22**, 169–186.

[36] Agresti, A. (1992) A survey of exact inference for contingency tables (with discussion). *Statistical Science*, **7**, 131–177.

[37] Cytel (2007) *StatXact 8 User Manual*, Cytel, Cambridge, MA.

[38] Gart, J.J. (1970) Point and interval estimation of the common odds ratio in the combination of $2 \times 2$ tables with fixed marginals. *Biometrika*, **57**, 471–475.

[39] Gart, J.J. (1971) The comparison of proportions: a review of significance tests, confidence intervals, and adjustments for stratification. *Review of the Indian Statistical Institute*, **39**, 148–169.

[40] Cleves, M., Gould, W., Guttierrez, R. *et al.* (2008) *An Introduction to Survival Analysis Using Stata*, 2nd edn, CRC Press, Boca Raton, FL.

[41] Cox, D.R. (1972) Regression models and life tables (with discussion). *Journal of the Royal Statistical Society, Series B*, **34**, 187–220.

[42] Carroll, K.J. (2007) Analysis of progression-free survival in oncology trials: Some common statistical issues. *Pharmaceutical Statistics*, **6**, 99–113.

[43] Gehan, E.A. (1965) A generalized Wilcoxon test for comparing arbitrarily singly-censored samples. *Biometrika*, **52**, 203–223.

[44] Prentice, R.L. and Marek, P. (1979) A qualitative discrepancy between censored data rank tests. *Biometrics*, **35**, 861–867.

[45] Cook, R.J. and Lawless, J.F. (2007) *Statistical Analysis of Recurrent Events*, Springer, New York.

[46] Sun, R.J. and Cotton, D. (2010) Analysis of Survival Data with Recurrent Events Using SAS, Statistics and Data Analysis – SAS Global Forum.

[47] Gould, A.L. (2007) Accounting for multiplicity in the evaluation of "signals" obtained by data mining from spontaneous report adverse event databases. *Biometrical Journal*, **49**, 151–165.

[48] Gould, A.L. (2008) Detecting potential safety issues in clinical trials by Bayesian screening. *Biometrical Journal*, **50**, 837–851.

[49] Berlin, J.A. (2008) Use of meta-analysis in drug safety assessments. Paper presented at Spring Statistical Meetings, International Biometric Society, ENAR, Arlington, VA.

[50] Ioannidis, J.P.A., Mulrow, C.D. and Goodman, S.N. (2006) Adverse events: the more you search, the more you find. *Annals of Internal Medicine*, **144**, 298–300.

Medication-related harms can be identified from many sources, typically case reports, observational studies, and randomized trials. How one defines and looks for problems affects the numbers of AEs that patients report. Patients' judgments about tolerable harm can depend on whether they felt they had effective therapeutic alternatives. It is important to follow appropriate guidelines specifying how and when harms-related information was collected. It is almost always inappropriate to make statements about no difference in adverse event rates based on non-significant *p*-values.

[51] Bridge, J.A., Iyengar, S., Salary, C.B. *et al.* (2007) Clinical response and risk for reported sucidal ideation and sucide attempts in pediatric antidepressant treatment: a meta-analysis of randomized controlled trials. *Journal of the American Medical Association*, **297**, 1683–1696.

[52] Claggett, B. and Wei, L.J. (2011) Analytical issues regarding rosiglitazone meta-analysis. *Archives of Internal Medicine*, **171**, 180.

[53] Hu, M., Cappelleri, J.C. and Lan, K.K.G. (2007) Applying the law of the iterated logarithm to control type I error in cumulative meta-analyses of binary outcomes. *Clinical Trials*, **4**, 329–340.

[54] Shuster, J.J., Jones, L.S. and Salman, D.A. (2007) Fixed vs random effects meta-analysis in rare event studies: the rosiglitazone link with myocardial and cardiac death. *Statistics in Medicine*, **26**, 4375–4385.

[55] Tian, L., Cai, T., Pfeiffer, M.A. *et al.* (2009) Exact and efficient inference procedures for meta-analysis and its application to the analysis of independent $2 \times 2$ tables with all available data but without artificial continuity correction. *Biostatistics*, **10**, 275–281.

[56] Liberati, A., Altman, D.G., Tetzlaff, J. *et al.* (2009) The PRISMA statement for reporting systematic reviews and meta-analyses of studies that evaluate health care interventions: explanation and elaboration. *Journal of Clinical Epidemiology*, **62**, e1–e34.

[57] Hammad, T.A., Neyarapally, G.A., Pinhiero, S.P. *et al.* (2013) Reporting of meta-analyses of randomized controlled trials with a focus on drug safety: an empirical assessment. *Clinical Trials*, **10**, 389–397.

[58] Simpson, E.H. (1951) The interpretation of interaction in contingency tables. *Journal of the Royal Statistical Society, Series B*, **13**, 238–241.

[59] Mantel, N. and Haenszel, W. (1959) Statistical aspects of the analysis of data from retrospective studies of disease. *Journal of the National Cancer Institute*, **22**, 719–748.

[60] Benjamini, Y. and Hochberg, Y. (1995) Controlling the false discovery rate: a practical and powerful approach to multiple testing. *Journal of the Royal Statistical Society, Series B*, **57**, 289–300.

[61] Benjamini, Y. and Yekutieli, D. (2005) False discovery rate-adjusted mulitple confidence intervals for selected parameters. *Journal of the American Statistical Association*, **100**, 81.

[62] Pounds, S. and Cheng, C. (2006) Robust estimation of the false discovery rate. *Bioinformatics*, **22**, 1979–1987.

[63] Pena, E.A., Habiger, J.D. and Wu, W. (2011) Power-enhanced multiple decision functions controlling family-wise and false discovery rates. *Annals of Statistics*, **39**, 556–583.

[64] Mehrotra, D.V. and Adewale, A.J. (2012) Flagging clinical adverse experiences: reducing false discoveries without materially compromising power for detecting true signals. *Statistics in Medicine*, **31**, 1918–1930.

[65] Berry, S.M. and Berry, D.A. (2004) Accounting for multiplicities in assessing drug safety: a three-level hierarchical mixture model. *Biometrics*, **60**, 418–426.

[66] Xia, H.A. (2012) Bayesian applications in drug safety evaluation. Paper presented at Spring Statistical Meetings, International Biometric Society, ENAR Washington, DC.

[67] Scott, J.G. and Berger, J.O. (2006) An exploration of aspects of Bayesian multiple testing. *Journal of Statistical Planning and Inference*, **136**, 2144–2162.

[68] Southworth, H. and O'Connell, M. (2009) Data mining and statistically guided clinical review of adverse event data in clinical trials. *Journal of Biopharmaceutical Statistics*, **19**, 803–817.

[69] Herson, J., Buyse, M. and Witte, J.S. (2012) On stopping a randomized clinical trial for futility, in *Designs for Clinical Trials: Perspectives on Current Issues*, Chapter 5 (ed D. Harrington), Springer, New York.

[70] Lan, K.K.G. and Wittes, J. (1988) The B-value: a tool for monitoring data. *Biometrics*, **44**, 579–585.

[71] Proschan, M.A., Lan, K.K.G. and Wittes, J. (2006) *Statistical Monitoring of Clinical Trials*, Springer, New York.

[72] Kubler, J., Vonk, R., Belmel, S. *et al.* (2005) Adverse event analysis and MedDRA: business as usual or challenge? *Drug Information Journal*, **39**, 63–72.

[73] Gray, R.J. (1988) A class of *k*-sample tests for comparing the cumulative incidence of a competing risk. *Annals of Statistics*, **16**, 1141–1154.

[74] Crowder, M.J. (2001) *Classical Competing Risks*, Chapman & Hall/CRC Press, Boca Raton, FL.

[75] Pintillie, M. (2006) *Competing Risks: A Practical Perspective*, John Wiley & Sons, Ltd, Chichester.

[76] Ibia, E.O. and Binkowitz, B. (2011) Proceedings of the DIA workshop on multiregional clinical trials. *Drug Information Journal*, **45**, 391–403.

[77] Piantadosi, S. (2005) *Clinical Trials: A Methodologic Perspective*, 2nd edn, Wiley-Interscience, Hoboken, NJ.

[78] Hosmer, D.W. and Lemeshow, S. (2000) *Applied Logistic Regression*, 2nd edn, Wiley-Interscience, Hoboken, NJ.

[79] Dragalin, V. and Fedorov, V. (2006) Multistage designs for vaccine safety studies. *Journal of Biopharmaceutical Statistics*, **16**, 539–553.

[80] Gallo, P. and Krams, M. (2006) PhRMA working group on adaptive designs: introduction to the full white paper. *Drug Information Journal*, **40**, 445–449.

[81] Cui, L., Hung, H.M.J. and Wang, S.-J. (1999) Modification of sample size in group sequential trials. *Biometrics*, **55**, 853–857.

[82] Chuang-Stein, C., Anderson, K., Gallo, P. *et al.* (2006) Sample size re-estimation: a review and recommendations. *Drug Information Journal*, **40**, 475–484.

[83] Korn, E.L., Freidlin, B., Abrams, J.S. *et al.* (2012) Design issues in randomized phase II/III trials. *Oncology*, **30**, 667–671.

[84] Califf, R.M., Filerman, G.L., Murray, R.K. *et al.* (2012) The clinical trials enterprise in the United States: a call for disruptive innovation. Institute of Medicine Discussion Paper, IOM Forum on Drug Discovery, Development and Translation.

# 12

# Sequential testing for safety evaluation

## Jie Chen

*Merck Serono (Beijing) R&D Hub, 9 Jian Guo Road, Chaoyang, Beijing 100022, China*

## 12.1 Introduction

Since the pioneering work by Wald [1] on the sequential probability ratio test (SPRT) that originated from the needs of sequential testing in the development of military and naval equipment, there have been many research and methodological developments in sequential analysis. Its applications have expanded to many applied fields including public health surveillance and clinical research. Comparing to the fixed sample size design, sequential tests have the merit of using a smaller expected sample size in order to reach the same statistical conclusions.

Sequential analysis is especially useful in safety evaluation of medical products, simply because (i) safety assessment is a continuous process during the application of medical products to human subjects; (ii) safety data are cumulated sequentially and there is a greater chance to detect potential safety issues earlier; (iii) sequential monitoring is essential for timely detection of any safety problems, which is critical from ethic and public health perspectives; and (iv) safety signals may appear any time, with known or unknown incubation period, after administration of medical products, and sequential looks of safety data increase the probability of detecting safety concerns right after their occurrence. In brief, sequential analysis of safety data ensure early detection of safety issues while minimizing the risk for patients who are exposed to the unsafe medical products.

*Statistical Methods for Evaluating Safety in Medical Product Development*, First Edition.
Edited by A. Lawrence Gould.
© 2015 John Wiley & Sons, Ltd. Published 2015 by John Wiley & Sons, Ltd.

## 12.2   Sequential probability ratio test (SPRT)

### 12.2.1   Wald SPRT basics

Wald presented the SPRTs in the framework of testing a simple null hypothesis against a simple alternative hypothesis [1]. We briefly describe the method here to provide a foundation for the discussion of a useful generalization later. Let $x_1, \ldots, x_N$ denote a sequence of observed independent random variables with a common probability density or mass function $f(x; \theta)$, where $\theta$ is the unknown parameter about which hypotheses are to be tested. The aim is to test the null hypothesis $H_0: \theta = \theta_0$ against the alternative hypothesis $H_1: \theta = \theta_1$, where both $\theta_0$ and $\theta_1$ are predefined known values. Suppose further that the $x_i$ are observed sequentially and $x_i$ follows the distribution $f(x_i; \theta_0)$ under the null hypothesis, and the distribution $f(x_i; \theta_1)$ under the alternative hypothesis. Let $\Lambda_n$ denote the likelihood ratio based on the observation sequence $x_1, \ldots, x_n$:

$$\Lambda_n = \prod_{i=1}^{n} \frac{f(x_i; \theta_1)}{f(x_i; \theta_0)} = \frac{f(\mathbf{x}; \theta_1)}{f(\mathbf{x}; \theta_0)}.$$

The Wald SPRT procedure stops sampling after $N$ observations are obtained, where

$$N = \inf_{n \geq 1} \{\Lambda_n \geq A \text{ or } \Lambda_n \leq B\}$$

and $A$ and $B$ $(0 < B < A < \infty)$ are critical values for the procedure to stop sampling. If $B < \Lambda_n < A$, the study is continued and no decision is made about accepting the null or alternative hypothesis. If $\Lambda_n \geq A$ or $\Lambda_n \leq B$, the study is terminated and the alternative hypothesis is accepted when $\Lambda_n \geq A$ or the null hypothesis is accepted when $\Lambda_n \leq B$.

The critical values $A$ and $B$ are determined so as to control both the Type I and Type II error rates at their respective levels. Let $\alpha$ denote the Type I error rate for rejection of the null hypothesis $H_0$ when it is true, that is, $\alpha = P_0\{\Lambda_n \geq A\}$, and let $\beta$ denote the Type II error rate for rejection of the alternative hypothesis $H_1$ when it is true, that is, $\beta = P_1\{\Lambda_n \leq B\}$, where $P_0(\cdot)$ and $P_1(\cdot)$ represent the probability under the null and alternative hypotheses, respectively. Let $A_n$ denote the subset of $n$-dimensional space where $B < \Lambda_{n-1} < A$ and $\Lambda_n \geq A$. Note that $\{N = k, \Lambda_k \geq A\} = (x_1, \ldots, x_n) \in A_n$. Since $\Lambda_n \geq A$ implies $f(\mathbf{x}; \theta_1) \geq Af(\mathbf{x}; \theta_0)$, it follows that

$$\alpha = \sum_{1 \leq k \leq \infty} P_0(N = k, \Lambda_k \geq A) = \sum_{1 \leq k \leq \infty} \int_{A_n} f(\mathbf{x}; \theta_0) dx$$

$$\leq A^{-1} \sum_{1 \leq k \leq \infty} \int_{A_n} f(\mathbf{x}; \theta_0) dx = A^{-1}(1 - \beta).$$

Consequently, the critical value $A$ must satisfy

$$A \leq (1 - \beta)/\alpha \tag{12.1}$$

and the lower limit of the lower critical value $B$ must satisfy

$$B \geq \beta/(1 - \alpha). \tag{12.2}$$

The critical values therefore can be approximated by $A \approx (1 - \beta)/\alpha$ and $B \approx \beta/(1 - \alpha)$. Alternatively, given the critical values $A$ and $B$, the Type I and Type II error probabilities can be approximated simply by

$$\alpha = (1-B)/(A-B) \quad \text{and} \quad \beta = B(A - 1)/(A - B).$$

The adjustment for multiple tests is automatic because the critical values are estimated using the Type I and Type II error rates. When both $\alpha$ and $\beta$ are small, the bounds can be usefully approximated by $A \approx 1/\alpha$ and $B \approx \beta$.

The sample size $N$ needed to reach a decision in an SPRT procedure is a random number and its distribution depends on the true state of the observed data. Since $N$ is finite with probability 1, it can take on values 1, 2, ... with probabilities $p_1, p_2, \ldots, \sum p_i = 1$.

If a decision to stop sampling is reached at the $n$th stage, then $\log(\Lambda_n)$ can be regarded as a two-valued random variable taking on the values $\log(A)$ and $\log(B)$, with approximate expectation

$$E[\log(\Lambda_N)] \approx \log(A)\, P\{\log(\Lambda_N) = \log(A)\} + \log(B)\, P\{\log(\Lambda_N) = \log(B)\}$$

$$= \log(A)P\{\text{reject } H_0\} + \log(B)P\{\text{accept } H_0\}. \tag{12.3}$$

Under $H_0$ and $H_1$, respectively, expression (12.3) is

$$E_0[\log(\Lambda_N)] \approx \log(A)\alpha + \log(B)(1 - \alpha),$$

$$E_1[\log(\Lambda_N)] \approx \log(A)(1 - \beta) + \log(B)\alpha.$$

Since $\log(\Lambda_N) = \sum_{i=1}^{N} Z_i$ where $Z_i = \log\{f(x_i; \theta_1)/f(x_i; \theta_0)\}$, it follows from Wald's likelihood identity, $E[\log(\Lambda_N)] = E(N)\, E(Z)$, and replacement of $\log(A)$ with $\log\{(1 - \beta)/\alpha\}$ and $\log(B)$ with $\log\{\beta/(1 - \alpha)\}$ that the expected sample sizes under $H_0$ and $H_1$ are given by

$$E_0(N) \approx \left\{ \alpha\, \log \left( \frac{1 - \beta}{\alpha} \right) + (1 - \alpha)\log \left( \frac{\beta}{1 - \alpha} \right) \right\} / \mu_0, \tag{12.4}$$

$$E_1(N) \approx \left\{ (1 - \beta)\, \log \left( \frac{1 - \beta}{\alpha} \right) + \beta\, \log \left( \frac{\beta}{1 - \alpha} \right) \right\} / \mu_1, \tag{12.5}$$

respectively, where $\mu_0 = E_{\theta_0}[\log(\Lambda_N)]$ under the null hypothesis and $\mu_1 = E_{\theta_1}[\log(\Lambda_N)]$ under the alternative. The SPRT method has the least expected sample size among all tests with error probabilities satisfying $P_0\{\text{reject } H_0\} \leq \alpha$ and $P_1\{\text{accept } H_0\} \leq \beta$ [2].

## 12.2.2    SPRT for a single-parameter exponential family

Suppose that the observed data $x_1, \ldots, x_n$ are independent and identically distributed with a distribution function in a single-parameter exponential family

$$f(x_i; \theta) = \exp[\theta T(x_i) - C(\theta)]\, h(x_i). \tag{12.6}$$

The goal is a sequential test of the null hypothesis $H_0: \theta = \theta_0$ against the alternative hypothesis $H_1: \theta = \theta_1$. Let $\ell_n$ denote the log likelihood ratio based on observations $x_1, \ldots, x_n$,

$$\ell_n = (\theta_1 - \theta_0)T(\mathbf{x}) - n[C(\theta_1) - C(\theta_0)],$$

where $T(\mathbf{x}) = \sum_{i=1}^{n} T(x_i)$. If the prespecified Type I and Type II error rates are $\alpha$ and $\beta$, respectively, and the corresponding critical values $A$ and $B$ are obtained from equations (12.1) and (12.2), then the "continue sampling" region for the Wald SPRT procedure consists of the values of $\mathbf{x}$ satisfying

$$B' = \frac{B + n[C(\theta_1) - C(\theta_0)]}{\theta_1 - \theta_0} < T(\mathbf{x}) < \frac{A + n[C(\theta_1) - C(\theta_0)]}{\theta_1 - \theta_0} = A'. \qquad (12.7)$$

Immediate consequences of the well-known property of exponential family distributions that $E[T(x_i)] = \partial C(\theta)/\partial\theta$ are that $\mu_0 = E_0(\ell_n)$ and $\mu_1 = E_1(\ell_n)$. Substituting these expressions into equations (12.4) and (12.5) provides estimates of the expected sample size under the null and alternative hypotheses, respectively.

### 12.2.3    A clinical trial example

Suppose that a data and safety monitoring committee (DSMC) for a trial of a new treatment would like to monitor the occurrence of a particular adverse event that might be associated with the administration of the new treatment. Let $x_i$ correspond to the $i$th observed event, taking the value 1 if the event occurs in the treatment group or 0 if it occurs in the control group. Let $\pi = P(x_i = 1)$ and $1 - \pi = P(x_i = 0)$. Each $x_i$ is a Bernoulli trial and the sequence of observations $\mathbf{x} = (x_1, \ldots, x_n)$ constitutes a sequence of independent Bernoulli trials with the likelihood function

$$f(\mathbf{x};\ \pi) = \pi^{\sum_{i=1}^{n} x_i}(1 - \pi)^{n - \sum_{i=1}^{n} x_i}. \qquad (12.8)$$

Just to make things interesting, suppose that the subject allocation ratio is $r : 1$, that is, $r$ subjects are assigned to the treatment group for every subject assigned to the control group. If the adverse event is not associated with the new treatment, then the number of events should be distributed between the two groups according to the subject allocation ratio $r : 1$, that is, $P\{x_i = 1\} = \pi = r/(r + 1)$ and $P\{x_i = 0\} = 1 - \pi = 1/(r + 1)$, assuming that all other factors (except for treatment difference) affecting the counting process (e.g., the pattern of missing data and drop-outs) are the same for both groups. On the other hand, if the treatment causes an increasing risk of the adverse event with a relative risk $\phi(>1)$ of the treatment over the control group, then for every event occurring in the control group, the number of events from the treatment group will increase from $r$ to $\phi r$. Hence, the probability $P\{x_i = 1\}$ becomes $\pi = \phi r/(\phi r + 1)$ and the probability $P\{x_i = 0\}$ becomes $1 - \pi = 1/(\phi r + 1)$.

The objective is to test, on an ongoing (sequential) basis, whether the treatment causes an increasing risk of the adverse event with prespecified relative risk $\phi > 1$ over the control. The null and alternative hypotheses can be written as

$$H_0^{\pi}\ :\ \pi = \pi_0 = r/(r + 1)\ \text{(i.e., } \phi = 1\text{),}$$
$$H_1^{\pi}\ :\ \pi = \pi_1 = \phi r/(\phi r + 1), \qquad (12.9)$$

respectively. If the parameter $\pi$ in equation (12.8) is expressed in terms of the relative risk $\phi$, the likelihood function (12.8) can be written in the form of (12.6) with

$$\theta = \log(\phi r), \quad C(\theta) = \log[1 + \exp(\theta)],$$

$$T_n(x) = \sum_{i=1}^{n} X_i, \quad h(x_i) \equiv 1.$$

Therefore, testing $H_0^\pi$ against $H_1^\pi$ in (12.9) is equivalent to testing the null hypothesis

$$H_0^\theta : \theta = \log(\phi_0 r) \quad (\phi_0 = 1) \tag{12.10}$$

against the alternative hypothesis

$$H_1^\theta : \theta = \log(\phi_1 r) \quad (\phi_1 > 1). \tag{12.11}$$

If $\alpha = 0.05$ and $\beta = 0.10$, then the corresponding critical values from (12.1) and (12.2) are

$$A = \log[(1 - \beta)/\alpha] = 2.89, \quad B = \log[\beta/(1 - \alpha)] = -2.25.$$

From (12.7), the Wald SPRT procedure stops sampling to reject the null hypothesis 12.10 and accept the alternative hypothesis 12.11 if

$$\sum_{i=1}^{n} X_i \geq A' = \frac{2.89 + n[\log(1 + \phi_1 r) - \log(1 + r)]}{\log(\theta_1)}$$

or to accept the null hypothesis 12.10 and reject the alternative hypothesis 12.11 if

$$\sum_{i=1}^{n} X_i \leq B' = \frac{-2.25 + n[\log(1 + \phi_1 r) - \log(1 + r)]}{\log(\theta_1)}.$$

The rejection bound $A'$ and the acceptance bound $B'$ both depend on the total observed number of events, $n$, the risk increase specified by the alternative hypothesis, $\phi_1$, and the allocation ratio, $r$. Figure 12.1 displays the bounds for $(\alpha, \beta) = (0.05, 0.1)$ and $(0.1, 0.01)$ and $\phi_1 = 2$ or 4. The bounds are rounded to the largest integers not exceeding the bounds. The rejection and acceptance bounds increase by steps because of their discreteness. The continuation region or the distance between $A'$ and $B'$ is relative stable across $n$ for fixed $\alpha, \beta$, and $\phi_1$. The continuation region becomes narrow as $\phi_1$ increases for a given $\alpha$ and $\beta$ because the difference between $A'$ and $B'$ is a decreasing function of the relative risk $\phi_1$,

$$A' \, B' = \frac{\log\left(\frac{1 - \beta}{\alpha}\right) - \log\left(\frac{\beta}{1 - \alpha}\right)}{\log(\phi_1)}$$

which does not depend on the total sample size, $n$.

The rejection and acceptance bounds $A'$ and $B'$ can be manipulated through the specification of the Type I and Type II error probabilities. One may choose to tolerate a higher proportion of false positives when monitoring a serious adverse event by using a larger Type I error rate $\alpha$ and smaller Type II error rate $\beta$ to ensure that a true safety issue will be discovered with a high statistical power. For instance, the rejection bounds $A'$ in parts (c) and (d) of Figure 12.1 are lower than those in (a) and (b).

## 12.2.4   Application to monitoring occurrence of adverse events

Although the Wald SPRT approach has been employed in many applied fields (e.g., process control) and in the design and analysis of clinical experiments almost since its inception [3], it has been applied only recently to monitoring human health concerns including surveillance of medical product safety. Among the earliest applications in adverse event monitoring, Spiegel-halter *et al.* applied a risk-adjusted SPRT to three longitudinal data sets for retrospective

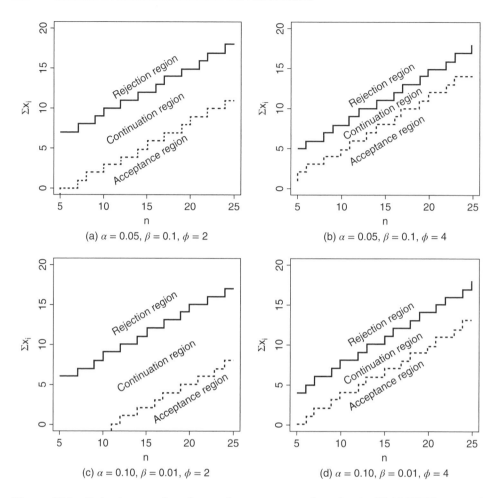

**Figure 12.1** Rejection, continuation, and acceptance regions for the Wald SPRT approach to monitoring Bernoulli trials with $(\alpha, \beta) = (0.05, 0.1)$ and $(0.1, 0.01)$, subject allocation ratio $r = 1$, and prespecified detectable risk ratio $\phi_1 = 2, 4$.

analyses of adverse clinical outcomes after cardiac surgery [4]. While there are many ways to estimate an individual's risk after adjusting for some risk factors (e.g., generalized linear models), the authors obtained the risks of death for individual patients after surgery by adjusting for risk factors at the provider level. A patient who either died or survived was treated as a Bernoulli trial and the aggregate death data of a group of patients from three medical centers were taken as a Poisson process. Different levels of the Type I and Type II error rates were employed for individual centers and for all the three centers as a whole to indicate different levels of urgency. For a single center, $\alpha = \beta = 0.1$ were used to derive an "alert" threshold, and $\alpha = \beta = 0.1$ for an "alarm." When applying the risk-adjusted SPRT approach to aggregate death data from all three centers, the authors employed Bonferroni-type adjustments to accommodate the multiple testing due to the increased number of deaths combined from the three centers. The authors also considered the SPRT reset method, that is, restarting the SPRT procedure when the lower limit is crossed, to avoid the possibility of building up excessive "credit" on the past data and hence to improve the sensitivity of event detection.

Davis *et al.* applied the Wald SPRT to a subset of the Centers for Disease Control and Prevention (CDC) Vaccine Safety Datalink (VSD) for surveillance of vaccine safety [5]. The motivation of this application was driven by the need to detect serious adverse events (e.g., intussusception in the rotavirus vaccine case) as soon as possible after the introduction of a new vaccine (e.g., rotavirus vaccine) using the CDC's dynamic VSD database. With rhesus-rotavirus vaccine as an example, Davis *et al.* first defined a time frame of nearly 5 years, and then segmented the chronological data into weekly cohorts of vaccinated children which were further partitioned into a baseline period before and a surveillance period after the introduction of the rotavirus vaccine. They employed risk-adjustment methods [6] to account for age, calendar time, season, and gender, to obtain strata with a unique combination of risk factors in each stratum. These risk factors were used in turn in a logistic model to estimate the probabilities of intussusception. The binomial likelihood function was chosen as a likelihood function for observing different numbers of intussusception cases each week in the database. *Davis et al.* were able to detect a 10-fold increased risk of intussusception in 10 weeks after introduction of the rotavirus vaccine, with the second reported case of intussusception among vaccine recipients using the SPRT method, a prespecified null hypothesis of no risk increase, and an alternative hypothesis of 10-fold increase (an effect size considered to be of public health importance) of intussusception risk among vaccinated children. They also applied the SPRT method to the detection of decreased risk of some adverse events associated with the changeover of diphtheria-tetanus-whole cell pertussis to diphtheria-tetanus-acellular pertussis vaccine.

## 12.3    Sequential generalized likelihood ratio tests

Although the Wald SPRT procedure has proven be a very useful tool for sequential testing, it does have some practical deficiencies. In addition to a potentially open continuation region for small log likelihood ratio values, the requirement of precise definitions a priori for simple null and alternative hypotheses makes testing composite hypotheses difficult. The open continuation region issue can be addressed by truncating the stopping rule or specifying the maximum sample size for specific applications, but tests of composite hypotheses require sequential generalized likelihood ratio (GLR) tests, which now are described.

### 12.3.1    Sequential GLR tests and stopping boundaries

The Wald SPRT may not be optimal in terms of expected sample size for testing composite hypotheses even though it does provide the minimum expected sample size under both simple null and simple alternative hypotheses among all tests satisfying the constraints of error probabilities. Kiefer and Weiss [7] showed that even though the SPRT has minimal expected sample sizes under $H_0$ and $H_1$ when testing a null hypothesis $H_0 : \theta < \theta_0$ against an alternative hypothesis $H_1 : \theta > \theta_1$ with $\theta_0 < \theta_1$ in the one-parameter exponential family (equation (12.6)) subject to the constraints of error probabilities, its expected sample size may not be optimal for other values of $\theta$, say, between $\theta_0$ and $\theta_1$. Lai [8] used 0–1 loss and absolute loss as special cases of a general loss function to provide a unified solution for one-sided hypotheses with an indifference zone $(\theta_1 - \theta_0 > 0)$ [9] and without an indifference zone $(\theta_1 - \theta_0 = 0)$

[10, 11]. In the context of a one-parameter exponential family, this unified treatment leads to simple sequential tests involving sequential GLR test statistics or mixture likelihood ratio test statistics [8, 12].

Consider a single-parameter exponential family density function (12.6). Let $\hat{\theta}_n$ denote the maximum likelihood estimate (MLE) of $\theta$ based on observations $x_1, \ldots, x_n$. The objective is a test of the composite null hypothesis $H_0 : \theta \leq \theta_0$ against the composite alternative hypothesis $H_1 : \theta \geq \theta_1 (> \theta_0)$. The sequential GLR test has the following stopping rule:

$$
\tau = \inf_{n \geq 1} \left\{
\begin{array}{l}
\displaystyle \prod_{i=1}^{n} \frac{f\left(x_i; \hat{\theta}_n\right)}{f(x_i; \theta_0)} \geq B_n^0 \quad \text{and} \quad \hat{\theta}_n > \theta_0, \\[3ex]
\text{or } \displaystyle \prod_{i=1}^{n} \frac{f(x_i; \hat{\theta}_n)}{f(x_i; \theta_1)} \geq B_n^1 \quad \text{and} \quad \hat{\theta}_n < \theta_1.
\end{array}
\right\}
\tag{12.12}
$$

The first test statistic in equation (12.12) is for testing $\theta \leq \theta_0$ versus $\theta > \theta_0$, while the second is for testing $\theta \geq \theta_1$ against $\theta < \theta_1$. A test rejects its corresponding null hypothesis when the corresponding test statistic exceeds the threshold $B_n^i$, $i = 0, 1$.

Let

$$
\ell_{n(i)} = \sum_{i=1}^{n} \log[f(x_i; \hat{\theta}_n)/f(x_i; \theta_i)]
$$

denote the logarithmic GLR under $H_i$ based on observations $x_1, \ldots, x_n$. A unified test of $H_0 : \theta \leq \theta_0$ against $H_1 : \theta \geq \theta_1 (> \theta_0)$ and of $H_0$ against $H_1' : \theta > \theta_0$ (without indifference zone), uses the stopping rule [8]

$$
\tau_c = \inf_{n \geq 1} \{\max(\ell_{n(0)}, \ell_{n(1)}) \geq g(cn)\},
\tag{12.13}
$$

where $g(\cdot)$ is the optimal stopping boundary for a continuous-time sequential testing problem associated with an approximate Brownian motion. In particular, when $\theta_0 = \theta_1$ the stopping rule (12.13) reduces to

$$
\tau_c' = \inf_{n \geq 1} \{\ell_{n(0)} \geq g(cn)\},
\tag{12.14}
$$

which rejects $H_0$ if and only if $\hat{\theta}_n > \theta_0$.

Let $I(\theta, \theta') = E_\theta \log[f(x_i; \theta)/f(x_i; \theta')]$ denote the Kullback–Leibler information number measuring the degree of divergence of the distributions for parameter values $\theta$ and $\theta'$. When $B_n^0 = B_n^1 = 1/c$, the stopping rule (12.12) is bounded above by $n^*$, the smallest integer satisfying $n^* I(\theta^*, \theta_0) \geq B_n^0 = B_n^1$, and $\theta^* \in (\theta_0, \theta_1)$ is the solution of the equation $I(\theta^*, \theta_0) = I(\theta^*, \theta_1)$. However, the stopping rule (12.12) does not have an upper bound for testing $H_0 : \theta \leq \theta_0$ against $H_1' : \theta > \theta_0$ with $B_n^0 = B_n^1 = B_n$ if a time-invariant threshold is used. The time-varying threshold $g(cn)$ in (12.13) or (12.14) has the property that $g(t) \to 0$ as $t \to \infty$ and $g(t) \sim \log(1/t)$ as $t \to 0$, thereby accounting for the time-varying uncertainty in the estimate $\hat{\theta}_n$ of $\theta$ as $t = cn$ varies from 0 to $\infty$ [8, 13].

The total number of observations often is constrained in practice to lie below an upper bound $N$ and/or a lower bound $n_L$. For instance, in clinical trials a maximum sample size is usually prespecified and the evaluation of safety events is most likely to start after observing some minimum number of adverse events. Bartroff et al. [14] replaced the time-varying boundary

$g(cn)$ by a constant $c$ and presented the constrained stopping rule for testing $H_0 : \theta = \theta_0$ as a "repeated GLR test,"

$$\tilde{\tau}'_C = \min(N, \hat{\tau}_C),$$  (12.15)

where

$$\hat{\tau}_C = \inf_{n \geq n_L} \{nI(\hat{\theta}, \theta_0 \geq C)\}.$$

The stopping rule (12.15) can be extended easily to testing composite null and composite alternative hypotheses by replacing $I(\hat{\theta}, \theta_0)$ with $I(\hat{\theta}_{H_1}, \hat{\theta}_{H_0})$, where $\hat{\theta}_{H_0}$ and $\hat{\theta}_{H_1}$ are the constrained MLEs of $\theta$ under $H_0 : \theta \leq \theta_0$ and $H_1 : \theta > \theta_0$, respectively.

## 12.3.2   Extension of sequential GLR tests to multiparameter exponential families

Lai and Shih [15] extended the sequential GLR tests to the multi-parameter natural exponential family with the probability density function

$$f(\mathbf{x}; \boldsymbol{\theta}) = \exp \left\{ \sum_{i=1}^{n} \eta_i(\boldsymbol{\theta}) \, T_i(\mathbf{x}_n) - C(\boldsymbol{\theta}) \right\} h(\mathbf{x}_n),$$  (12.16)

where $\boldsymbol{\theta} = (\theta_1, \ldots, \theta_k) \in \Theta$, $\mathbf{x}_n = (\mathbf{x}_{1n}, \ldots, \mathbf{x}_{kn})$, and $\mathbf{x}_{in} = (x_{i1}, \ldots, x_{in_i})$. The $\eta_i$ and $C$ are real-valued functions of the parameters $\theta$, and the $T_i$ are real-valued statistics. Expression (12.16) can be reparameterized by using $\eta_i$ as the parameters, leading to a convenient expression in canonical form,

$$f(\mathbf{x}; \boldsymbol{\theta}) = \exp \left\{ \sum_{i=1}^{n} \eta_i T_i(\mathbf{x}_n) - G(\boldsymbol{\eta}) \right\} h(\mathbf{x}_n).$$  (12.17)

The natural parameter space for equation (12.17) is the set of $\boldsymbol{\theta}$ values for which $[\eta_1(\boldsymbol{\theta}), \ldots, \eta_k(\boldsymbol{\theta})]$ is in $\Omega$.

Suppose now that the objective is to test the null hypothesis $H_0^{\theta} : \boldsymbol{\theta} \in \Theta_0$ against the alternative hypothesis $H_1^{\theta} : \boldsymbol{\theta} \in \Theta_1$, where $\Theta_0 \cap \Theta_1 = \emptyset$ and $\Theta_0 \cup \Theta_1 = \Theta$. That is, $\Theta_0$ and $\Theta_1$ represent a disjoint partition of the entire parameter space $\Theta$. Testing $H_0^{\theta}$ against $H_1^{\theta}$ is equivalent to testing $H_0^{\eta} : \boldsymbol{\eta} \in \Omega_0$ against the alternative hypothesis $H_1^{\eta} : \boldsymbol{\eta} \in \Omega_1$ where $\Omega_0$ implies $\Theta_0$, $\Omega_1$ implies $\Theta_1$, $\Omega_0 \cap \Omega_1 = \emptyset$, and $\Omega_0 \cup \Omega_1 = \Theta$. The sequential GLR test statistic based on the observations $\mathbf{x}_n$ then becomes

$$\ell_n(\boldsymbol{\eta}) = \sum_{i=1}^{n} \hat{\eta}_i T_i(\mathbf{x}_n) - G(\hat{\boldsymbol{\eta}}) - \sup_{\eta \in \Omega_0} \left\{ \sum_{i=1}^{n} \eta_i T_i(\mathbf{x}_n) - G(\boldsymbol{\eta}) \right\} = \inf_{\eta \in \Omega_0} I(\hat{\boldsymbol{\eta}}, \boldsymbol{\eta}),$$

where $\ell_n$ is a multivariate version of the Kullback–Leibler information number; see also [14].

## 12.3.3   Implementation of sequential GLR tests

The Type I and Type II error rates, and the stopping rule (12.12) or (12.15) must be specified before using the sequential GLR approach for testing safety hypotheses. As an example, the following steps are needed to determine the stopping rule (12.12):

1. Calculate the MLE of the parameter of interest, say, $\hat{\theta}_n$ of $\theta$, and the log generalized likelihood ratio $\Lambda_n$, based on the observations $\mathbf{x}_n = (x_1, \ldots, x_n)$;

2. Determine the upper bound $n^*$ of $n$ by solving the equation $I(\theta^*, \theta_0) = I(\theta^*, \theta_1)$ the smallest integer satisfying $n^* I(\theta^*, \theta_0) \geq B_n^0 = B_n^1$ and $\theta^* \in (\theta_0, \theta_1)$.

3. Determine the stopping rule (12.12) by calculating

$$\alpha = P_0\{\ell_{\tau(0)} \geq b_0\} = \sum_{n=1}^{n^*} P_0\{\tau = n, \Lambda_{\tau(0)} \geq b_0, \hat{\theta} > \theta_0\},$$

$$\beta = P_0\{\ell_{\tau(1)} \geq b_1\} = \sum_{n=1}^{n^*} P_1\{\tau = n, \Lambda_{\tau(1)} \geq b_0, \hat{\theta} > \theta_1\},$$

where $\Lambda_{n(i)} = \sum_{i=1}^{n} \log[f(x_i; \hat{\theta})/f(x_i; \theta_i)]$. The calculation can be carried out recursively [13] or iteratively [16] by starting with the initial values $b_0^{(0)} = \log(1/\alpha)$ and $b_1^{(0)} = \log(1/\beta)$ and increasing or decreasing the $i$th critical values, $b_0^{(i)}$ and $b_1^{(i)}$ by an amount $\delta$, depending on whether $P_0(\Lambda_{\tau(0)} \geq b_0) > \alpha$[or $P_1(\Lambda_{\tau(1)} \geq b_1)$], to get new critical values $b_0^{(i+1)}$ and $b_1^{(i+1)}$. This calculation also can be carried out using the R package pmvnorm to calculate $b_0$ and $b_1$ after obtaining $n^*$.

Shih *et al.* [13] used Bernoulli trials as an example to demonstrate how the stopping boundaries in equation (12.12) are derived and also presented calculations for power and expected sample size or number of events for sequential GLR tests, SPRT, and the maximized SPRT [17].

## 12.3.4  Example from Section 12.2.3, continued

In this example, each adverse event is assumed to be generated from a Bernoulli distribution with parameter $\pi = \phi r/(\phi r + 1)$ denoting the probability that the event occurred in the treatment group, where $r$ denotes the allocation ratio and $\phi$ denotes the risk for the treatment relative to the control. The objective is to test the null hypothesis $H_0 : \phi \leq \phi_0 = 1$ against the alternative $H_1 : \phi = \phi_1 > 1$. These hypotheses can be reformulated with respect to the natural parameter $\theta$ in the one-parameter exponential family (equation (12.6)) as $H_0 : \theta \leq \theta_0 = \log(\phi_0 r)$ against $H_1^\theta : \theta \geq \theta_1 = \log(\phi_1 r)$. The sequential GLR test statistic for testing $\theta_i (i = 0, 1)$ can then be written as

$$\ell_{n(i)}^\theta = (\hat{\theta} - \theta_i) T_n(\mathbf{x}) - n \log\left\{\frac{1 + \exp\left(\hat{\theta}\right)}{1 + \exp(\theta_i)}\right\},$$

where $T_n(\mathbf{x}) = \sum_i x_i$ denotes the total number of events from treatment group and $\hat{\theta}$ denotes the MLE of the parameter $\theta$ as given by $\hat{\theta} = \log\{T(\mathbf{x})/[n - T(\mathbf{x})]\}$. Let $\theta^* \in (\theta_0, \theta_1)$ be the solution of the equation

$$I(\theta^*, \theta_1) = I(\theta^*, \theta_0), \tag{12.18}$$

where

$$I(\theta^*, \theta_i) = (\theta^* - \theta_i)\exp(\theta^*)/(1 + \exp(\theta^*)) - \log\{(1 + \exp(\theta^*))/(1 + \exp(\theta_i))\}, \quad i = 0, 1,$$

or simply

$$\theta^* = \log\{[C(\theta_1) - C(\theta_0)]/[\theta_1 - \theta_0]\} = \log\left\{\frac{\log\left[(1 + \exp(\theta_1))/(1 + \exp(\theta_0))\right]}{\theta_1 - \theta_0}\right\}.$$

Let $I(\theta^*)$ denote the value of either side of equation (12.18). Then the stopping rule (12.12) of the sequential GLR test is given by

$$\tau = \inf_{n \geq 1}\{\Lambda^\theta_{n(0)} \geq b^\theta_0 \text{ and } \hat{\theta} > \theta_0, \text{ or } \Lambda^\theta_{n(1)} \geq b^\theta_1 \text{ and } \hat{\theta} < \theta_1\},$$

which is bounded above by $n^*$, the smallest integer $n$ such that $n^* I(\theta^*) \geq \max(b_0, b_1)$.

The log likelihood function also can be expressed in terms of the relative risk $\phi$ as

$$\ell_n^{\eta\theta} = T_n(\mathbf{x})\log(r\phi) = n\log(1 + r\phi),$$

which corresponds to equation (12.6) with $\theta(\phi) = \log(r\phi)$ and $C(\phi) = \log(1 + r\phi)$. The log likelihood ratio for testing $\phi_i$ is then given by

$$\ell_{n(i)}^{\eta\theta} = T_n(\mathbf{x})\log(\hat{\phi}/\phi_i) - n\log\{(1 + r\hat{\phi})/(1 + r\phi_i)\}.$$

Note that $E[T(\mathbf{x})] = \theta'(\phi)/C'(\phi) = nr\phi/(1 + r\phi)$ and hence the MLE of $\phi$ is given by $\hat{\phi} = T_n(\mathbf{x})/[r(n - T_n(\mathbf{x}))]$. The stopping rule (12.12) still applies but with $\phi^*$ being the solution of the equation

$$I(\phi^*, \phi_1) = I(\phi^*, \phi_0), \tag{12.19}$$

where

$$I(\phi^*, \phi_1) = \frac{r\phi^*}{1 + r\phi^*}\log\left(\frac{\phi^*}{\phi_i}\right) - \log\left(\frac{1 + r\phi^*}{1 + r\phi_i}\right), \quad i = 0, 1$$

or, equivalently, $\phi^*$ is the solution of

$$\frac{\theta'(\phi^*)}{C'(\phi^*)} = \frac{C(\phi_1) - C(\phi_0)}{\theta(\phi_1) - \theta(\phi_0)}. \tag{12.20}$$

Both (12.19) and (12.20) lead to the solution

$$\phi^* = \frac{C(\phi_1) - C(\phi_0)}{r[\theta(\phi_1) - C(\phi_1)] - [\theta(\phi_0) - C(\phi_0)]} = \frac{\log\{(1 + r\phi_1)/(1 + r\phi_0)\}}{r\{\log[\phi_1(1 + r\phi_0)/\phi_0(1 + r\phi_1)]\}}. \tag{12.21}$$

Figure 12.2 presents the stopping boundaries for the sequential GLR tests for detection of an adverse event in Bernoulli trials obtained using this algorithm as step functions for various combinations of Type I and Type II errors, and hypothetical values of the relative risk $\phi_0 = 1$ and $\phi_1 = 5$, 10. The stopping boundaries clearly rely heavily on the hypothetical values of the alternative relative risk $\phi_1$ for acceptance of the safety concern regarding the particular adverse event. The higher the alternative relative risk $\phi$, the earlier stopping is likely to occur. Also, unlike the SPRT procedure, the rejection boundary and acceptance boundary are closer to each other as the surveillance continues, and eventually reach the same stopping point.

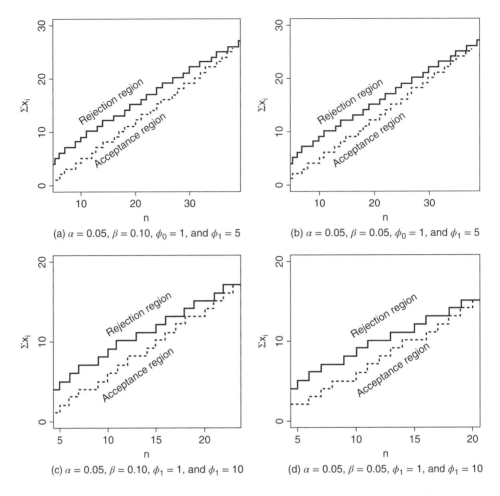

**Figure 12.2** Rejection, continuation, and acceptance regions for a sequential GLR test for monitoring Bernoulli trials with $\alpha = 0.05$, $\beta = 0.05$ or $0.10$, and $\phi_1 = 5$ or $10$.

## 12.4  Concluding remarks

Sequential tests are useful tools for early detection of deviations of a process from its target. The SPRT has been employed since its inception in biomedical applications [3], but only relatively recently for sequentially monitoring unwanted medical outcomes, for example, adverse clinical events after surgery [4], and vaccine safety surveillance [18]. The most important deficiency of the SPRT method is its incapability of handling composite hypotheses. Kulldorff *et al.* [17] proposed an SPRT approach that maximizes the (log) likelihood ratio by posting a constraint on the MLE of the parameter of interest within the domain of the alternative hypothesis, while the sequential GLR approach of Lai [8] calculates the (log) likelihood ratio without any constraint and its stopping rule is determined jointly by the magnitude of the (log) likelihood ratio and the MLE of the parameter. The sequential GLR approach has smaller expected sample size (earlier detection of safety signals) as compared with either the SPRT or the maximized SPRT method, while still maintaining satisfactory power under a variety of circumstances [13].

# References

[1]  Wald, A. (1947) *Sequential Analysis*, John Wiley & Sons, Inc., New York.

[2]  Wald, A. and Wolfowitz, J. (1948) Optimum character of the sequential probability ratio test. *Annals of Mathematical Statistics*, **19**, 326–339.

[3]  Bartholomay, A. (1957) The squential probability ratio test applied to the design of clinical experiments. *New England Journal of Medicine*, **256**, 498–505.

[4]  Spiegelhalter, D., Grigg, O., Kinsman, R. and Treasure, T. (2003) Risk-adjusted sequential probability ratio tests: applications to Bristol, Shipman, and adult cardiac surgery. *International Journal for Quality in Health Care*, **15**, 7–13.

[5]  Davis, R., Kolczak, M., Lewis, E. *et al.* (2005) Active surveillance of vaccine safety: a system to detect early signs of adverse events. *Epidemiology*, **16**, 336–341.

[6]  Steiner, S., Cook, R., Farewell, V. and Treasure, T. (2000) Monitoring surgical performance using risk-adjusted cumulative sum charts. *Biostatistics*, **1**, 441–452.

[7]  Kiefer, J. and Weiss, L. (1957) Some properties of generalized sequential probability ratio tests. *Annals of Mathematical Statistics*, **28**, 57–74.

[8]  Lai, T. (1988) Nearly optimal sequential tests of composite hypotheses. *Annals of Statistics*, **16**, 856–886.

[9]  Schwarz, G. (1962) Asymptotic shapes of Bayes sequential testing regions. *Annals of Mathematical Statistics*, **33**, 224–236.

[10]  Chernoff, H. (1965) Sequential test for the mean of a normal distribution III (small $t$). *Annals of Mathematical Statistics*, **36**, 54.

[11]  Chernoff, H. (1965) Sequential tests for the mean of a normal distribution IV (discrete case). *Annals of Mathematical Statistics*, **36**, 55–68.

[12]  Lai, T. (1997) On optimal stopping problems in sequential hypothesis testing. *Statistica Sinica*, **7**, 33–52.

[13]  Shih, M.-C., Leung, T.L., Heyse, J.F. and Chen, J. (2010) Sequential generalized likelihood ratio tests for vaccine safety evaluation. *Statistics in Medicine*, **29**, 2698–2708.

[14]  Bartroff, J., Lai, T. and Shih, M. (2013) *Sequential Experimentation in Clinical Trials*, Springer, New York.

[15]  Lai, T. and Shih, M. (2004) Power, sample size, and adaptation considerations in the design of group sequential trials. *Biometrika*, **91**, 507–528.

[16]  Jennison, C. and Turnbull, B.W. (1999) *Group Sequential Methods with Applications to Clinical Trials*, Chapman & Hall/CRC Press, Boca Raton, FL.

[17]  Kulldorff, M., Davis, R., Kolczak, M. *et al.* (2011) A maximized sequential probability ratio test for drug and vaccine safety surveillance. *Sequential Analysis*, **30**, 58–78.

[18]  Lieu, T., Kulldorff, M., Davis, R. *et al.* (2007) Real-time vaccine safety surveillance for the early detection of adverse events. *Medical Care*, **45**, 889.

# 13

# Evaluation of post-marketing safety using spontaneous reporting databases

**Ismaïl Ahmed,[1] Bernard Bégaud,[2] and Pascale Tubert-Bitter[1]**

[1]*Biostatistics Team, Centre for Research in Epidemiology and Population Health, UMRS U1018, Inserm-Université Paris Sud, F-94807 Villejuif, France*

[2]*U657 – Pharmacoepidemiology, Inserm – Université de Bordeaux, F-33000 Bordeaux, France*

## 13.1 Introduction

Active drugs have multiple pharmacological properties that can interact with various human genotypes and other attributes of patients such as diet, current diseases, age, and other treatments. Consequently, there is a potential risk, however small, of adverse reactions to any active drug. Adverse effects of drugs are very often not identified until after their marketing approval for at least two reasons. First, the adverse effects can be rare, specific to some subcategories of the population, or occur a long period of time after the beginning of exposure. The "rule of three," based on a Poisson model for event occurrence, states that if no events occur among $N$ treated patients, then there is reasonable (95%) confidence that the true incidence is less than $3/N$. For instance, if no event is observed among 3000 treated patients, event incidences larger than $1/1000$ are statistically unlikely. Another reason is that the conditions of utilization of a drug by patients once it is on the market can differ from those studied during pre-approval

*Statistical Methods for Evaluating Safety in Medical Product Development*, First Edition.
Edited by A. Lawrence Gould.
© 2015 John Wiley & Sons, Ltd. Published 2015 by John Wiley & Sons, Ltd.

clinical trials. Post-marketing pharmacovigilance systems aim to detect as quickly as possible the potential existence of adverse effects of marketed drugs. They generally rely on the analysis of spontaneous reports by healthcare providers or patients of adverse events that are suspected to be induced by a drug. Definite conclusions about the causal or associative role of a drug in the occurrence of an adverse event seldom can be drawn from a single spontaneous report. Several spontaneous reports mentioning a drug and an adverse event generally need to be accumulated in order to identify a potential adverse drug effect.

The accumulation of huge numbers of spontaneous reports at transnational or even national levels has motivated the development over the past two decades of automatic signal detection tools to identify drug–event associations that may represent potential toxicity. These tools identify signals, that is, adverse event–drug pairs that are statistically overrepresented, deserving further evaluation by pharmacovigilance experts or additional pharmacoepidemiologic study. The tools have limitations, however. The main limitations lie in the spontaneous character of the data that introduces several sources of bias, the most obvious being underreporting [1], and the fact that no causal or even real associative relationship can be directly deduced from adverse event–drug associations pointed out by such systems without further evaluation. However, despite such limitations, pharmacovigilance reporting system databases are unique resources that make data quickly available and thus allow the discovery of potential toxicity of new marketed drugs. The interest in such methods is grounded in several retrospective studies [2, 3, 4, 5]. Automatic signal detection tools currently are applied routinely to the largest pharmacovigilance databases. The main tools currently in use are the Bayesian Component Propagation Neural Network method (BCPNN) used to screen the World Health Organization (WHO) safety database [6–8], the gamma Poisson shrinkage (GPS) method used by the Food and Drug Administration (FDA) adverse event reporting systems [9, 10], and the proportional reporting ratio (PRR) methods for the European Medicines Agency EudraVigilance database [3, 11].

These automated signal detection methods differ according to the statistical model used and the decision rule that defines a "signal." The purpose of this chapter is to provide a description of the automated methods that have been proposed or are currently in use for evaluating reports in spontaneous reporting databases, including their limitations and issues with the signal detection rules.

## 13.2    Data structure

In principle, a spontaneous reporting database that mentions $I$ drugs and $J$ adverse events populates a sparse $I \times J$ contingency table in which the $(i, j)$th entry consists of the number of reports mentioning drug $i$ and adverse event $j$. Since spontaneous reports may include several events and/or drugs, any report can contribute to the count in more than one cell of this large table. Consequently, the sum of all of the table entries will exceed the total number of spontaneous reports. However, the table is sparse because many of the possible drug–event combinations will not be reported, so that many of the cells of the table will have a zero count.

In practice, the full $I \times J$ table never is considered. Instead, attention generally is focused on the $2 \times 2$ subtables corresponding to individual drug–event pairs. For drug $i$ and event $j$, this table is Table 13.1, where $n$ is the total number of reports, $n_{ij}$ is the number of reports mentioning drug $i$ and event $j$, $n_{i.}$ is the total number of reports mentioning drug $i$, and $n_{.j}$ is the total number of reports mentioning event $j$.

**Table 13.1**   Numbers of reports mentioning a specific drug and event

|                 | Event $j$             | All other events                     | Total       |
|-----------------|-----------------------|--------------------------------------|-------------|
| Drug $i$        | $n_{ij}$              | $n_{i\cdot} - n_{ij}$                | $n_{i\cdot}$ |
| All other drugs | $n_{\cdot j} - n_{ij}$ | $n - n_{i\cdot} - n_{\cdot j} + n_{ij}$ | $n - n_{i\cdot}$ |
| Total           | $n_{\cdot j}$         | $n - n_{\cdot j}$                    | $n$         |

All of the signal detection methods commonly used rely on a three-step strategy: for all (drug, event) pairs $(i, j)$, (1) determine the number of reports mentioning drug $i$ and event $j$ if the mention of event $j$ is independent of (does not depend on) whether drug $i$ was mentioned or not; (2) construct a measure of the degree to which the observed count $n_{ij}$ exceeds the count expected if independence applies (the "disproportionality" measure); and (3) decide that a "signal" has occurred if this measure exceeds a specified critical value.

## 13.3   Disproportionality methods

All of the disproportionality methods described below use a variation of the same metric, namely,

$$T_{ij} = n_{ij}/E_{n_{ij}},\qquad(13.1)$$

where $E_{n_{ij}}$ denotes the expected number of reports mentioning drug $i$ and event $j$ if drug $i$ and event $j$ occur independently in the database.

### 13.3.1   Frequentist methods

The PRR and the reporting odds ratio (ROR) are the metrics used most commonly by frequentist-based methods. For drug $i$ and event $j$, these metrics are calculated as

$$\text{PRR} = \frac{n_{ij}(n - n_{ij})}{n_{i\cdot}(n_{i\cdot} - n_{ij})} \quad \text{and} \quad \text{ROR} = \frac{n_{ij}(n - n_{i\cdot} - n_{\cdot j} + n_{ij})}{(n_{i\cdot} - n_{ij})(n_{\cdot j} - n_{ij})}$$

so that $E_{n_{ij}} = \frac{(n_{i\cdot} - n_{ij})n_i}{(n - n_{i\cdot})}$ for the PRR and $E_{n_{ij}} = \frac{(n_{i\cdot} - n_{ij})(n_{\cdot j} - n_{ij})}{(n - n_{i\cdot} - n_{\cdot j} + n_{ij})}$ for the ROR. If the mention of event $j$ in a report is independent of the mention of drug $i$, then the expected value of both of these metrics is 1.

The signal detection strategy proposed by van Puijenbroek *et al.* [12] identifies a signal for a drug–event pair if the lower bound of a 95% two-sided confidence interval for the true odds ratio calculated assuming that the logarithm of the odds ratio is normally distributed exceeds 1, that is, if

$$\log(\text{ROR}_{ij}) - 1.96\sqrt{1/n_{ij} + 1/(n_{i\cdot} - n_{ij}) + 1/(n_{\cdot j} - n_{ij}) + 1/(n - n_{i\cdot} - n_{\cdot j} + n_{ij})} > 0.$$

Two detection strategies have been proposed using the PRR metric. The strategy proposed by Evans *et al.* [11] combines three criteria: an observed relative risk (PRR value) $\geq 2$, a corrected $\chi^2$ statistic value greater than 4, and $n_{ij} \geq 3$. Requiring more than three reports of a drug–event pair reduces the likelihood of highlighting many possibly spurious signals.

An alternative to the Evans *et al.* approach based on a one-sided version of Fisher's exact test is proposed by Ahmed *et al.* [12]. Although this approach is computationally more intensive, it removes the requirement of assuming normality and can be implemented by standard statistical software.

In the literature, usage of the terms PRR and ROR very often refers to the whole detection strategy, including the association measure of interest and the signal detection criteria. In practice, the values (and the asymptotic distributions) of both disproportionality measures ($PRR_{ij}$ and $ROR_{ij}$) are very close, and the main differences lie in the signal detection strategies.

## 13.3.2 Bayesian methods

Two Bayesian methods currently are used to explore spontaneous reporting databases. The FDA uses an empirical Bayes method [9] and the WHO uses a purely Bayesian method [6, 14–16]. In general, the Bayesian methods seek to assess the likelihood of a reporting association between a drug and an adverse event that combines the observed number of reports of the drug and event and prior information or belief about the likelihood that an association exists. More specifically, suppose that the likelihood of an observed report count $n_{ij}$ for drug $i$ and event $j$ has the form $f(n_{ij}; \boldsymbol{\theta}_{ij})$, where $\boldsymbol{\theta}_{ij}$ denotes a corresponding vector of parameters that will be used to express the degree of association. What is commonly known or believed about the value of any of the $\boldsymbol{\theta}_{ij}$ before observing the corresponding report counts is expressed in terms of a *prior distribution* $g_0(\boldsymbol{\theta}; \boldsymbol{\Theta})$, where the values of $\boldsymbol{\Theta}$ are known. This assumption implies *exchangeability* of the $\boldsymbol{\theta}$ values across the population of reports, which may or may not be justified in practice. When it is not justified, then stratification may be considered, or the analyses may be undertaken in separate subgroups of the population such as children or the elderly [17, 18]. The information about the degree of association between drug $i$ and event $j$ that combines the observation and the prior assumptions is provided by the posterior distribution of $\boldsymbol{\theta}_{ij}$,

$$g(\boldsymbol{\theta}_{ij}; n_{ij}, \boldsymbol{\Theta}) = f(n_{ij}; \boldsymbol{\theta}_{ij})g_0(\boldsymbol{\theta}_{ij}; \boldsymbol{\Theta})/h(n_{ij}; \boldsymbol{\Theta}),$$

where

$$h(n_{ij}; \boldsymbol{\Theta}) = \int f(n_{ij}; \boldsymbol{\theta})g_0(\boldsymbol{\theta}; \boldsymbol{\Theta})\mathrm{d}\boldsymbol{\theta}$$

denotes the *marginal likelihood* of the observations given the value of $\boldsymbol{\Theta}$, the parameter vector for the prior distribution. The specification of the prior information/belief, that is, of the functional form of $g_0$ and the value of $\boldsymbol{\Theta}$, is the key component of a Bayesian approach. The two methods just mentioned provide this specification differently. The empirical Bayes method [9] determines the value of $\boldsymbol{\Theta}$ by maximizing the product of the marginal likelihoods, $\prod_{ij} h(n_{ij}; \boldsymbol{\Theta})$.

### 13.3.2.1 Empirical Bayes Method (FDA)

The empirical Bayes approach [9] assumes that an observed event count $n_{ij}$ is generated from a Poisson distribution with parameter $\theta_{ij} = \lambda_{ij}E_{ij}$, where $E_{ij} = n_i.n_{.j}/n$ denotes the number of reports expected if there is no association between the drug and the event, and $\lambda_{ij}$ denotes the inflation (if any) of the reporting risk corresponding to the drug and the event, so that $\lambda_{ij}$ is a variation of metric (13.1). The likelihood corresponding to $n_{ij}$ is

$$f(n_{ij}; \theta_{ij}) = f(n_{ij}; \lambda_{ij}, E_{ij}) = \frac{\theta_{ij}^{n_{ij}} e^{-\theta_{ij}}}{n_{ij}!}.$$

This definition of $E_{ij}$ is not the same as the definitions for the PRR or ROR. The parameter in this representation is the quantity $\lambda_{ij}$. The prior distribution for $\lambda_{ij}$ is assumed to be a mixture of gamma distributions,

$$g_0(\lambda; a_0, b_0, a_1, b_1, \gamma) = (1 - \gamma)f_{\text{gam}}(\lambda; a_0, b_0) + \gamma f_{\text{gam}}(\lambda; a_1, b_1), \tag{13.2}$$

where

$$f_{\text{gam}}(\lambda; a, b) = \frac{b(b\lambda)^{a-1}e^{-b\lambda}}{\Gamma(a)}.$$

The gamma distribution is chosen primarily for mathematical convenience; it is a *natural conjugate prior distribution* for the Poisson distribution in the sense that when it is used, the posterior distribution for the Poisson parameter also is a gamma distribution. The choice of a natural conjugate prior, while convenient, is not essential; other prior distributions could be used as well.

The marginal likelihood $h(n_{ij}; \Theta)$ is a mixture of negative binomial distributions,

$$h(n_{ij}; \Theta) = h(n_{ij}; a_0, b_0, a_1, b_1, \gamma) = (1 - \gamma)f_{\text{negbin}}(\lambda; a_0, b_0, E_{ij}) + \gamma f_{\text{negbin}}(\lambda; a_1, b_1, E_{ij}),$$

where

$$f_{\text{negbin}}(n; a, b, E) = \frac{\Gamma(a+n)}{n!\Gamma(a)}\left(\frac{E}{E+b}\right)^n\left(\frac{b}{E+b}\right)^a.$$

The values of $a_0, b_0, a_1, b_1,$ and $\gamma$ are obtained by maximizing the product of the marginal likelihoods. Since the gamma distribution is the natural conjugate prior for the Poisson distribution, the posterior distribution of $\lambda_{ij}$ also is a mixture of gamma distributions,

$$g(\lambda_{ij}; n_{ij}, a_0, b_0, a_1, b_1, \gamma) = (1 - \gamma_{ij})f_{\text{gam}}(\lambda_{ij}; a_0 + n_{ij}, b_0 + 1) + \gamma_{ij}f_{\text{gam}}(\lambda_{ij}; a_1 + n_{ij}, b_1 + 1),$$

where

$$\gamma_{ij} = \frac{\gamma f_{\text{negbin}}(\lambda; a_1, b_1, E_{ij})}{(1 - \gamma)f_{\text{negbin}}(\lambda; a_0, b_0, E_{ij}) + \gamma f_{\text{negbin}}(\lambda; a_1, b_1, E_{ij})}.$$

None of the parameters in these expression have natural interpretations.

Current practice in implementing the empirical Bayes method defines a "signal" if the lower 5% quantile of the posterior distribution of $\lambda_{ij}$ (commonly referred to as the "EBGM05," where EBGM stands for "empirical Bayes gamma mixture") exceeds 2 [10]. However, the statistical/diagnostic properties of this rule are not clear. There is a considerable literature on evaluating the effectiveness of automated signaling systems, but no definitive guidance (see also the discussion below).

### 13.3.2.2   Bayesian approach (WHO)

This approach assumes that the four cells of Table 13.1 follow a multinomial distribution,

$$f(\mathbf{n};\mathbf{p}) = \frac{n!}{n_{ij}!(n_{i\cdot} - n_{ij})!(n_{\cdot j} - n_{ij})!(n - n_{i\cdot} - n_{\cdot j} + n_{ij})!}$$

$$\times p_{ij}^{n_{ij}}(p_{i\cdot} - p_{ij})^{n_{i\cdot} - n_{ij}}(p_{\cdot j} - p_{ij})^{n_{\cdot j} - n_{ij}}(1 - p_{i\cdot} - p_{\cdot j} + p_{ij})^{n - n_{i\cdot} - n_{\cdot j} + n_{ij}}$$

where $\boldsymbol{n} = (n_{ij}, n_{i\cdot} - n_{ij}, n_{\cdot j} - n_{ij}, n - n_{i\cdot} - n_{\cdot j} + n_{ij})$ and $\boldsymbol{p} = (p_{ij}, p_{i\cdot} - p_{ij}, p_{\cdot j} - p_{ij}, 1 - p_{i\cdot} - p_{\cdot j} + p_{ij})$ As before, it is convenient to use a natural conjugate prior which for a multinomial likelihood is a Dirichlet distribution, $[\boldsymbol{a} = (a_1, a_2, a_3, a_4)]$

$$g_0(\boldsymbol{p}; \boldsymbol{a}) = \text{Dirichlet}(\boldsymbol{a}) \propto p_{ij}^{a_1}(p_{i\cdot} - p_{ij})^{a_2}(p_{\cdot j} - p_{ij})^{a_3}(1 - p_{i\cdot} - p_{\cdot j} + p_{ij})^{a_4}$$

so that the posterior distribution of the multinomial parameters also is a Dirichlet distribution,

$$g(\boldsymbol{p}; \boldsymbol{n}, \boldsymbol{a}) = \text{Dirichlet}(a_1 + n_{ij}, a_2 + n_{i\cdot} - n_{ij}, a_3 + n_{\cdot j} - n_{ij}, a_4 + n - n_{i\cdot} - n_{\cdot j} + n_{ij})$$

The "information criterion" used by the WHO method is defined by

$$\text{IC}_{ij} = \log_2\left(\frac{p_{ij}}{p_{i\cdot} p_{\cdot j}}\right),$$

which is the logarithm to the base 2 of the metric (13.1) expressed in terms of the multinomial probabilities. The prior and posterior distributions of the marginal probabilities are immediate from the joint distribution of the table probabilities. The posterior distribution of the information criterion does not have a closed form, so the WHO criterion for a "signal" is that the expectation of $\text{IC}_{ij}$ minus twice its posterior standard deviation exceeds a predefined critical value, for example, 0. The original paper used an approximation to these statistics; exact expressions were provided in [18].

The calculations required for these approaches (and some others) can be carried out using the R (http://cran.r-project.org/) package PhViD, which incorporates a graphical interface to simplify its use.

## 13.4   Issues and biases

All methods for analyzing findings from spontaneous reporting databases suffer from limitations that are inherent in these databases. A key limitation is that reports (cases) recorded in a pharmacovigilance database are by no means a random or even representative sample of all adverse events that occurred in the source population. Several studies conducted in various countries have shown that no more than 5% of observed cases, even serious, were actually reported by health professionals or patients to pharmacovigilance systems [19]. Even worse, this reporting is anything but random because it is affected by many subjective biases [19, 20]. For example, since the pioneering work of Weber and Griffin [21] it is well known that an adverse drug reaction (ADR) has more chance of being reported if it is severe or serious, previously unknown or unlabeled or involves a drug recently marketed, or the reporting rate for a given drug–event pair decreasing over time since launch. Moreover, media attention may induce a transient, but possibly spectacular, increase in the reporting rate, the drug–event pair being in fact less underreported during this period. Therefore, a disproportionality identified in a database does not necessarily reflect what would be measured in the whole source population.

### 13.4.1   Notoriety bias

Overrepresentation of a given drug–event pair in the database may ensue simply from better reporting (i.e., less massive underreporting) because of media attention or particular attention to a specific association. This could lead to an apparent "signal" that would not be detected without such a distortion in the reporting intensity. A safe practice before concluding that an apparent signal truly is real therefore would be a search for a marked change in the reporting rate over time, for example, by examining the numbers of cases reported within regular time intervals. An increase in the number of reported cases could indicate the occurrence of this notoriety bias. There are subtler manifestations of non-uniform reporting intensity. One such manifestation is *indication bias* or *prescription channeling*, where a drug could be overrepresented if systematically or preferentially co-prescribed or used with the drug causing the effect. An example of this process is illustrated by the apparent association between angiotensin converting enzyme inhibitors (ACEIs) and hypoglycemia [21]. This drug class was presented as safer than other antihypertensive agents in diabetic patients. The excess number of episodes of hypoglycemias observed with ACEIs was in fact related to antidiabetic drugs co-prescribed in those patients as shown when the assessment was done separately in diabetic and non-diabetic patients [21, 22].

### 13.4.2   Dilution bias

Not all drugs are equally likely to generate signals. Drugs that have been on the market for a long time will be mentioned in many more reports than will more recently marketed drugs. The drugs with longer tenure will be less prone to generate disproportionality signals. This is an example of *dilution bias* because the difference between the observed and expected numbers of drug–event reports for these drugs will be diluted by the large number of reports mentioning the drug that will have been accumulated. The experience with selective serotonin reuptake inhibitors (SSRIs) in the United Kingdom illustrates this bias [23]. This class of antidepressant drugs was presented as causing suicides during a TV program. A transient peak of reports of suicide cases involving SSRIs was observed after the program was broadcast, generating a signal for the most recently marketed one, escitalopram: 4 reports for a total of 281 versus 146/25 197 for other SSRIs. The consequence of this prompted reporting was quite apparent for this drug because of the dilution of the apparent risk for the older drugs due to the many reports that had mentioned them. This type of bias may be minimized by using appropriate time intervals and dates of occurrence of the events rather than the reporting dates.

### 13.4.3   Competition bias

A disproportionality signal also can arise because of an atypical distribution of adverse events that are reported for a given drug, either with respect to the target event of interest or to other events. For example, if a specific event represents the vast majority of events mentioned in reports that mention a specific drug (or therapeutic class), then it may be difficult to detect potential associations of other events with the drug simply because of the masking effect due to the first event [17, 18, 24].

To illustrate the point, suppose that only bleeding or haemorrhage is mentioned in 75% of the reports that mention antithrombotic drugs (as a class), but in only 4% of the reports that do not mention antithrombotic drugs. All other adverse events reported for antithrombotics are assumed to occur in the 25% of reports mentioning these drugs that do not also mention bleeding. This is unrealistic, of course, but useful for illustration. A table of proportions corresponding to Table 13.1 summarizing these findings would look like

|                    | Bleeding | All Other Events |
|--------------------|----------|------------------|
| Antithrombotics    | 0.75     | 0.25             |
| All Other Drugs    | 0.04     | 0.96             |

The PRR for bleeding events is the ratio $0.75/0.04 = 18,8$, while the PRR for events other than bleeding is $0.25/0.96 = 0.26$. Detection of a 'signal' for events other than bleeding is unlikely unless the disproportionality for these events also is extreme.

In circumstances when the existence of confounding drugs or classes or the existence of confounding events may affect the value of metrics such as the PRR, there may be some value in removing cases involving the confounders to reveal previously masked signals [25].

## 13.5    Method comparisons

Several studies have been performed to compare the performances of the different automated detection methods, generally using one of two strategies. One strategy uses actual data, usually from a spontaneous reporting database, and evaluates the methods by how well they detect "true positives," which can be well-known adverse reactions, events listed in drug labels, or pharmacovigilance signals [3, 5, 10, 26–29]. An issue with these strategies is that there is no unique definition of "gold standard."

The other strategy uses simulation studies to compare the methods [30–32]. These approaches generate by simulation data sets that include "true" signals and then evaluate the sensitivity and specificity of the various methods for detecting the known true signals. The advantage of such approaches is that the definition of the true signal is unambiguous. On the other hand, these approaches assume that the simulated datasets accurately reflect actual spontaneous reporting data, and validation of this assumption can be difficult.

The comparative studies do, however, support some general conclusions. The crucial determinant of the number of signals detected by the frequentist methods (PRR and ROR) is the detection threshold as long as there are at least three reports mentioning a drug and event. The empirical Bayes method using a detection threshold of 2 for the EBGM05 tends to generate substantially fewer signals than the frequentist methods; consequently, it tends to generate fewer false and true positive signals. Simulation studies show that both current Bayesian methods tend to rank the drug–event combinations very similarly. In addition, they seem to prioritize signals with more support of the data (large $n_{ij}$) in comparison with frequentist methods.

The properties of the various methods all depend crucially on the detection threshold. In practice, each signal generated by a method has to be further investigated by pharmacovigilance experts. Eventually, this task can become burdensome enough to govern the choice of a detection rule.

## 13.6    Further refinements

### 13.6.1    Recent improvements on the detection rule

All these methods, as they are currently used, share the common limitation of arbitrary detection thresholds that are not defined by any error-limiting constraint. In particular, the thresholds do not account for the multiplicity that occurs because of the very large number of drug–event combination evaluations (potentially $I \times J$). Even if there are no reporting associations between any of the drugs and events in a database, it is entirely possible that by chance alone some fraction of the association metrics will be large enough to exceed any threshold. If the threshold is set so that, for example, 5% of the values would be expected to exceed the threshold in the absence of any association then, if a million comparisons (drug–event combinations) are made, about 50 000 of these would be detected as "signals," all false positives, which clearly would be unacceptable. The multiplicity issue has received considerable attention in the statistical literature over the past 20 years, and a number of new error rate criteria such as the false discovery rate (FDR) [33] have been proposed. All the previously described methods have all been revisited in the light of the multiple comparison framework [13, 34, 35], by considering each combination $(i, j)$ decision (signal/not signal) as a comparison.

A number of alternative ranking statistics also have been proposed. For the frequentist methods, the use of the $p$-values represents the optimal choice. As usual, a small $p$-value means that there is a good chance that there is some disproportionality in the data for that combination. Therefore all combinations can be ranked from the smallest $p$-value (high likelihood for a signal) to the largest (no likelihood for a signal). One advantage is that the methodology allows one to estimate the FDR error rate corresponding to any threshold applied to those $p$-values and therefore to provide that FDR estimate for any set of signals resulting from the application of a threshold on the $p$-values. Regarding the Bayesian methods, the proposed ranking statistics are simply defined as the posterior probability for $\lambda_{ij}$ to be less than 1 for GPS and as the posterior probability for $IC_{ij}$ to be less than 0 for the information criterion.

## 13.6.2   Bayesian screening approach

Both of the methods described above provide a way to identify potential 'signals', essentially using hypothesis-testing techniques expressed in terms of credible intervals, but without consideration of the effects of multiplicity and their statistical properties. An alternative approach casts the detection of 'signals' into the context of a screening process, where the objective is to choose between two explicit choices [35]. The approach uses the model (13.2), but is purely Bayesian: the parameters of the prior distributions are defined so that the distribution of metric values (l) corresponding to $(a_0, b_0)$ is what would be anticipated or acceptable from a clinical/regulatory point of view if there were no reporting association and the distribution of metric values corresponding to $(a_1, b_1)$ is what is of interest to detect, similar in concept to defining the noncentrality parameter in a conventional hypothesis-testing context. The other key difference is that the quantity $\gamma$ in (13.2) is regarded as a random variable instead of a fixed quantity, with its own prior distribution, e.g., $g_0(\gamma; \xi) = \xi^{-1} \gamma^{\xi-1}$. Adding this additional level of randomness turns out to remove the influence of multiplicity [36]. The calculations provide posterior probabilities for each drug-event combination that the corresponding value of $\gamma$ is zero, i.e., that the reporting frequency $n_{ij}$ is consistent with an assertion of no reporting relationship. A 'signal' occurs when this posterior probability is sufficiently low, which could depend on the particular adverse event. The usual diagnostic properties (sensitivity, specificity, and positive and negative predictive values) can be calculated directly because the alternatives are identified explicitly. A SAS® macro to perform the calculations for this method and for the other methods mentioned above is available from the website associated with this book.

### 13.6.3    Confounding and interactions

The methods described so far used only information related to drug exposure and adverse event occurrence. However, spontaneous reports often include additional information such as the patient's age and sex, the year of the report, and the country/region of origin. One way of accounting for such variables is through stratification, each association measure being calculated for a subcategory defined by these variables. When proposed, the GPS method suggested accounting for such variable via the Mantel–Haenszel technique. In practice, this means using as expected number the average of the expected number calculated for each stratum. Some useful guidance is provided in [17].

### 13.6.4    Comparison of two signals

All of the methods presented above aim to derive at a given time a set of detected signals among all possible drug–effect pairs that exist in the spontaneous reporting database under study. Eventually, pharmacovigilance experts will have to sort out those signals and to assess to which extend they may flag a real safety issue. The signal strength cannot be taken as a risk measure *per se*. Signal assessment relies on a thorough examination of reported cases, literature search, and pharmacological expertise. For the latter, the plausibility of the ADR in terms of potential underlying mechanisms is analyzed and investigation of a possible therapeutic class is one way to tackle this task. Accordingly, it might be useful in some circumstances and with sensitivity to potential biases to compare two signals for drugs belonging to the same class that may induce the same adverse event. Methods for carrying out this comparison are described in [37].

### 13.6.5    An alternative approach

A potential important limit of current signal detection methods, largely imposed by computational considerations, is the simplistic representation of the data as a large contingency table crossing all the adverse events and all the drugs mentioned at least once in a spontaneous report. Recently, the idea has emerged of building statistical models using the individual spontaneous reports rather than the aggregated form of the data, which consists of the number of spontaneous reports for each adverse event–drug combination in the contingency table [38]. Disaggregating data could address two specific issues that are consequences of the contingency table representation: the masking effect (a phenomenon whereby the background relative reporting rate of an ADR is distorted by massive reporting on the ADR with a particular drug or drug group) and confounding effect by co-reported drugs [17, 39]. With this new approach, the *individual spontaneous report* becomes the observation, the outcome is the presence/absence (coded by 1/0) of a given adverse reaction and the covariates are all the drugs, coded by 1 if they are present in the spontaneous report and 0 otherwise. This approach casts the problem as a multivariate logistic regression with very many regressors: for example, about 12 000 different drug categories when using the fifth level, chemical subgroup of the Anatomical Therapeutic Chemical (ATC) Classification for drugs [40, 41]. The pharmacovigilance objective is then to select the few drugs that could be statistically linked to a given adverse event from this very large set of regressors. Bayesian multivariate logistic regression techniques seek parsimonious models by shrinking the coefficients of the regression toward zero, some to exactly zero [38, 42]. Caster *et al.* [38] first applied Bayesian binary regression [43] to the WHO VigiBase and compared it to the information component method.

This is an example of *variable selection* amongst a very large number of covariates, a statistical field currently the object of many methodological advances, which have mainly been applied so far to genetic and genomic studies. These approaches impose a very heavy computational burden because separate multivariate logistic regressions are applied for each of the adverse event types. The advantages of such innovative approaches in comparison to the classical detection methods have not been fully explored [44].

# References

[1] Moride, Y., Haramburu, F., Requejo, A.A. and Begaud, B. (1997) Under-reporting of adverse drug reactions in general practice. *Br.J Clin.Pharmacol*, **43**, 177–181.

[2] Ahmed, I., Thiessard, F., Miremont-Salame, G. *et al.* (2012) Early detection of pharmacovigilance signals with automated methods based on false discovery rates: a comparative study. *Drug Safety*, **35**, 495–506.

[3] Alvarez, Y., Hidalgo, A., Maignen, F. and Slattery, J. (2010) Validation of statistical signal detection procedures in eudravigilance post-authorization data: a retrospective evaluation of the potential for earlier signalling. *Drug Safety*, **33**, 475–487.

[4] Hauben, M. and Reich, L. (2005) Potential utility of data-mining algorithms for early detection of potentially fatal/disabling adverse drug reactions: A retrospective evaluation. *Journal of Clinical Pharmacology*, **45**, 378–384.

[5] Hochberg, A.M. and Hauben, M. (2009) Time-to-signal comparison for drug safety data-mining algorithms vs traditional signaling criteria. *Clinical Pharmacology & Therapeutics*, **85**, 600–606.

[6] Bate, A., Lindquist, M., Edwards, I.R. *et al.* (1998) A Bayesian neural network method for adverse drug reaction signal generation. *Eur.J Clin.Pharmacol*, **54**, 315–321.

[7] Noren, G.N., Bate, A., Orre, R. and Edwards, I.R. (2006) Extending the methods used to screen the WHO drug safety database towards analysis of complex associations and improved accuracy for rare events. *Statistics in Medicine*, **25**, 3740–3757.

[8] Orre, R., Lansner, A., Bate, A. and Lindquist, M. (2000) Bayesian neural networks with confidence estimations applied to data mining. *Computational Statistics and Data Analysis*, **34**, 473–493.

[9] DuMouchel, W. (1999) Bayesian data mining in large frequency tables, with an application to the FDA spontaneous reporting system (Disc: p190-202). *The American Statistician*, **53**, 177–190.

[10] Szarfman, A., Machado, S.G. and O'Neill, R.T. (2002) Use of screening algorithms and computer systems to efficiently signal higher-than-expected combinations of drugs and events in the USFDA's spontaneous reports database. *Drug Safety*, **25**, 381–392.

[11] Evans, S.J.W., Waller, P.C. and Davis, S. (2001) Use of proportional reporting ratios (PRRs) for signal genertion from spontaneous adverse drug reaction reports. *Pharmacoepidemiology and Drug Safety*, **10**, 483–486.

[12] van Puijenbroek, E.P., Bate, A., Leufkens, H.G. *et al.* (2002) A comparison of measures of disproportionality for signal detection in spontaneous reporting systems for adverse drug reactions. *Pharmacoepidemiology and Drug Safety*, **11**, 3–10.

[13] Ahmed, I., Dalmasso, C., Haramburu, F. *et al.* (2010) False discovery rate estimation for frequentist pharmacovigilance signal detection methods. *Biometrics*, **66**, 301–309.

[14] Bate, A., Lindquist, M. and Edwards, I.R. (2008) The application of knowledge discovery in databases to post-marketing drug safety: example of the WHO database. *Fundamental & Clinical Pharmacology*, **22**, 127–140.

[15] Caster, O., Juhlin, K., Watston, S. and Norén, G.N. (2014) Improved statistical signal detection in pharmacovigilance by combining multiple strength-of-evidence aspects in vigiRank. *Drug Safety*, **37**, 617–628.

[16] Norén, G.N., Hopstadius, J. and Bate, A. (2013) Shrinkage observed-to-expected ratios for robust and transparent large-scale pattern discovery. *Statistical Methods in Medical Research*, **22**, 57–69.

[17] Almenoff, J., Tonning, J.M., Gould, A.L. *et al.* (2005) Perspectives on the use of data mining in pharmacovigilance. *Drug Safety*, **28**, 981–1007.

[18] Gould, A.L. (2003) Practical pharmacovigilance analysis strategies. *Pharmacoepidemiology and Drug Safety*, **12**, 559–574.

[19] Bégaud, B., Martin, K., Haramburu, F. and Moore, N. (2002) Rates of spontaneous reporting of adverse drug reactions in France. *Journal of the American Medical Association*, **288**, 1588.

[20] Fletcher, A.P. (1991) Spontaneous adverse drug reactions reporting vs event monitoring: A comparison. *Journal of the Royal Society of Medicine*, **84**, 341–344.

[21] Weber, J.C.P. and Griffin, J.P. (1984) Epidemiology of adverse drug reactions to non-steroidal antiinflammatory drugs, in *Advances in Inflammatory Research* (eds K.D. Rainsford and G.P. Velo), Raven Press.

[22] Grégoire, F., Pariente, A., Fourrier-Reglat, A. *et al.* (2008) A signal of increased risk of hypoglycaemia with antiotensin receptor blockers caused by confounding. *British Journal of Clinical Pharmacology*, **66**, 142–145.

[23] Pariente, A., Daveluy, A., Laribière-Bénard, A. *et al.* (2009) Effect of date of drug marketing on disproportionality measures in pharmacovigilance: The example of suicide with SSRIs using data from the UK MHRA. *Drug Safety*, **32**, 441–447.

[24] Wang, D.L., Cheung, Y.B., Arezina, R. *et al.* (2010) A nonparametric approach to QT interval correction for heart rate. *Journal of Biopharmaceutical Statistics*, **20**, 508–522.

[25] Pariente, A., Avillach, P., Salvo, F. *et al.* (2012) Effect of competition bias in safety signal generation: Analysis of a research database of spontaneous reports in France. *Drug Safety*, **35**, 855–864.

[26] Hochberg, A.M., Hauben, M., Pearson, R.K. *et al.* (2009) An evaluation of three signal-detection algorithms using a highly inclusive reference event database. *Drug Safety*, **23**, 533–542.

[27] Lehman, H.P., Chen, J., Gould, A.L. *et al.* (2007) An evaluation of computer-aided disproportionality analysis for post-marketing signal detection. *Clinical Pharmacology & Therapeutics*, **82**, 173–180.

[28] Lindquist, M., Stahl, M., Bate, A. *et al.* (2000) A retrospective evaluation of a data mining approach to aid finding new adverse drug reaction signals in the WHO international database. *Drug Safety*, **23**, 533–542.

[29] Pizzoglio, V., Ahmed, I., Auriche, P. and Tubert-Bitter, P. (2012) Implementation of an automated signal detecction method in the French pharmacovigilance database: a feasibility study. *European Journal of Clinical Pharmacology*, **69**, 793–799.

[30] Ahmed, I., Thiessard, F., Miremont-Salamé, G. *et al.* (2010) Pharmacovigilance data mining with methods based on false discovery rates: a comparative simulation study. *Clinical Pharmacology & Therapeutics*, **88**, 492–498.

[31] Matsushita, Y., Kuroda, Y., Niwa, S. *et al.* (2007) Criteria revision and performance comparison of three methods of signal detection applied to the spontaneous reporting database of a pharmaceutical manufacturer. *Drug Safety*, **30**, 715–726.

[32] Roux, E., Thiessard, F., Fourrier, A. *et al.* (2005) Evaluation of statistical association measures for the automatic signal generation in pharmacovigilance. *IEEE TRans.Inf.Technol.Biomed*, **9**, 518–527.

[33] Benjamini, Y. and Hochberg, Y. (1995) Controlling the false discovery rate: A practical and powerful approach to multiple testing. *Journal of the Royal Statistical Society, Series B: Methodological*, **57**, 289–300.

[34] Ahmed, I., Haramburu, F., Fourrier-Reglat, A. *et al.* (2009) Bayesian pharmacovigilance signal detection methods revisited in a multiple comparison setting. *Statistics in Medicine*, **28**, 1774–1792.

[35] Gould, A.L. (2007) Accounting for multiplicity in the evaluation of "signals" obtained by data mining from spontaneous report adverse event databases. *Biometrical Journal*, **49**, 151–165.

[36] Scott, J.G. and Berger, J.O. (2010) Bayes and empirical-Bayes multiplicity adjustment in the variable-selection problem. *Annals of Statistics*, **38**, 2587–2619.

[37] Tubert-Bitter, P., Bégaud, B., and Ahmed, I. "Comparison of two drug safety signals in a pharmacovigilance data mining framework", Statistical Methods in Medical Research. (2012). Accessed 1-30-2013.

[38] Caster, O., Norén, G.N., Madigan, D. and Bate, A. (2010) Large-scale regression-based pattern discovery.: The example of screening the WHO global drug safety database. *Statistical Analysis and Data Mining*, **3**, 197–208.

[39] Evans, S.J.W. (2005) Statistics: Analysis and Presentation of Safety Data, in *Stephens' Detection of New Adverse Drug Reactions*, 5th edn (eds J. Talbot and P. Waller), John Wiley & Sons, Chichester, UK.

[40] Miller, G.C. and Britt, H. (1995) A new drug classification for computer systems: the ATC extension code. *International Journal of Bio-Medical Computing*, **40**, 121–124.

[41] Thiessard, F., Roux, E., Miremont-Salame, G. *et al.* (2005) Trends in spontaneous adverse drug reaction reports to the French pharmacovigilance system (1986-2001). *Drug Safety*, **28**, 731–740.

[42] An, L., Fung, K.Y. and Krewski, D. (2010) Mining pharmacovigilance data using Bayesian logistic regressiion with James-Stein type shrinkage estimation. *Journal of Biopharmaceutical Statistics*, **20**, 998–1012.

[43] Genkin, A., Lewis, D.D. and Madigan, D. (2007) Large-scale Bayesian logistic regression for text categorization. *Technometrics*, **49**, 291–304.

[44] Harpaz, R., DuMouchel, W., LePendu, P. *et al.* (2013) Performance of pharmacovigilance signal-detection algorithms for the FDA adverse event reporting system. *Clinical Pharmacology & Therapeutics*, **93**, 539–546.

# 14

# Pharmacovigilance using observational/longitudinal databases and web-based information

## A. Lawrence Gould

*Merck Research Laboratories, 770 Sumneytown Pike, West Point, PA, 19486 USA*

## 14.1   Introduction

The previous chapter (see also [1, 2]) described statistical methods for identifying potential associations between medical products (drugs, vaccines, devices) and adverse events (AEs)using data from spontaneous reporting databases. Spontaneous reporting databases are convenient sources of information for identifying potential toxicities of medical products, but are subject to deficiencies that limit the interpretability of analyses based on the data they contain [2].

Other sources of information, especially insurance claim databases and various kinds of electronic health record (EHR) databases, can be used to identify potential AE risks. Insurance companies or other agencies concerned with payment or reimbursement for medical expenses generally maintain claims databases. More recently, text mining of web-based information has been used to evaluate drug AE risks.

The best use of the substantial amount of information about patients' medical events contained in claims databases needs careful consideration. Claims databases do not ordinarily provide information about AEs as such (nor about prescribed or unprescribed over-the-counter

*Statistical Methods for Evaluating Safety in Medical Product Development*, First Edition.
Edited by A. Lawrence Gould.
© 2015 John Wiley & Sons, Ltd. Published 2015 by John Wiley & Sons, Ltd.

medications or unfilled prescriptions), so that the occurrence of an AE reflecting possible product-related harm must be inferred from the information about physician visits, diagnosis codes, medical indications, or dispensed medications that the database provides. There also may be some uncertainty about the reliability of the information provided because the reporting incentive for a claims database is payment or reimbursement for medical services or prescriptions, and not necessarily an accurate description of the medical events or procedures, or of whether the patient took a reimbursed medication as prescribed (or even at all). Claims usually will be reasonably accurate for drugs and vaccines because billing is often made for the particular therapy dispensed, but the same may not be true for medical devices [1].

EHR databases in principle capture patient records within a healthcare system, including records of results of laboratory tests, vital signs measurements, diagnoses, medications, and so on, so that a longitudinal picture of patient experience can be obtained. However, this is true only as long as the patient stays in the healthcare system. EHR databases provide an opportunity to study the temporal pattern of occurrence of AEs, for example, whether they occur soon after initiating treatment or after extended exposure, or whether they are transient or persistent. However, only whether a medicine was prescribed generally is recorded, not whether it actually was taken as prescribed. Also, information about the occurrence of potential AEs generally needs to be inferred from the record unless the occurrence of an AE as such has been recorded because EHR databases are designed for patient care management, not for detection of harm. How AEs (more accurately, "health outcomes of interest") are defined can materially affect the ability of any algorithm to detect their occurrence [3].

The Observational Medical Outcomes Partnership (OMOP) was established in 2008 to study how information from disparate databases, typically observational, claims, and EHR databases, could best be used to expedite the detection of potential harm. The project has considered, and continues to consider, a number of issues including database combination, data accessibility, and statistical and epidemiological approaches for identifying potential harm. Information about the completed first phase of the work is available (as of this writing) at http://omop.org. The OMOP Research Lab, a central computing resource developed to facilitate methodological research, has been rebranded as the IMEDS (Innovation in Medical Evidence Development and Surveillance) Lab (http://imeds.reaganudall.org/). Observational Health Data Sciences and Informatics (OHDSI) has been established as a multi-stakeholder, interdisciplinary collaborative to create open-source solutions that bring out the value of observational health data through large-scale analytics (http://ohdsi.org/). A recent review of the ongoing work of the OMOP project addresses a number of statistical issues associated with the evaluation of data from observational databases [4].

The US FDA launched the "Sentinel Initiative" in May 2008 to track the safety of drugs (http://www.fda.gov/safety/fdassentinelinitiative/ucm149340.htm). The associated "Mini Sentinel" active surveillance program analyzes claims data from more than 100 million patients (as of early 2014) and has provided the basis for a number of FDA actions (http://www.mini-sentinel.org/).

The European ADR (Adverse Drug Reaction) project [5] (http://www.euadr-project.org) seeks to supplement spontaneous report systems for detecting AEs by using a variety of text mining, epidemiological, and other computational techniques to detect "signals" using EHR data of over 30 million patients from the Netherlands, Denmark, United Kingdom, and Italy.

There are two commercially available databases in Japan. One is an insurance claim database called the Japan Medical Data Center (www.jmdc.co.jp/en/). The other is an HER database called Medical Data Vision (www.mdv.co.jp). The Japan Pharmaceutical and Medical Devices Agency (PMDA) (www.pmda.go.jp/english/) recently opened a spontaneous reporting database called JADER, and a national insurance claim database currently is under construction.

## 14.2    Methods based on observational databases

A number of approaches have been described for identifying potential drug–AE associations using observational (claims, EHR) databases, a number of which are described briefly here. A broader discussion of methods that may be applied is provided in [6]. Many of the methods described here were evaluated as part of the OMOP project using a common data substrate consisting of five observational healthcare databases (four claims, one EHR) and six simulated data sets. All of the data sets were used to evaluate the predictive accuracy in terms of the area under the curve (AUC) of the various methods for detecting four specific AEs: acute liver failure, acute renal failure, acute myocardial infarction, and upper gastrointestinal bleeding. A "signal" of a drug–event association occurred if the element of $\beta$ corresponding to the drug for the event exceeded a threshold value. An indicator was set to 1 if there really was an association or 0 if there really was not an association, and the fractions of "true event" cases for which a "1" was recorded, and of "true non-event" cases for which a "0" was recorded (the "sensitivity" and "specificity," respectively) were determined for each threshold values. The area under a receiver operating characteristic curve plotting 1 minus sensitivity against specificity for each threshold value (AUC) was used to assess the diagnostic accuracy of the method in each design scenario. The simulated data sets were used to estimate the bias of estimates of AE risk and to evaluate the coverage probabilities of confidence intervals for the risk estimates. Details of the considerations underlying the construction of the data sets used to evaluate the various approaches are provided in [7–9].

### 14.2.1    Disproportionality analysis with redefinition of report frequency table entries

This approach [10] applies methods for assessing findings from spontaneous reporting databases to longitudinal or observational databases by redefining the entries of the typical $2 \times 2$ reporting table such as Table 14.1. Any analysis method that uses input as in Table 14.1 can be used for the calculations. The definitions of the $w$ values depend on how event occurrences and drug exposures are counted. A patient could have multiple intervals of continuous exposure to a drug separated by intervals when the patient was not exposed to the drug; the on-drug intervals are called "drug eras" in [10]. The entries in spontaneous report databases consist of reports that mention the occurrence of events when there is no drug exposure, and there certainly are no reports that mention exposure to a drug when no events occur. Longitudinal databases do (or may) provide this information, and so some modification of the methods used for assessing spontaneous report databases would be appropriate to capture this information and possibly obtain a more accurate estimate of potential drug toxicity. Table 14.2 summarizes three strategies for mapping longitudinal database outcomes described in [8].

The term "reported" is used in these definitions rather than the term "experienced" to emphasize that the analyses deal with events that were recorded. Events that may have occurred but were not recorded do not enter the analyses.

**Table 14.1**    Generic form of input to methods commonly used to assess findings from spontaneous reporting system databases.

| Target drug | Target AE | | Total |
|---|---|---|---|
| | Yes | No | |
| Yes | $w_{DE}$ | $w_{D\bar{E}}$ | $w_D$ |
| No | $w_{\bar{D}E}$ | $w_{\bar{D}\bar{E}}$ | $w_{\bar{D}}$ |
| Total | $w_E$ | $w_{\bar{E}}$ | $w$ |

**Table 14.2**    Strategies for mapping longitudinal database findings to Table 14.1 entries.

| Strategy Counted | Distinct patients Number of patients | SRS Number of time points in $T$ | Modified SRS Number of time points in $T$ |
|---|---|---|---|
| $w_{DE}$ | Reporting event $E$ while on drug $D$ at least once in $T$ | When a patient reported event $E$ while on drug $D$ | When a patient reported event $E$ while on drug $D$ |
| $w_{D\bar{E}}$ | Observed to be on drug $D$ at least once in $T$, but did not report event $E$ then | When a patient reported any event other than $E$ while on drug $D$ | When a patient reported any event other than $E$ while on drug $D$ plus the number of event-free intervals of exposure to $D$ |
| $w_{\bar{D}E}$ | Reporting event $E$ at least once in $T$ while not on drug $D$ | When a patient reported event $E$ while on any drug $D' \neq D$ | When a patient reported event $E$ while on any drug $D' \neq D$ plus the number of time points when the patient reported event $E$ while on no drug |
| $w_{\bar{D}\bar{E}}$ | Not on drug $D$ in $T$ who did not report event $E$ in $T$ | When a patient reported any event $E' \neq E$ while on any drug $D' \neq D$ | When a patient reported any event $E' \neq E$ while on any drug $D' \neq D$ plus the number of event-free intervals to any drug other than $D$ plus the number of time points when a patient reported any event $E' \neq E$ while on no drug |

**Table 14.3**   Indicator variables used to define alternative mappings of the entries Table 14.1.

| Vector | Indicator variables | Definition (value $= 0$ if condition is not met) |
|---|---|---|
| $\overrightarrow{x}_i^{(d)}$ | $(x_{i1}^{(d)}, x_{i2}^{(d)}, \ldots, x_{iT}^{(d)})$ | $x_{it}^{(d)} = 1$ if patient $i$ is exposed to drug $D$ at time $t$ |
| $\overrightarrow{y}_i^{(e)}$ | $(y_{i1}^{(e)}, y_{i2}^{(e)}, \ldots, y_{iT}^{(e)})$ | $y_{it}^{(e)} = 1$ if patient $i$ experiences the onset of an episode of event $E$ at time $t$ |
| $\overrightarrow{y}_i^{(e)*}$ | $(y_{i1}^{(e)*}, y_{i2}^{(e)*}, \ldots, y_{iT}^{(e)*})$ | $y_{it}^{(e)*} = 1$ if $y_{it}^{(e)} = 1$ and $y_{is}^{(e)} = 1$ for all $s < t$ (that is, the first (only) occurrence of event $E$ is at time $t$) |

The different models can be defined formally using indicator variables defined in Table 14.3.

For example, the value of $w_{DE}$ is calculated as

$$w_{DE} = \sum_i I\left(\overrightarrow{x}_i^{(d)\prime} \overrightarrow{y}_i^{(e)}\right) = \sum_i \overrightarrow{x}\overrightarrow{x}_i^{(d)\prime} \overrightarrow{y}_i^{(e)*}$$

for the distinct patients model, and

$$w_{DE} = \sum_i \overrightarrow{x}_i^{(d)\prime} \overrightarrow{y}_i^{(e)}$$

for the spontaneous reporting system (SRS) and modified SRS models, where $I(x) = 1$ if $x > 0$ or 0 otherwise. The other entries are defined analogously. The mapping is termed a "prevalent condition" mapping if the $\overrightarrow{y}_i^{(e)}$ outcome vectors are used, or an "incident condition" if the $\overrightarrow{y}_i^{(e)*}$ outcome vectors are used. The $w_{DE}$ definitions are the same for both mappings, but the other definitions differ according to the mapping.

The performance of these approaches to defining the entries to Table 14.1 was evaluated via simulation in terms of a "mean average precision" score. Larger values of this score indicated "better" performance of the combination of entry definition strategy and analysis method; the details are described in [10]. The key finding from this evaluation was that the SRS and modified SRS approaches performed similarly, and both generally performed better than the distinct patients approach regardless of whether incident or prevalent events were considered. However, a subsequent evaluation of the predictive accuracy of the approach applied to five real observational databases and six simulated databases using various conventional metrics (proportional reporting ratio, reporting odds ratio, etc.) demonstrated poor diagnostic accuracy, with AUC values mostly in the range (0.35, 0.6), suggesting that the methods evaluated did not discriminate true positives from true negatives using healthcare data [11]. The authors of that article concluded that "adapting disproportionality methods, designed for analysis of spontaneous report databases, and applying them to longitudinal healthcare data may be unfruitful."

## 14.2.2   LGPS and LEOPARD

The Longitudinal Gamma Poisson Shrinker (LGPS) calculates a disproportionality measure based on the entries in Table 14.1 [12]. The expected value of $w_{DE}$ under the assumption of no drug-event association is

$$E_{DE} = t_D \times w_{\overline{DE}}/t_{\overline{D}}$$

where $t_D$ denotes the total time patients are exposed to drug $D$ and $t_{\overline{D}}$ denotes the total time that patients were included in the database but not exposed to $D$. The article appears to use the Gamma Poisson Shrinker (GPS) [13] as the metric for disproportionality, although any metric based on Table 14.1 could in principle be used. A potential defect of the LGPS approach (or, for that matter, any approach that considers temporal relationships between prescription of a drug and manifestation of an AE) is the possibility of *protopathic bias,* where a drug is pre-scribed for a symptom or manifestation of a condition before the condition itself is diagnosed so that the initial prescription appears to cause the condition. The Longitudinal Evaluation of Observational Profiles of Adverse Events Related to Drugs (LEOPARD) approach seeks to identify cases of protopathic bias and so avoid false positive signals of potential drug-related AEs. The approach proceeds in outline as follows. Let $t^{(E)}$ denote the index date for event $E$, that is, the date on which event $E$ is reported. Starting at some point $t_a^{(E)}$ days before $E$ ($t_a^{(E)}$ is a parameter of the method), count the cumulative number of prescriptions on relative days $-t_a^{(E)}, -t_a^{(E)} + 1, \dots, 0$ (corresponding to $t^{(E)}$), 1, 2, $\dots, t_a^{(E)}$. A sudden increase in the cumula-tive number of prescriptions (just) before day 0 would be an indicator of possible protopathic bias. A steady increase in the cumulative number of prescriptions before day 0 followed by a plateau or continued steady increase after day 0 might indicate possible toxicity. Schuemie proposed comparing relative risk during exposure with relative risk just prior to exposure by performing an LGPS analysis followed by a "reverse" LGPS, that is, starting from time $t^{(E)} + t_a^{(E)}$ and working backward [12]. Application to a simulated database suggested that the LEOPARD approach could be valuable for filtering out cases of protopathic bias while still retaining reasonable sensitivity for detecting potential drug–event relationships. However, a subsequent more extensive application of the LGPS and LEOPARD approaches to five real observational healthcare databases and six simulated databases found weak discrimination between positive and negative controls, biased estimates of relative risk, and confidence inter-vals with poor coverage, leading to a conclusion that these methods may not be "designs of choice" for risk identification [14].

## 14.2.3   Self-controlled case series (SCCS)

The self-controlled case series (SCCS) approach uses conditional Poisson regression to esti-mate the relative risk of exposures to possibly multiple drugs over sequences of days of observation of each patient [15]. In principle, a patient can be exposed on any day to one or more of $J$ possible drugs, and can experience on any day one or more, or possibly no, AEs. Let $\mathbf{x}_d$ denote a vector of $J$ elements whose values can be 0 or 1 accordingly as the patient was not or was exposed to the $J$th drug ($j = 1, \dots, J$) on day $d$. Let $y_d$ denote the number of AEs reported for the patient on that day. Suppose that $\beta_0$ denotes the patient's unknown exposure-free event rate so that $\lambda_0 = \exp(\beta_0)$ denotes the parameter for a Poisson distribu-tion for the number of events the patient would experience on any day. Let $\boldsymbol{\beta} = (\beta_1, \dots, \beta_J)$ denote the relative risk multipliers for the event rate that are due to exposure to drugs 1, $\dots, J$

on any day, so that the Poisson parameter for day $d$ would be $\lambda_d = \lambda_0 \times \exp(\mathbf{x}_d'\boldsymbol{\beta})$. If one conditions on the value of $n = y_1 + y_2 + \ldots$, the total number of AEs experienced by the patient over the period of observation, then the logarithm of the likelihood considered as a function of the elements of $\boldsymbol{\beta}$ does not contain any contribution due to $\beta_0$, and only patients with at least one drug exposure and one AE contribute to the joint likelihood of the observations. This formulation assumes that exposure is independent of when events occur, and is biased when this assumption does not hold, which may occur often in practice [16]. Multiple drug exposures on any day ($J > 1, \mathbf{1}'\mathbf{x}_d > 1$) are possible, which casts the inference about the elements of $\boldsymbol{\beta}$ into the context of a high-dimensional regression problem. The authors recommend the use of a regularized regression approach to avoid issues of overfitting and numerical instability [17]. The performance of the method was evaluated by application to five observational databases and six simulated databases, with 64 choices of design combinations: (i) consideration of all occurrences or only the first occurrence of an AE (all/first only); (ii) adjusting for concurrent exposures through a "multiple SCCS extension" (yes/no); (iii) choice of "time at risk" window during which the occurrence of an AE may be related to drug exposure (30 days/no limit); (iv) including drug effects that may occur on the day of initial exposure (yes/no); and (v) the minimum observation length for observing an individual's experience (none/180 days). The diagnostic accuracy of the method varied among the AEs and the various databases; at best the AUC was about 0.7 for acute liver failure and greater than 0.8 for the other AEs. However, for estimating coverage probabilities based on the simulated data, the method returned substantially lower coverage (generally less than 65%) than the nominal 95%.

## 14.2.4    Case–control approach

This approach compares the exposures to drug $D$ of patients demonstrating the event $E$ (cases) within a defined period of time with the exposures during the same period of time of (usually, one or more matched) patients not demonstrating the event $E$ (controls) [18]. The occurrence of $E$ that identifies a case also establishes an index date; the observation period for the case is an interval of time preceding the index date, for example, 180 days previously. The index date for one or more controls, who may be matched to a case by, for example, age and gender, usually is the same date as for the control, and the same observation period usually applies. The observations consist of the numbers of cases of $E$ who were exposed to $D$ in the observation period ($x_{DE}$) and who were not exposed to $D(x_{\overline{D}E})$, and the numbers of controls who were exposed to $D(x_{D\overline{E}})$ and who were not exposed to $D(x_{\overline{D}\overline{E}})$, along with the total person-time of exposure to $D(t_D)$ and the total person-time in the period of observation of cases and controls who were not exposed to $D(t_{\overline{D}})$. The metric of interest is the odds ratio,

$$\text{OR} = \frac{x_{DE}x_{\overline{D}\overline{E}}}{x_{\overline{D}E}x_{D\overline{E}}}.$$

If controls are selected independently of exposure, then the number of exposed controls per unit time should be about the same as the number of unexposed controls per unit time, that is, $x_{D\overline{E}}/t_D \approx x_{\overline{D}\overline{E}}/t_{\overline{D}}$, so that the odds ratio can be approximated by

$$\text{OR} \approx \frac{x_{DE}/t_D}{x_{\overline{D}E}/t_{\overline{D}}},$$

that is, by the incidence rate ratio (IRR) among the cases. The diagnostic operating characteristics (AUC), bias, and confidence interval coverage were evaluated by applying the method to five observational healthcare databases and six simulated data sets. The predictive accuracy varied considerably, depending on the database and the target AE, but generally was fairly poor, with AUC values usually at or below 0.5. Estimates of the true odds ratio also generally were positively biased, and the confidence interval coverage probabilities were substantially lower than the nominal 95% level; none of the scenarios achieved a coverage probability greater than 76%, and many were substantially lower.

## 14.2.5   Self-controlled cohort

This method is similar, but not identical, to the SCCS method [15, 19]. The essential differences are that this approach does not condition on the individual patients to estimate effect size, and that it makes use of the exposed and unexposed times for all patients exposed to the target drug rather than only to patients with the target event. The analysis uses only patients with at least one exposure to the target drug ($D$). A distinction for these patients is made between periods of time during which a patient is exposed to $D$ and periods of time when the patient is not exposed to $D$. Let $x_{DE}$ denote the number of events among the patients exposed to $D$, and let $t_D$ denote the total exposure time to $D$. Likewise, let $x_{\overline{DE}}$ denote the number of events among the patients before they were exposed to $D$, and let $t_{\overline{D}}$ denote their total time under observation before exposure to $D$. The incidence rates for the exposed and non-exposed eras are, respectively,

$$r_{DE} = x_{DE}/t_D \quad \text{and} \quad r_{\overline{DE}} = x_{\overline{DE}}/t_{\overline{D}}.$$

The metric of interest is the IRR, given by $r_{DE}/r_{\overline{DE}}$. Under the assumption that $x_{DE}$ and $x_{\overline{DE}}$ are generated from Poisson distributions with respective rate parameters $t_D\lambda_{DE}$ and $t_{\overline{D}}\lambda_{\overline{DE}}$, (frequentist) inference about the IRR can be carried out using a score-based method with a normal approximation [20]. It is worth noting, and trivial to establish, that a simple Bayesian argument gives an "exact" interval for the ratio $\rho = \lambda_{DE}/\lambda_{\overline{DE}}$ (which is what IRR estimates). If $\lambda_{DE}$ has a gamma prior distribution with parameters $(a_D, b_D)$, and $\lambda_{\overline{DE}}$ has a gamma prior distribution with parameters $(a_{\overline{D}}, b_{\overline{D}})$, then the posterior distribution of

$$\pi = \frac{(b_D + t_D)\rho}{(b_D + t_D)\rho + b_{\overline{D}} + t_{\overline{D}}}$$

is a beta distribution with parameters $(a_D + x_{DE}, a_{\overline{D}} + x_{\overline{DE}})$. Inference about $\rho$ is immediate from the fact that $\rho = (b_{\overline{D}} + t_{\overline{D}})\pi/(b_D + t_D)(1 - \pi)$. Setting the prior distributions to small values (e.g., all equal to $1/2$) will make the inference essentially completely dependent on the observations. The method was applied to the detection of four kinds of AEs using five observational databases and six replications of a simulated database. The diagnostic properties turned out to be quite good, with the best analysis specification having an average AUC of 0.83 and with the AUC $\geq 0.7$ in all cases. However, the estimates of the true IRR turned out to be positively biased, and the coverage probability was substantially lower than the nominal 95%, in fact always less than 60%. The conclusion was that the self-controlled cohort method had some promise as a tool for detecting potential "signals," but was unlikely to be satisfactory tor estimating relative risk.

## 14.2.6  Temporal pattern discovery

This approach was designed for use with EHR databases consisting of records of medical events, clinic/doctor visits, and prescriptions for individual patients over time [21–23]. There are two kinds of events: index events and focus or target events. Index events (denoted by $x$ in what follows) typically are initial prescriptions for various drugs, so that for a patient there may be index events $x_1, x_2, \ldots$ . A patient could have more than one index event of a specific kind (e.g., more than one initial prescription for the same drug), depending on how much time had elapsed between the events. Let $t_x$ denote the real (calendar) time at which index event $x$ occurs. Successive intervals of time $t_{x1}, t_{x2}, \ldots$ of possibly varying durations following the index event can be defined, as can intervals of time $t_{x,-1}, t_{x,-2}, \ldots$ preceding the index event. Focus, or target, events (denoted by $y$ in what follows) usually correspond to AEs, and can occur more than once for any patient. Index and focus events are related through an event history defined by the index event. Thus, given an index event $x$, focus events can be (or have been) recorded after (or before) the index event. Each focus event occurs in one of the intervals of time preceding or succeeding the index event. Let $t$ denote an interval of time relative to a focus event. Define $n_{xy}^t$ as the observed number of event histories where (i) the index event is $x$ and (ii) the focus event $y$ occurs in interval $t$ at least once. Let $n^t$ denote the total number of event histories that at least partially cover the interval $t$, let $n_x^t$ denote the number of event histories corresponding to the index event $x$ that at least partially cover $t$, and let $n_y^t$ denote the number of event histories where the focus event $y$ occurs at least once in interval $t$. The expected number of event histories $E_{xy}^t$ where $x$ is the index event and the focus event $y$ occurs in interval $t$ under the assumption that the proportion of index events $x$ with focus event $y$ in $t$ is the same for all other index events is

$$E_{xy}^t = n_x^t n_y^t / n^t.$$

Histogram plots of the values of $n_{xy}^t$ along with line plots of the corresponding values of $E_{xy}^t$ for each time interval $t$ before and after the index event comprise a "chronograph." Inspection of all chronographs when there are many index–focus event pairs is not practical, so numeric measures of disproportionality are needed. Various measures of disproportionality that estimate the ratio of the observed to expected event counts $\lambda_{xy}^t = n_{xy}^t / E_{xy}^t$ can be defined. Norén *et al.* use a modified "information component" (IC) metric, $\mathrm{IC}_{xy}^t = \log_2 \left( n_{xy}^t + \frac{1}{2} \right) / \left( E_{xy}^t + \frac{1}{2} \right)$ [22, 23]. Temporal association is expressed by relating the value of $\lambda_{xy}^t$ corresponding to an interval of interest $t$ to the value at some predefined control interval $v$ of fairly long duration at some time prior to the index event. This provides a modified expression for the expectation $E_{xy}^{t*}$, namely, $E_{xy}^{t*} = n_{xy}^v E_{xy}^t / E_{xy}^v$. Expressing the disproportionality relative to a control period provides a way to express the temporal associations as opposed to the general tendencies of index and focus events to occur in the same event histories. The corresponding modified IC metric is $\mathrm{IC}_{xy}^{t*} = \log_2 \left( n_{xy}^t + \frac{1}{2} \right) / \left( E_{xy}^{t*} + \frac{1}{2} \right)$. Plotting the value of this metric as a function of the interval $t$ can provide insight into the occurrence of AEs. The method with this refinement subsequently was termed "calibrated self-controlled cohort analysis within temporal pattern discovery." [21] The original publications provided a number of examples to illustrate how chronographs and IC plots could be used to identify characteristics of AE occurrence [22, 23]. A subsequent empirical evaluation of the method based on its application to four claims databases and an EHR database demonstrated generally good predictive accuracy (average AUC $= 0.75$, AUC $> 0.7$ for all but one of the combinations of data source and target AE cases) [21]. Further details and software for performing the calculations can be downloaded from http://omop.org.

### 14.2.7   Unexpected temporal association rules

The MUTARA (Mining the Unexpected Temporal Association Rules Given the Antecedent) [24] and HUNT [25] algorithms were developed for implementation on linked healthcare data sets from Queensland, Australia [24, 25]. Both methods use a dependency measure called leverage that calculates the temporal dependency of a medical event $E$ consequent to administration of a drug $D$ within a time period of $T$ days. Both are essentially case–control methods consisting of cases (patients prescribed $D =$ users) and controls (patients who never used $D =$ non $-$ users), who provide an estimate of the background rate of $E$. In its simplest form, assuming that each included patient provides only one hazard interval, the algorithm proceeds as follows. The hazard interval length, $T_h$, for a case either is a specified number of days, $T_e$, following prescription of $D$ if $D$ is not represcribed within $T_e$ days of the initial prescription, or $T_e + s$ if $D$ is represcribed within $s < T_e$ days of the initial prescription. A corresponding constrained interval $T_c$ for non-users is randomly chosen from the interval of observation of a non-user corresponding to the case.

The notation in the original papers is unconventional so a simpler expression of the model using conventional notation is described here under the assumption that each case provides only one hazard interval. The observations corresponding to a particular event $E$ and users of a particular drug $D$ can be arranged in a table similar to Table 14.1. The essential difference from Table 14.1 besides the labels is the inclusion of information about the occurrence of event $E$ in a reference interval preceding the hazard interval for the cases.

There are $n_U$ users (cases) and $n_{\overline{U}}$ non-users (there could be multiple controls corresponding to each case) for a total of $n = n_U + n_{\overline{U}}$ patients (Table 14.4). The event $E$ occurs in the hazard interval $(T_h)$ for $n_{UE}$ of the $n_U$ users following the initiation of $D$, and in the control interval $(T_c)$ for $n_{\overline{U}E}$ of the $n_{\overline{U}}$ non-users (controls). The support for the occurrence of $E$ following initiation of $D$ is the fraction of all patients consisting of cases where the event occurs in the hazard interval,

$$\text{support} = p_{UE} = n_{UE}/n$$

The confidence is the fraction of all cases consisting of cases where the event occurs in the hazard interval,

$$\text{confidence} = p_{E|U} = p_{UE}/p_U,$$

**Table 14.4**   Generic form of input to the MUTARA and HUNT algorithms.

| | Event $E$ in Hazard or Control Interval | | | | |
|---|---|---|---|---|---|
| | Yes | Yes | Yes | No | Total |
| *E* In Ref. Interval | Yes | No | – | – | – |
| Cases | $m_{UE}$ | $n_{UE} - m_{UE}$ | $n_{UE}$ | $n_{\overline{U}E}$ | $n_U$ |
| Controls | – | – | $n_{\overline{U}E}$ | $n_{\overline{U}E}$ | $n_{\overline{U}}$ |
| Total | – | – | $n_E$ | $n_{\overline{E}}$ | $n$ |

where $p_U = n_U/n$. The leverage, which can be interpreted as the difference between the observed number of cases with event $E$ and the expected number of cases if the probability of an event is the same as the marginal probability in the entire data set, is defined as

$$\text{lev} = p_{UE} - p_U p_E,$$

where $p_E = (n_{UE} + n_{\overline{U}E})/n$. Potential toxicities can be identified by ranking the leverage values. A shortcoming of this metric is that it does not distinguish between true AEs and events that are a consequence of an underlying illness. An adjustment designed to mitigate this situation (the MUTARA approach) proceeds by incorporating "user-based exclusions," that is, by decreasing the counts of cases experiencing event $E$ during their hazard intervals by the number of these cases that also experienced the event during a prior reference interval (because these cases no longer would be considered "unexpected"). The calculations are almost the same:

$$\text{support}^* = q_{UE} = (n_{UE} - m_{UE})/n,$$

$$\text{confidence}^* = q_{E|U} = q_{UE}/p_U,$$

and unexpected leverage

$$\text{unexlev} = q_{UE} - p_U q_E,$$

where $q_E = (n_{UE} - m_{UE} + n_{\overline{U}E})/n$. The HUNT algorithm uses both the leverage and unexpected leverage values to calculate a quantity called rankRatio corresponding to a drug $D$ and an event $E$. First, one determines the rank of the lev value corresponding to drug $D$ and event $E$ relative to the lev values for all drugs and all events ($\text{rank}_{\text{lev}}(D, E)$), and the rank of the unexlev values for drug $D$ and event $E$ among all unexlev values ($\text{rank}_{\text{unexlev}}(D, E)$). The rank ratio statistic is

$$\text{rankRatio}(D, E) = \text{rank}_{\text{lev}}(D, E)/\text{rank}_{\text{unexlev}}(D, E)$$

The details required for implementation of the method are complex, and omitted here for brevity.

The MUTARA and HUNT approaches, although fundamentally disproportionality-based, incorporate the concept of "expectedness" of an AE. The original publications suggest that they have some advantages over conventional methods [24, 25]. Reps *et al.* [26] compared the performance of these methods with the temporal pattern discovery [23] and modified reporting odds ratio [10, 27] methods by application to the THIN (The Health Improvement Network, www.thin-uk.com) database. The AUCs depended on where thresholds were set to reduce the proportion of false positives but, at best, the AUCs for all of the variations of the methods that were studied ranged between 0.5 and 0.6. The general conclusion was that "none of the existing algorithms is able to rank rare ADRs highly and currently the existing algorithms tend to focus on detecting more common ADRs."

## 14.2.8   Time to onset for vaccine safety

Using information about time to onset of an AE following immunization can lead to better sensitivity and positive predictive value when evaluating vaccine safety [28]. The idea is to look at the distribution of time to onset of event for a particular vaccine–event pair and compare it to the distribution of time to onset for all other vaccine–event pairs using a Kolmogoroff–Smirnov two-sample test. The recommendation is to combine this approach with a standard disproportionality analysis such as the empirical Bayes gamma Poisson method [13]. However, the statistical properties of an approach using time to onset with or without the empirical Bayes procedure remain to be established.

## 14.3   Web-based pharmacovigilance (infodemiology and infoveillance)

The approaches described in the previous section are variations of traditional epidemiologic and pharmacovigilance approaches for systematically exploring conventional databases of accumulated health information. A growing body of internet-based information that includes patient inquiries about health-related issues presents some potentially useful avenues for early detection of potential drug toxicities. Methods for exploiting this information tend to be described in the informatics literature, rather than the statistical or epidemiologic literature. The terms *infoepidemiology* and *infosurveillance* [29, 30] are used in the literature to describe methods for identifying and using electronic information, especially internet content, to inform public health policy or for surveillance.

These approaches differ from conventional analyses of spontaneous reporting databases and analyses (not yet conventional) of observational databases primarily in the source of the informational substrate used for the analyses and in the techniques needed to put this material into a form amenable to signal-detection analysis. The current literature uses essentially the same signal-detection methods used for conventional disproportionality analyses. Their prediction accuracy, especially for later-onset AEs, seems promising, although the statistical properties of metrics expressing relative risk still need to be explored.

Medical discussion boards may be especially useful for identifying possible drug toxicity, although (at least recently) there were "few reports in the medical or social science literature that apply methods to extract information from the text of medical discussion board content to identify and analyze reports of adverse drug events" [31]. A project undertaken to characterize AEs associated with hormonal medications commonly used in breast cancer treatment by text-mining medical discussion boards entailed a considerable effort to extract useful information. A number of pre-analysis processing steps were required, including extracting over 1 million messages from the discussion boards of 11 websites, removing content unrelated to the posts, de-identifying the messages, developing a controlled vocabulary, and removing terms not indicative of the drug or event/symptom (by hand). A key finding from the project was that about 23% of the drug–event rules identified by the method were undocumented in the labels of the drugs of interest [31].

Records of search queries (search logs) provide another source of information that can be used for identifying possible toxicity relationships. A project aimed at evaluating a potential interaction between the antidepressant paroxetine and the lipid-lowering product pravastatin with respect to the occurrence of hyperglycemia used search logs of "millions of consenting web users" incorporating all of their searches during 2010 on three search engines (Google®, Bing®, and Yahoo!®) [32]. A conventional disproportionality analysis was used to identify potential "signals." The diagnostic accuracy of the method (AUC) was about 0.82, which is fairly high.

**Table 14.5**  Counts of symptom queries before and after.

| Group | Frequency symptom queried | |
|---|---|---|
| | Before day 0 | After day 0 |
| Users | $n_{UB}$ | $n_{UA}$ |
| Non-users | $n_{NB}$ | $n_{NA}$ |

Yom-Tov and Gabrilovich presented an automated method for continuous monitoring of AE for drugs singly and in combination based on aggregated search data from large populations of internet users that they described as complementary to conventional pharmacovigilance approaches [33]. The method uses a "Query Log Reaction Score" (QLRS) that amounts to the usual Pearson chi-square statistic applied to a count table (Table 14.5) corresponding to a particular drug and AE (symptom) to identify AEs associated with widely used drugs and vaccines on the basis of queries to the Yahoo!® US web search engine during 6 months in 2010 provided by 176 million unique users. The findings corresponding to 20 of the top 100 best-selling drugs were presented (limited to non-generic versions); 195 symptoms from the ICD-10 collection of the International Classification of Disease (see http://www.icd10data.com) were considered, with up to 50 of the most frequently mentioned symptoms for any drug. Users were defined as individuals who had made a query about the drug in question, with day 0 defined as the day of their initial query. Day 0 for non-users consisted of the day at the midpoint of their observed query history. Two reference sets were used to assess the validity of the proposed approach: FAERS (FDA Adverse Event Reporting System) reports submitted between January 2004 and June 2010, and the SIDER (side Effect Resource) list [34]. A distinction was made between the AEs (symptoms) that were and were not consistently found by the proposed method and standard signal detection methods applied to FAERS. The AEs more likely to be reported to regulatory agencies were those that occurred shortly after starting treatment (acute onset), while the AEs identified by the proposed method tended to appear much later after starting treatment.

## 14.4  Discussion

Evaluating drug safety using observational/longitudinal databases or other large-scale data collections is currently a work in progress. Evaluations of the performance of various approaches for evaluating drug safety using observational or longitudinal databases have not clearly identified which, if any, of the currently proposed methods should be considered for routine use, nor is it clear how they should be used. An evaluation of various detection methods (proportional reporting ratio [35], reporting odds ratio [27, 36], GPS [13], temporal pattern discovery [22, 23], IRR, LGPS [12], hierarchical Bayes [37], case–control, and SCCS [38]) applied to seven European electronic health databases with prespecified positive and negative controls (known drug–event associations and known non-associations) demonstrated AUCs in the range of 0.7–0.8 [39]. Post-filtering the findings using the LEOPARD method [12] improved the AUC values to over 0.8. However, an evaluation carried out by the OMOP project of the performance of seven methods (new user cohort [40], case–control [18], SCCS

[15], self-controlled cohort [19], disproportionality analysis [11], temporal pattern discovery [21–23], and LGPS [12]) applied to four claims and one EHR database to detect four AEs (acute liver failure, acute myocardial infarction, acute renal failure, and upper gastrointestinal bleeding) concluded that although some of the methods, especially the self-controlled cohort approach, could consistently (across the databases and AEs) achieve reasonable predictive accuracy (AUC > 0.7), all of the methods gave biased estimates of the actual risk increase metric and all provided poor coverage for the estimates of relative risk [41]. A replication of the OMOP evaluation applied to six European databases yielded a similar finding and conclusions [42].

Taken together, the findings suggest that the self-controlled cohort approach provides the best (or nearly best) predictive accuracy, although accuracy may be improved by using combinations of methods [41]. The bias and poor coverage may reflect systematic errors due to confounding or misclassification, which conventional calculations do not address. Including negative and, if possible, positive controls in observational studies would be helpful for identifying those elevated risk measures that represent true adverse effects.

Text mining approaches applied to web-based queries and message boards provide an alternative approach that could be a useful complement to conventional epidemiologic methods. Text mining approaches can be carried out more nearly in real time than conventional approaches and, therefore, might provide more timely warning of possible drug toxicities. In addition, text mining approaches may be useful for identifying late-onset AEs that would be difficult to detect using spontaneous reporting systems or even observational databases.

# References

[1] Gould, A. L., Lystig, T.C., Lu, Y., Fu, H., and Ma, H., (2014) Methods and isues to consider for detection of safety signals from spontaneous reporting databases. Report of the DIA Bayesian Safety Signal Detection Working Group. *Therapeutic Innovation and Regulatory Science.* Published online 8 May 2014.

[2] Hauben M, Madigan D, Gerrits C, Walsh L, van Puijenbroek EP. The role of data mining in pharmacovigilance. *Expert Opinion in Drug Safety* 2005; **4**:929–948.

[3] Hansen RA, Gray MD, Fox BI, Hollingsworth JC, Gao J, Zeng P. How well do various health outcome definitions identify appropriate cases in observational studies? *Drug Safety* 2013; **36**:S27–S32.

[4] Madigan D, Stang PE, Berlin JA, Schuemie MJ, Overhage JM, Suchard MA, DuMouchel W, Hartzema AG, Ryan PB. A systematic statistical approach to evaulating evidence from observational studies. *Annual Review of Statistics* 2014; **1**:11–39.

[5] Trifiro G, Fourrier-Reglat A, Sturkenboom MC, *et al.*, The EU-ADR project: preliminary results and perspective. *Studies in Health Technologies and Informatics* 2009; **148**:43–49.

[6] Harpaz R, Vilar S, DuMouchel W, Salmasian H, Haerian K, Shah NH, Chase HS, Friedman C. Combing signals from spontaneous reports and electronic health records for detection of adverse drug reactions. *Journal of the American Medical Informatics Association* 2013; **20**:413–419.

[7] Reich CG, Ryan PB, Schuemie MJ. Alternative outcome definitions and their effect on the performance of methods for observational studies. *Drug Safety* 2013; **36**:S181–S193.

[8] Ryan PB, Schuemie MJ, Welebob E, Duke J, Valentine S, Hartzema AG. Defining a reference set to support methodological research in drug safety. *Drug Safety* 2013; **36**:S33–S47.

[9] Ryan PB, Schuemie MJ. Evaluating performance of risk identification methods through a large-scale simulation of observational data. *Drug Safety* 2013; **36**:S171–S180.

[10] Zorych I, Madigan D, Ryan P, Bate A. Disproportionality methods for pharmacovigilance in longitudinal observational databases. *Statistical Methods in Medical Research* 2013; **22**:39–56.

[11] DuMouchel W, Ryan PB, Schuemie MJ, Madigan D. Evaluation of disproportionality safety signaling applied to healthcare databases. *Drug Safety* 2013; **36**:S123–S132.

[12] Schuemie MJ. Methods for drug safety signal detection in longitudinal observational databases: LGPS and LEOPARD. *Pharmacoepidemiology and Drug Safety* 2011; **20**:292–299.

[13] DuMouchel W. Bayesian data mining in large frequency tables, with an application to the FDA spontaneous reporting system (Disc: p190–202). *American Statistician* 1999; **53**:177–190.

[14] Schuemie MJ, Madigan D, Ryan PB. Empirical performance of LGPS and LEOPARD: lessons for developing a risk identification and analysis system. *Drug Safety* 2013; **36**:S133–S142.

[15] Suchard MA, Zorych I, Simpson SE, Schuemie MJ, Ryan PB, Madigan D. Empirical performance of the self-controlled case series design: lessons for developing a risk identification and analysis system. *Drug Safety* 2013; **36**:S83–S93.

[16] Nicholas JM, Grieve AP, Gulliford MC. Within-person study designs had lower percision and greather susceptibility to bias because of trends in exposure than cohort and nested case-control designs. *Journal of Clinical Epidemiology* 2012; **65**:384–393.

[17] Simpson SE, Madigan D, Zorych I, Schuemie MJ, Ryan PB, Suchard MA. Multiple self-controlled case series for large-scale longitudinal observational databases. *Biometrics* 2013; **69**:893–902.

[18] Madigan D, Schuemie MJ, Ryan PB. Empirical performance of the case-control method: lessons for developing a risk identification and analysis system. *Drug Safety* 2013; **36**:S73–S82.

[19] Ryan PB, Schuemie MJ, Madigan D. Empirical performance of a self-controlled cohort method: lessons for developing a risk identification and analysis system. *Drug Safety* 2013; **36**:S95–S106.

[20] Graham PL, Mengerson K, Morton AP. Confidence limits for the ratio of two rates based on likelihood scores. *Statistics in Medicine* 2003; **22**:2071–2083.

[21] Noren GN, Bergvall T, Ryan PB, Juhlin K, Schuemie MJ, Madigan D. Empirical performance of the calibrated self-controlled cohort analysis within temporal pattern discovery: lessons for developing a risk identification and analysis system. *Drug Safety* 2013; **36**:S107–S121.

[22] Norén, G. N., Bate, A., Hopstadius, J., Star, K., and Edwards, I. R. *Temporal Pattern Discovery for Trends and Transient Effects: Its Application to Patient Records*, ACM, Washington, DC, 2008.

[23] Norén GN, Hopstadius J, Bate A, Star K, Edwards IR. Temporal pattern discovery in longitudinal electronic patient records. *Data Mining and Knowledge Discovery* 2010; **20**: 361–387.

[24] Jin H, Chen J, Kelman C, He H, McAullay D, O'Keefe CM. Mining unexpected associations for signalling potential adverse drug reactions from administrative health databases. In Ng, W.K., Kutsuregawa, M., and Li, J. eds. *Advances in Knowledge Discovery and Data Mining: 10th Pacific-Asia Conference, PADKK 2006*, Lecture Notes in Artificial Intelligence 3918, Springer-Verlag, Berlin, 2006, pp. 867–876.

[25] Jin H, Chen J, He H, Kelman C, McAullay D, O'Keefe CM. Signaling potential adverse drug reactions from administrative health databases. *IEEE Transactions on Knowledge and Data Engineering* 2010; **22**:839–852.

[26] Reps JM, Garibaldi JM, Aickelin U, Soria D, Gibson J, Hubbard R. Comparison of algorithms that detect drug side effects using electronic healthcare databases. *Soft Computing* 2013; **17**:2381–2397.

[27] van Puijenbroek EP, Bate A, Leufkens HG, Lindquist M, Orre R, Egberts AC. A comparison of measures of disproportionality for signal detection in spontaneous reporting systems for adverse drug reactions. *Pharmacoepidemiology and Drug Safety* 2002; **11**:3–10.

[28] Van Holle L, Bauchau V. Signal detection on spontaneous reports of adverse events following immunisation: a comparison of the performance of a disproportionality-based algorithm and a time-to-onset based algorithm. *Pharmacoepidemiology and Drug Safety* 2014; **23**:178–185.

[29] Eysenbach G. Infodemiology and infoveillancd: framework for an emerging set of public health informatics methods to analyze search, communication and publication behavior on the internet. *Journal of Medical Internet Research* 2009; **11**:e11.

[30] Eysenbach G. Infodemiology and infoveillance. Tracking online health information and cyberbehavior for public health. *American Journal of Preventive Medicine* 2011; **40**:S154–S158.

[31] Benton A, Ungar L, Hill S, Hennessy S, Mao J, Chung A, Leonard CE, Holmes JH. Identifying potential adverse effects using the web: a new approach to medical hypothesis generation. *Journal of Biomedical Informatics* 2011; **44**:989–996.

[32] White RW, Tatonetti NP, Shah NH, Altman RB, Horvitz E. Web-scale pharmacovigilance: listening to signals from the crowd. *Journal of the American Medical Informatics Association* 2013; **20**:404–408.

[33] Yom-Tov E, Gabrilovich E. Postmarket drug surveillance without rrial costs: discovery of adverse drug reactions rhrough large-scale analysis of web search queries. *Journal of Medical Internet Research* 2013; **15**:e124.

[34] Kuhn M, Campillos M, Letunic I, Jensen LJ, Bork P. A side effect resource to capture phenotypic effects of drugs. *Molecular Systems Biology* 2010; **6**:343.

[35] Evans SJW, Waller PC, Davis S. Use of proportional reporting ratios (PRRs) for signal genertion from spontaneous adverse drug reaction reports. *Pharmacoepidemiology and Drug Safety* 2001; **10**:483–486.

[36] Rothman KJ, Lanes S, Sacks ST. The reporting odds ratio and its advantages over the proportional reporting ratio. *Pharmacoepidemiology and Drug Safety* 2004; **13**:519–523.

[37] Berry SM, Berry DA. Accounting for multiplicities in assessing drug safety: a three-level hierarchical mixture model. *Biometrics* 2004; **60**:418–426.

[38] Whitaker HJ, Farrington CP, Spiessens B, Musonda P. Tutorial in biostatistics: The self-controlled case series method. *Statistics in Medicine* 2006; **25**:1768–1797.

[39] Schuemie MJ, Coloma PM, Straatman H, Herings RMC, Trifiro G, Matthews JN, Prieto-Merino D, Molokhia M, Pedersen L, Gini R, Innocenti F, Mazzaglia G, Picelli G, Scotti L, van der Lei J, Starkenboom MCJM. Using electronic health care records for drug safety signal detection. *Medical Care* 2012; **50**:890–897.

[40] Ryan PB, Schuemie MJ, Gruber S, Zorych I, Madigan D. Empirical performance of a new user cohort method: lessons for developing a risk identifcation and analysis system. *Drug Safety* 2013; **36**:S59–S72.

[41] Ryan PB, Stang PE, Overhage JM, Suchard MA, Hartzema AG, DuMouchel W, Reich CG, Schuemie MJ, Madigan D. A comparison of the empirical performance of methods for a risk identification system. *Drug Safety* 2013; **36**:S143–S158.

[42] Schuemie MJ, Gini R, Coloma PM, Straatman H, Herings RMC, Pedersen L, Innocenti F, Mazzaglia G, Picelli G, van der Lei J, Sturkenboom MCJM. Replication of the OMOP experiment in Europe: evaluating methods for risk identification in electronic health record databases. *Drug Safety* 2013; **36**:S159–S169.

# Index

Note: Page numbers in italics denote figures and page numbers in bold denote tables.

*Statistical Methods for Evaluating Safety in Medical Product Development*, First Edition.
Edited by A. Lawrence Gould.
© 2015 John Wiley & Sons, Ltd. Published 2015 by John Wiley & Sons, Ltd.

# Statistics in Practice

## *Human and Biological Sciences*

Berger – Selection Bias and Covariate Imbalances in Randomized Clinical Trials

Berger and Wong – An Introduction to Optimal Designs for Social and Biomedical Research

Brown, Gregory, Twelves and Brown – A Practical Guide to Designing Phase II Trials in Oncology

Brown and Prescott – Applied Mixed Models in Medicine, Third Edition

Campbell and Walters – How to Design, Analyse and Report Cluster Randomised Trials in Medicine and Health Related Research

Carpenter and Kenward – Multiple Imputation and its Application

Carstensen – Comparing Clinical Measurement Methods

Chevret (Ed.) – Statistical Methods for Dose-Finding Experiments

Cooke – Uncertainty Modeling in Dose Response: Bench Testing Environmental Toxicity

Eldridge – A Practical Guide to Cluster Randomised Trials in Health Services Research

Ellenberg, Fleming and DeMets – Data Monitoring Committees in Clinical Trials: A Practical Perspective

Gould (Ed.) – Statistical Methods for Evaluating Safety in Medical Product Development

Hauschke, Steinijans and Pigeot – Bioequivalence Studies in Drug Development: Methods and Applications

Källén – Understanding Biostatistics

Lawson, Browne and Vidal Rodeiro – Disease Mapping with Win-BUGS and MLwiN

Lesaffre, Feine, Leroux and Declerck – Statistical and Methodological Aspects of Oral Health Research

Lesaffre and Lawson – Bayesian Biostatistics

Lui – Binary Data Analysis of Randomized Clinical Trials with Noncompliance

Lui – Statistical Estimation of Epidemiological Risk

Marubini and Valsecchi – Analysing Survival Data from Clinical Trials and Observation Studies

Millar – Maximum Likelihood Estimation and Inference: With Examples in R, SAS and ADMB

Molenberghs and Kenward – Missing Data in Clinical Studies

Morton, Mengersen, Playford and Whitby – Statistical Methods for Hospital Monitoring with R

O'Hagan, Buck, Daneshkhah, Eiser, Garthwaite, Jenkinson, Oakley and Rakow – Uncertain Judgements: Eliciting Expert's Probabilities

O'Kelly and Ratitch – Clinical Trials with Missing Data: A Guide for Practitioners

Parmigiani – Modeling in Medical Decision Making: A Bayesian Approach

Pintilie – Competing Risks: A Practical Perspective

Senn – Cross-over Trials in Clinical Research, Second Edition

Senn – Statistical Issues in Drug Development, Second Edition

Spiegelhalter, Abrams and Myles – Bayesian Approaches to Clinical Trials and Health-Care Evaluation

Walters – Quality of Life Outcomes in Clinical Trials and Health-Care Evaluation

Welton, Sutton, Cooper and Ades – Evidence Synthesis for Decision Making in Healthcare

Whitehead – Design and Analysis of Sequential Clinical Trials, Revised Second Edition

Whitehead – Meta-Analysis of Controlled Clinical Trials

Willan and Briggs – Statistical Analysis of Cost Effectiveness Data

Winkel and Zhang – Statistical Development of Quality in Medicine

Zhou, Zhou, Lui, and Ding – Applied Missing Data Analysis in the Health Sciences

## *Earth and Environmental Sciences*

Buck, Cavanagh and Litton – Bayesian Approach to Interpreting Archaeological Data

Chandler and Scott – Statistical Methods for Trend Detection and Analysis in the Environmental Statistics

Christie, Cliffe, Dawid and Senn (Eds) – Simplicity, Complexity and Modelling

Gibbons, Bhaumik and Aryal – Statistical Methods for Groundwater Monitoring, 2nd Edition

Haas – Improving Natural Resource Management: Ecological and Political Models

Haas – Introduction to Probability and Statistics for Ecosystem Managers

Helsel – Nondetects and Data Analysis: Statistics for Censored Environmental Data

Illian, Penttinen, Stoyan and Stoyan – Statistical Analysis and Modelling of Spatial Point Patterns

Mateu and Muller (Eds) – Spatio-Temporal Design: Advances in Efficient Data Acquisition

McBride – Using Statistical Methods for Water Quality Management

Ofungwu – Statistical Applications for Environmental Analysis and Risk Assessment

Okabe and Sugihara – Spatial Analysis Along Networks: Statistical and Computational Methods

Webster and Oliver – Geostatistics for Environmental Scientists, Second Edition

Wymer (Ed.) – Statistical Framework for RecreationalWater Quality Criteria and Monitoring

## *Industry, Commerce and Finance*

Aitken – Statistics and the Evaluation of Evidence for Forensic Scientists, Second Edition

Balding – Weight-of-evidence for Forensic DNA Profiles

Brandimarte – Numerical Methods in Finance and Economics: A MATLAB-Based Introduction, Second Edition

Brandimarte and Zotteri – Introduction to Distribution Logistics

Chan – Simulation Techniques in Financial Risk Management

Coleman, Greenfield, Stewardson and Montgomery (Eds) – Statistical Practice in Business and Industry

Frisen (Ed.) – Financial Surveillance

Fung and Hu – Statistical DNA Forensics

Gusti Ngurah Agung – Time Series Data Analysis Using EViews

Jank and Shmueli – Modeling Online Auctions

Jank and Shmueli (Ed.) – Statistical Methods in e-Commerce Research

Lloyd – Data Driven Business Decisions

Kenett (Ed.) – Operational Risk Management: A Practical Approach to Intelligent Data Analysis

Kenett (Ed.) – Modern Analysis of Customer Surveys: With Applications using R

Kenett and Zacks – Modern Industrial Statistics: With Applications in R, MINITAB and JMP, Second Edition

Kruger and Xie – Statistical Monitoring of Complex Multivariate Processes: With Applications in Industrial Process Control

Lehtonen and Pahkinen – Practical Methods for Design and Analysis of Complex Surveys, Second Edition

Mallick, Gold, and Baladandayuthapani – Bayesian Analysis of Gene Expression Data

Ohser and Mücklich – Statistical Analysis of Microstructures in Materials Science

Pasiouras (Ed.) – Efficiency and Productivity Growth: Modelling in the Financial Services Industry

Pfaff – Financial Risk Modelling and Portfolio Optimization with R

Pourret, Naim and Marcot (Eds) – Bayesian Networks: A Practical Guide to Applications

Rausand – Risk Assessment: Theory, Methods, and Applications

Ruggeri, Kenett and Faltin – Encyclopedia of Statistics and Reliability

Taroni, Biedermann, Bozza, Garbolino, and Aitken – Bayesian Networks for Probabilistic Inference and Decision Analysis in Forensic Science, Second Edition

Taroni, Bozza, Biedermann, Garbolino and Aitken – Data Analysis in Forensic Science